Blood Pressure Measurements

W. Meyer-Sabellek, M. Anlauf,
R. Gotzen, L. Steinfeld (Eds.)

Blood Pressure Measurements

New Techniques in Automatic and 24-hour Indirect Monitoring

Steinkopff Verlag Darmstadt
Springer-Verlag New York

The Editors:

Priv.-Doz. Dr. med. W. Meyer-Sabellek
Prof. Dr. med. R. Gotzen
Medizinische Klinik und Poliklinik
Klinikum Steglitz der Freien Universität Berlin
Hindenburgdamm 30
1000 Berlin 45, FRG

Prof. Dr. med. M. Anlauf
Medizinische Klinik und Poliklinik
der Universität Essen (GHS)
Abt. für Nieren- und Hochdruckkranke
Hufelandstraße 55
4300 Essen 1, FRG

Prof. Dr. med. Leonard Steinfeld
Division of Cardiology
Mount Sinai School of Medicine
The Mount Sinai Hospital
One Gustav L. Levy Place
New York, NY 10029-6574
USA

CIP-Titelaufnahme der Deutschen Bibliothek

Blood pressure measurements : new techniques in automatic and 24-hour indirect monitoring / W. Meyer-Sabellek ... (eds.). – Darmstadt : Steinkopff ; New York : Springer, 1989
ISBN-13: 978-3-642-72425-1 e-ISBN-13: 978-3-642-72423-7
DOI: 10.1007/978-3-642-72423-7
NE: Meyer-Sabellek, Wolfgang [Hrsg.]

Softcover reprint of the hardcover 1st edition 1990
Medical Editorial: Sabine Müller — Copy Editing: James C. Willis — Production: Heinz J. Schäfer

Printed on aced-free paper

Preface

In addition to standardized casual blood pressure readings, ambulatory blood pressure monitoring (ABPM) — using automatic noninvasive (= indirect) devices for home readings and fully automated monitors for 24-h profiles — have become a widely used necessary tool in clinical research.

This book summarizes the state of the art in the whole field of indirect blood pressure monitoring. It is based on two international meetings and on invited papers. We have divided the subject matter into two main areas:

1) Automatic blood pressure devices for discontinuous registration, and
2) Portable, fully automated programmable monitors for continuous monitoring.

The availability of all new technologies is described in detail and current technical and physiological problems have been covered in depth. Both topics have been subdivided into

a) Methods and Techniques, and
b) Clinical Applications. Both parts are updated and have critically evaluated available automatic sphygmomanometers and portable computers equipped with different techniques (e.g., auscultation, oscillometry, plethysmography). Reliability in the intensiv Care unit as well as in outpatients management, common clinical problems, clinical relevance compared to casual blood pressure are described in the first part. In the second part, ten years of experience on fully automated noninvasive methodology - compared to intraarterial techniques - have been elaborated by international experts; the possibilities and limitations are clearly demonstrated. Analyses in different clinical fields in the diagnosis of primary and secondary hypertension are given. Different statistical analyses of blood pressure variability and circadian rhythms are discussed. Blood pressure variability and profiles have been evaluated in the natural environment, in different diseases (e.g., cardiac transplant, hemodialysis), in pregnancy, and in athletics. Blood pressure profiles are described in normotension and hypertension. The effect of antihypertensive treatment on blood pressure profile has been studied under nonpharmacological and pharmacological (established versus new antihypertensive agents) treatment. The prediction of cardiovascular morbidity from ambulatory blood pressure is finally discussed.

In conclusion we hope that this book will serve as a useful guide and reference and will contribute to a critical use of different new expensive and highly sophisticated techniques of blood pressure measurements. Blood pressure monitoring enables us to evaluate the patient by short-term and long-term repetitive monitoring, to do so more individually, and to differentiate "white coat hypertension"; thus it may contribute to a more detailed diagnosis of elevated blood pressure and at the same time rather, lower costs and reduce side effects of antihypertensive treatment.

W. Meyer-Sabellek
R. Gotzen

M. Anlauf
L. Steinfeld

Contents

2. Ambulatory 24-h Blood Pressure Monitoring

Methods and Techniques

Clinical Application for Diagnosis

Clinical Application for Therapy

Referees and participants of the discussions

Dr. H.-H. Abel
Freie Universität Berlin
Institut für Physiologie
Arnimallee 22
1000 Berlin 33

Prof. Dr. M. Anlauf
Abt. für Nieren- und Hochdruckkranke
Med. Klinik und Poliklinik der
Universitätsklinik Essen
Hufelandstraße 55
4300 Essen 1

Dr. P. Baumgart
Medizinische Poliklinik
Universität Münster
Albert Schweitzer Str. 33
D 4400 Münster

Prof. Dr. H. Brunner
Centre Hospitalier Universitaire Vaudois
Département de médecine interne
CH 1011 Lausanne
Switzerland

Dr. J. Conway
Department of Cardiovascular Medicine
John Radcliffs Hospital
Headington
Oxford
UK (England)

Prof. Dr. I. Franz
Klinik Wehrawald
7865 Todtmoos

Dr. U. Frucht
Klinik für Anaesthesiologie und
Operative Intensivmedizin
Klinikum Steglitz der Freien Universität Berlin
1000 Berlin 45

Dr. Gould
Department of Cardiology
Northwick Park Hospital
Harrow
Middlesex/HA 1 3 VJ
UK (England)

Prof. Dr. R. Gotzen
Medizinische Klinik und Poliklinik
Klinikum Steglitz der Freien Universität Berlin
Hindenburgdamm 50
1000 Berlin 45

F. Halberg, M. D.
Chronobiology Laboratories
University of Minnesota
5-187 Lyon Laboratories
420 Washington Ave. S.E.
Minneapolis, MN 55455
USA

G. A. Harshfield, Ph. D.
The Hypertension Center
Department of Medicine
Mail Point 11
The Charles P. Drew Post-graduate Medical
School
1621, East 120th Street
Los Angeles A 90059
USA

Prof. Dr. T. Kenner
Physiologisches Institut der Universität Graz
Harrachgasse 21
A-8010 Graz
Austria

Prof. Dr. B. Krönig
Innere Medizin
Ev. Elisabeth Krankenhaus
Theobaldstr. 12
5500 Trier

Doz. Dr. D. Magometschnigg
I. Med. Univ. Klinik
Abt. für Klinische Pharmakologie
Lazarettgasse 14
1090 Wien
Austria

F. H. Messerli, M. D.
Ochsner Clinic
1514 Jefferson Highway
New Orleans
Louisiana 70121
USA

Priv. Doz. Dr. W. Meyer-Sabellek
Medizinische Klinik und Poliklinik
Klinikum Steglitz der Freien Universität Berlin
Hindenburgdamm 30
1000 Berlin 45

Dr. S. Mieke
Physikalisch-Technische Bundesanstalt
Braunschweig und Berlin
Institut Berlin
Abbestraße 2-12
1000 Berlin 10

Dr. W. Nitsche
Dept. of Aeronautics and
Astronautics
Technical University of Berlin
Marchstraße 14
1000 Berlin 10

Prof. Dr. T. Öney
Frauenklinik und Poliklinik
Klinikum Steglitz der
Freien Universität Berlin
Hindenburgdamm 30
1000 Berlin 45

P. Palatini, M. D.
Medical Clinic I
University of Padova
Via Giustiniani 2
I 35126 Padova
Italy

T. G. Pickering, M. D.
Cardiovascular Center, Starr-4
New York Hospital-Cornell
Medical Center
25 East 8th Street
New York, New York 10021
USA

Dr. E. B. Raftery, B. Sc., M.B.F.A.C.C.,
F.R.C.P.
Consultant Cardiologist
Department of Cardiology
Northwick Park Hospital
Harrow/Middlesex/HA 1 3 UJ
U.K. (England)

M. Ramsey III, M.D. Ph.D.
Critikon Inc.
P.O. Box 22800
Tampa, Florida 33630
USA

Dr. U. Scherrer
Centre Hospitalier Universitaire
Vaudois
Départment de medicine interne
CH-1011 Lausanne
Switzerland

Priv.-Doz. Dr. K.-L. Schulte
Medizinische Klinik und Poliklinik
Klinikum Steglitz der
Freien Universität Berlin
Hindenburgdamm 30
1000 Berlin 45

PD Dr. J. Sehested
Rudolf-Virchow-Krankenhaus
Deutsches Herzzentrum Berlin
Augustenburger Platz 1
1000 Berlin 65

Leonard Steinfeld, M.D.
Mount Sinai Medical Center
1, Gustav L. Levy Place
New York, New York 10029
USA

Prof. Dr. B. Streitberg
Institut für Statistik
Universität Hamburg
von Mellepark 5
2000 Hamburg 13

Prof. Dr. H. Vetter
Wilhelmstr. 35-35
Universitätspoliklinik
Medizinische Klinik
5300 Bonn 1

Prof. Dr. W. Vetter
Dept. of Internal Medicine
University Hospital Zürich
Rämistraße 100
8091 Zürich
Switzerland

M. A. Weber, M. D.
VA Medical Center
Department of Medicine
Hypertension Center
5901 East Seventh Street
Long Beach, California 90822
USA

Dr. K. H. Wesseling
TNO Biomedical Instrumentation
AMC, Suite G1-111
Meibergdreef 9
1105 AZ Amsterdam
The Netherlands

1. Automatic Blood Pressure Devices

Automatic detection of Korotkoff sounds, markers for systolic and diastolic blood pressure in automated instruments

S. Mieke[1], D. Neubert[1], R.W. Gülch[2]

[1] Physikalisch-Technische Bundesanstalt, Berlin
[2] Physiologisches Institut II, FRG

Introduction

Since 1905, when Korotkoff developed the auscultatory method to measure blood pressure, this technique has evolved to become the standard method for non-invasive blood pressure determination. When in the late 1960s manufacturers started designing automated sphygmomanometers, they tried to implement the experience of physicians using sphygmomanometers and stethoscopes. As a consequence of the human threshold of audibility and the transmission characteristics of stethoscopes for low frequencies, the microphone-filter combination used for most automated sphygmomanometers have their maximum sensitivity in the range of 60 Hz to 80 Hz.

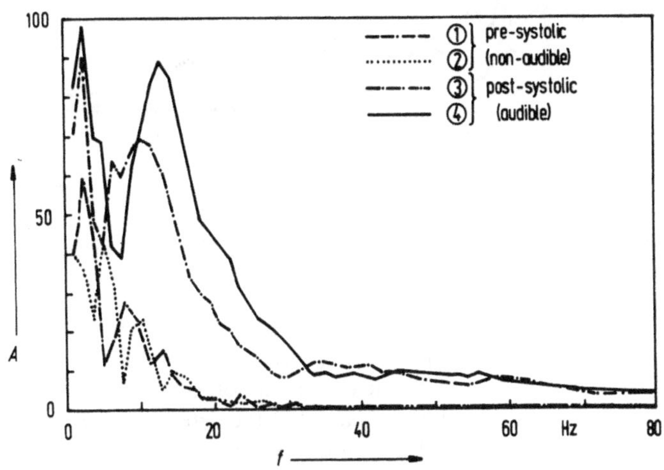

Fig. 1. Frequency spectra of Korotkoff-sounds two and one heartbeats before (no. 1 and 2) and one and two heartbeats after (no. 3 and 4) the systolic blood pressure.

Figure 1 shows the frequency spectra of typical Korotkoff-sounds (1) before and after the systolic blood pressure. The curves numbered 1 and 2 represent non-audible signals; curve number 1 measured two heartbeats, curve number 2 one heartbeat before the systolic blood pressure. The curves numbered 3 and 4 represent the frequency spectra of the first and second audible Korotkoff sound. Around 30 Hz to 80 Hz one sees an abrupt increase from curve number 2 to curve number 3, due to the first Korotkoff sound. Another much stronger change occurs around 10 Hz to 30 Hz, the magnitude of the increase makes the detection of the Korotkoff sound in this range less sensitive to artifacts.

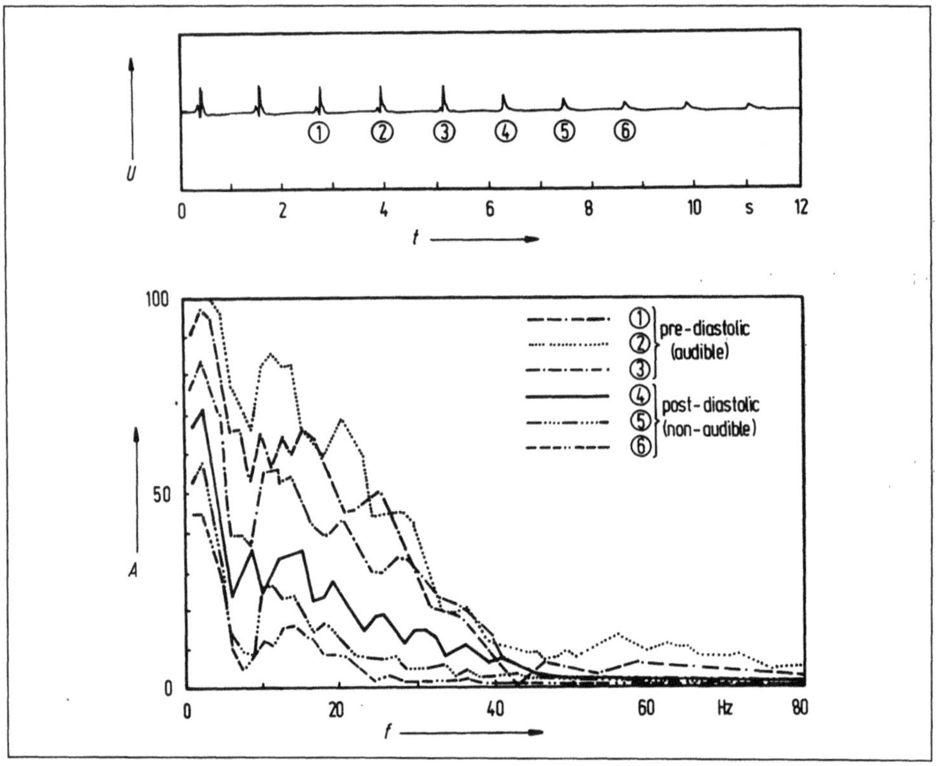

Fig. 2. Upper part: Microphone-signal of Korotkoff sounds.
Lower part: Frequency spectra of the Korotkoff-sounds shown in the upper part.

Contrary to these marked changes for the systolic pressure the frequency spectra around the diastolic pressure (phase V) change continuously, as seen in Fig. 2. Due to the absence of prominent changes, the criteria for the determination of the diastolic blood pressure have been discussed in great detail in the past. For the determination of diastolic blood pressure it is very important to find a generally accepted threshold.

At present, at least in Germany, no automated sphygmomanometers are available on the market having two filters with different characteristics for the determination of systolic and diastolic blood pressure. Only for NASA's skylab program did Golden, Wolthuis and Hoffler (2) develop an instrument with two filters, one from 18 Hz to 26 Hz for systolic and the other from 40 Hz to 60 Hz for diastolic blood pressure. Apart from this non-commercial instrument, there are only a few commercial instruments with a bandpass at a low frequency. One commercial instrument is equipped with a filter selecting frequencies in the range of 10 Hz to 50 Hz for the determination of systolic and diastolic blood pressure; for another, the manufacturer claims to use even lower frequencies than 10 Hz.

Especially for the determination of diastolic blood pressure, another method (3) has been picked up recently by Lange and Schoknecht (1) of the Federal Health Office in Germany and by Yamori et al. (4) and Blank et al. (5). Here the shape of the microphone signal (upper part of Fig. 2) is analyzed. The disappearance of the negative spike is the criteria for the diastolic blood pressure. This very characteristic criteria was found to be in good agreement with auscultatory measurements. A similar criteria exists for systolic blood pressure. The disappearing negative spike might be the first clear criteria for the determination of the diastolic blood pressure and worth further investigations. So far there are no commercial instruments available using this method, only special instruments with modified ECG-recorders.

For the automatic detection of Korotkoff sounds, a good signal-to-noise ratio is also an important factor. In the following examples are given for different ways to improve this ratio:

Using two microphones in the cuff allows to discriminate Korotkoff signals from noise. One microphone picks up the Korotkoff signal plus the artifact noise, the second microphone picks up only the artifact noise. The two microphones should be placed in close proximity in order to ensure that the artifact noise is registrated by both as nearly identically as possible and hence is cancelled by their substraction in the following network. This technique is often chosen for automated sphygmomanometers designed for measurements during exercise stress testing.

Another more frequently used technique to improve the signal-to-noise ratio employs an electronic time window for the Korotkoff signal, which is controlled by the pulse wave. Parallel to the Korotkoff signal, pressure oscillations are present in the occluding cuff deriving from the pulse wave. The oscillations can be used for the determination of systolic and diastolic blood pressure, as has been discussed in the contribution of Ramsey (5) in this book. Here we are only interested in the time relation between the oscillation and the Korotkoff signal. Figure 3 shows the time delay between the oscillations and the Korotkoff signal, which is not constant but continuously decreasing from about 200 ms for systolic to almost no delay for diastolic blood pressure.

Using an electronic time window, open only for the time when the Korotkoff signal occurs, will improve the signal-to-noise ratio. So far all instruments equipped with this technique are using a constant window, open for about 200 ms after the beginning of the oscillation. This technique will probably become standard for all instruments, detecting the Korotkoff signal.

Instruments with smaller but dynamic electronic time windows would improve the signal-to-noise ratio, too. They are more complicated to realize because one needs information about whether the cuff pressure is close to the systolic, respectively diastolic, value. More sophisticated hard- and software is required to solve this problem in the future.

The third technique improving the signal-to-noise ratio uses also an electronic time window, but in this approach it is controlled by the time delay with respect to the R-wave of the ECG. Figure 3 shows the relationship of R-wave, oscillation and Korotkoff signal. Besides the time delay between the R-wave and the oscillation, which is only slightly changing, there is the time delay between the R-wave and the Korotkoff signal, which is dynamically changing. Although the R-wave is easy to detect, this technique requires additional effort by handling ECG electrodes. This might be the reason why this method is used only for special applications such as measurements during exercise stress testing or 24-h monitoring with portable instruments.

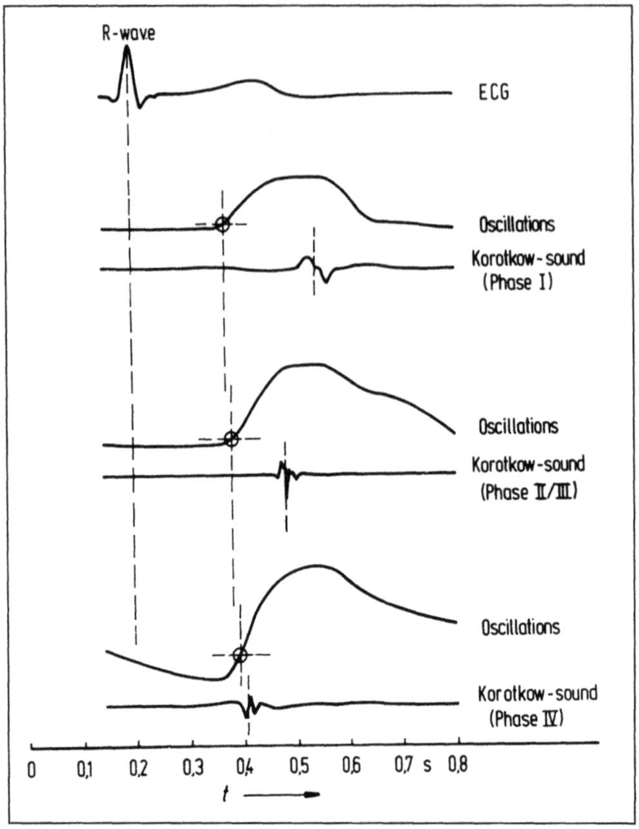

Fig. 3 Relationship between R-wave, oscillations and Korotkoff-sound, plotted for different phases.

In the late 1970s the oscillometric method has become a serious competitor in the market for automated sphygmomanometers. As a consequence, sphygmomanometers after Korotkoff are now mainly designed for special applications, such as measurements during exercise stress testing or for private use. Since sphygmomanometers for private use based on the oscillometric method are already available and are even cheaper than the Korotkoff instruments, the oscillometric method might become the favourable method also for this application. On the other hand, there seems to be enough potential for an improvement in the Korotkoff-method and some new techniques are expected to be implemented in the near future.

References

1. Lange Th, Schoknecht G (1985) Graphische und audiometrische Blutdruckmessung — Fourier-Analyse von Korotkoff-Geräuschen. Med. Phys. 16
2. Golden D, Wolthuis R, Hoffler W, Gowen R (1974) Development of a Korotkoff Sound Processor for Automatic Identification of Auscultatory Events — Part I and II. IEEE Transactions on Biomedical Engineering, Vol. BME-21, No. 2

3. Irnich W (1970) Zur Problematik der unblutigen Blutdruckmessung. Arch. Kreislaufforsch. 61
4. Yamori Y, Fukuoka M, Nara Y, Mancia G, Zanchetti A (1986) Accuracy of an objective indirect blood pressure determination with a newly developed semi-automated device; 11th Scientific Meeting of the International Society of Hypertension
5. Blank SG, West JE, Müller FB, Cody RJ, Harshfield GA, Laragh JH, Pickering ThG (1986) The Nature of the Korotkow Signal and its Application for Blood Pressure Measurement. 11th Scientific Meeting of the International Society of Hypertension
6. Ramsey M (1989) Automatic oscillometric noninvasive blood pressure: theory and practice. In Meyer-Sabellek W, Anlauf M, Gotzen R, Steinfeld L (eds.): Blood pressure measurements. New techniques in automatic indirect monitoring. p. 15—21, Steinkopff/Springer, Darmstadt/New York.

Testing the accuracy of automated and semi-automated sphygmomanometers designed for home use

L. Steinfeld, M. Cohen, S. Kurtz, O.D. Almeida
Mt. Sinai Medical Center New York, New York, USA

Measuring blood pressure at home has become very popular among those who feel they are at risk because of the perils of hypertension. This has resulted in a proliferation on the consumer market of various types of inexpensive sphygmomanometers designed for home use. Virtually all these instruments implicitly or explicitly allege to measure arterial blood pressure with a reasonable degree of accuracy, but whether this is so remains to be proven. It is not widely appreciated that there are no governmental regulations regarding performance standards for home-use sphygmomanometers, and not unexpectedly there is a paucity of unbiased published data attesting to their efficacy.
The purpose of this investigation was to evaluate in an adult population the accuracy and reliability of a variety of automated and semi-automated sphygmomanometers marketed for home use.

65 different sphygmomanometers were obtained for testing primarily from sources in the United States, Germany and Japan. The 65 instruments could be divided into three subtypes:
The simplest system employed a stethoscope for detecting Korotkoff sounds. The stethoscope head was housed on the undersurface of the occluding cuff, and Korotkoff sounds served to discriminate systolic and diastolic points.
A second type of sphygmomanometer housed a microphone on the undersurface of the occluding cuff, but the Korotkoff sounds were processed electronically, enabling either an audio or light signal to indicate systolic and diastolic points.
The third type of instrument employed the principles of oscillometry. Arterial pulsewaves were transmitted via the occluding cuff and tubing to an electronic box which processed the signals for digital display of pressures.

Each instrument was evaluated by measuring an instrument blood pressure simultaneously with a direct arterial pressure. Instrument blood pressures were obtained from the left arm. The direct blood pressure was recorded with either a fluid-filled catheter coupled to a strain gauge or with a micromanometer tip catheter, the tip of which was positioned at the aortic origin of the left subclavian artery. The 65 instruments were randomly tested in 162 patients whose ages ranged between 20 and 75 years (Fig. 1—3). For each instrument, duplicate blood pressure measurements were always taken on three different patients.

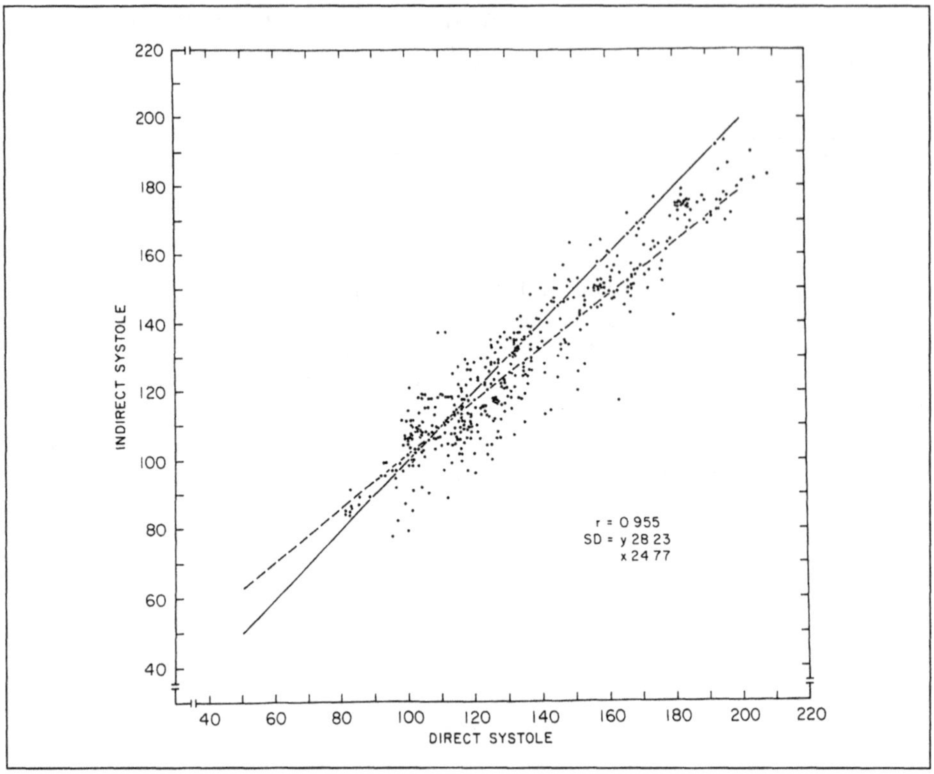

Fig. 1. The aggregated data for systolic pressure are detailed. Instrument systolic pressure measurements are shown on the ordinate and the direct systolic measurements are shown on the abscissa. The correlation coefficient is 0.95 and there is a relatively narrow spread of data points about the line of identity.

In Fig. 6 there is a minor difference between the two groups of instruments in the measurement of systolic pressure, but there is a conspicuous difference in the measurement of diastolic pressure. The stethoscopic devices measured systolic and diastolic blood pressure more accurately than the electronic instruments. It is important to recognize that doctors familiar with Korotkoff sounds performed these tests, and results might be different for non-professionals.

Since an objective of this investigation was to identify instruments which would measure blood pressure with reasonable accuracy at home, the original 65 instruments were screened for accuracy. Each device was graded on a scale of 1—4. Grade 1 was considered the most accurate and grade 4 the least accurate. 25 devices graded either 1 or 2 were selected for re-evaluation (Fig. 4). The format for testing was the same as that previously described.

In a continuing effort to identify those sphygmomanometers from which the home user can expect a reasonably accurate blood pressure measurement, five devices were specially selected for more intensive evaluation (Fig. 6). The choice of instruments were made on the basis of previously demonstrated favorable correlative studies, in conjunction with certain preferred design and engineering features. All were electronic devices, and of the

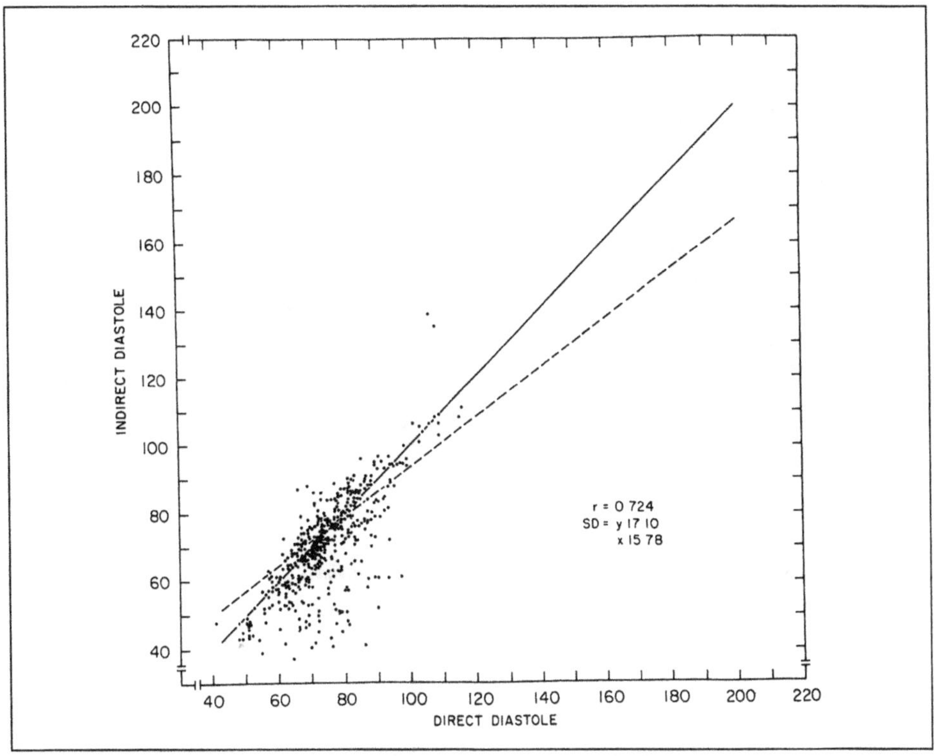

Fig. 2. The aggregated data for diastolic pressure are shown. The correlation coefficient is 0.72, but here is a wide dispersion of values around the line of identity. When the data from the 65 instruments were thus considered in the aggregate, the accuracy of measuring systolic blood pressure was regarded as acceptable, whereas diastolic blood pressure measurement was unacceptable.

five, four used Korotkoff sounds, and one oscillometric technology as the measurement discriminator. Simultaneous instrument, direct and auscultatory blood pressure measurements were made on the left arm. The blood pressure measurements were obtained from a representative adult population consisting of 44 subjects. The study was performed within the framework of a statistically valid factorial design which considered the measurement accuracy of the five units the effects of age, sex and arm circumference on blood pressure measurement. To assess these variables, two analyses of variance were conducted, one for systolic and one for diastolic blood pressure. The inaccuracy of a device was defined as a difference between the device measurement and the direct or auscultatory measurement. The accuracy of each device was evaluated against the proposed AAMI standards for electronic sphygmomanometers.

AAMI is the acronym for the Association for the Advancement of Medical Instrumentation. The proposed AAMI standard for sphygmomanometers states that the mean pressure difference obtained by the system shall be within 5 mmHg mean difference, with a standard deviation of 8 mmHg, of the mean measurements obtained by the direct or auscultatory measurements.

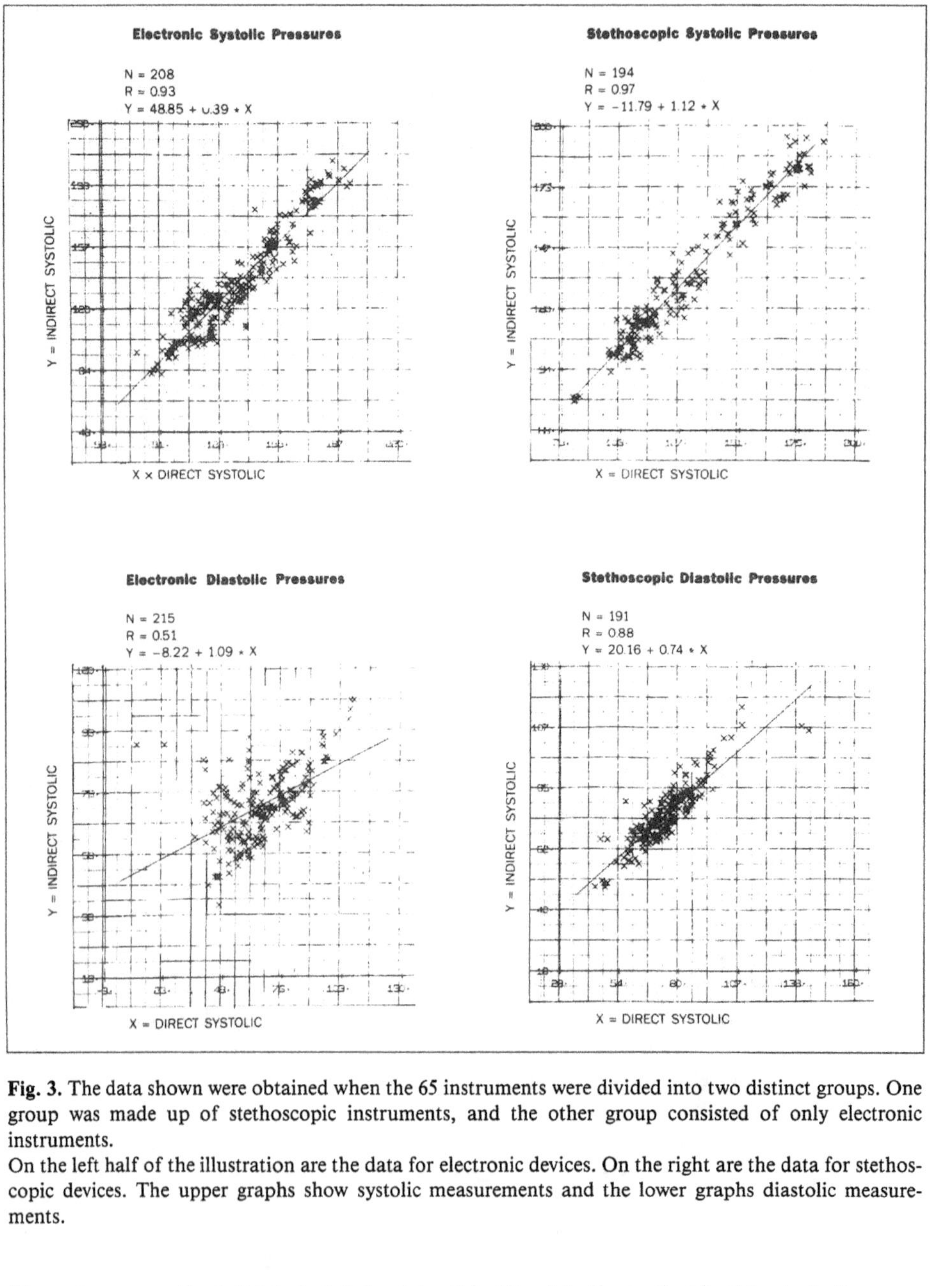

Fig. 3. The data shown were obtained when the 65 instruments were divided into two distinct groups. One group was made up of stethoscopic instruments, and the other group consisted of only electronic instruments.
On the left half of the illustration are the data for electronic devices. On the right are the data for stethoscopic devices. The upper graphs show systolic measurements and the lower graphs diastolic measurements.

The columns on the left labeled "physician" in Fig. 6 indicate that in this study the conventional sphygmomanometer or auscultatory measurements, compared with direct arterial pressure, conform to AAMI standards. It is clear from the five instruments' bar graphs that, when comparisons were made between instrument measurements and direct measurements, none of the five selected devices met the AAMI standards for both mean pressure difference and standard deviation, with respect to both systole and diastole (Fig. 7).

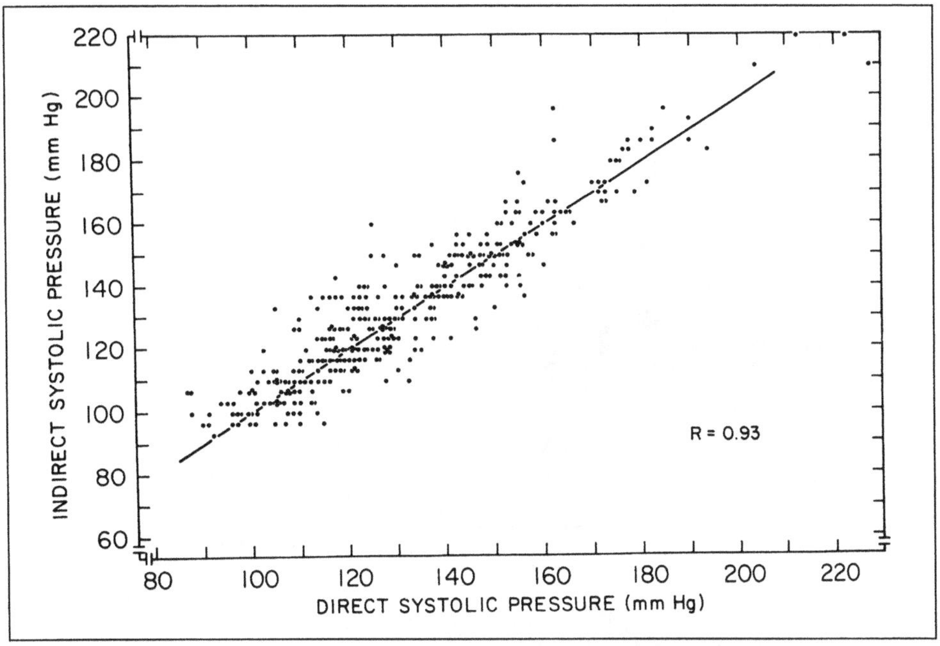

Fig. 4. For the 25 selected instruments, the R value for systolic blood pressure was 0.93.

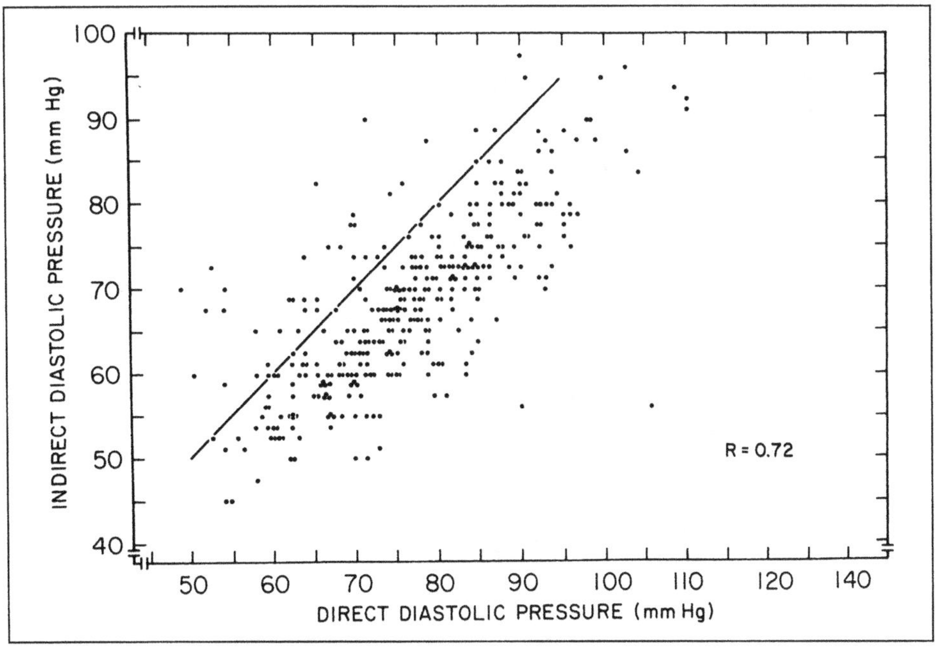

Fig. 5. The R value for diastolic blood pressure was 0.72. For reasons yet to be explained, the R values for the 25 selected instruments were similar to those of the larger unselected series.

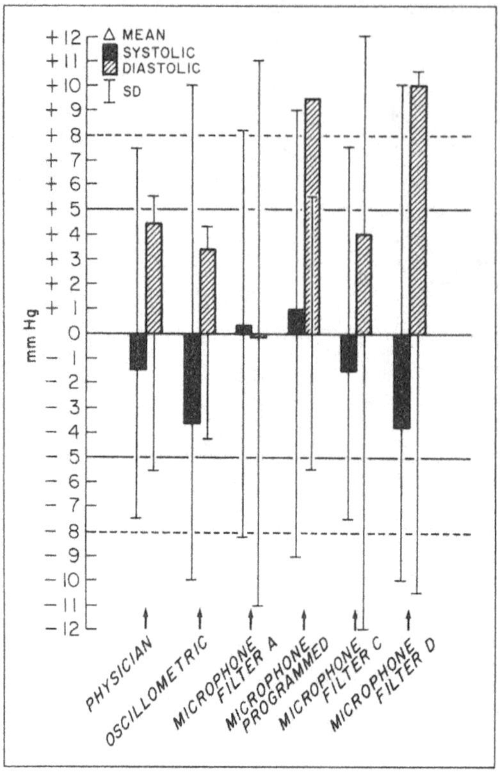

Fig. 6. This illustration summarizes the results of testing of the five specially selected sphygmomanometers. The wide bars represent the difference in mean pressure between instrument and direct pressure measurements. The solid bars are the systolic and the striped bars the diastolic mean pressure differences. The vertical linear bars represent the standard deviations. The horizontal lines at 5 mmHg are the AAMI limits for the mean difference in pressure, and the horizontal interrupted lines at 8 mmHg represent the AAMI limits for standard deviation.

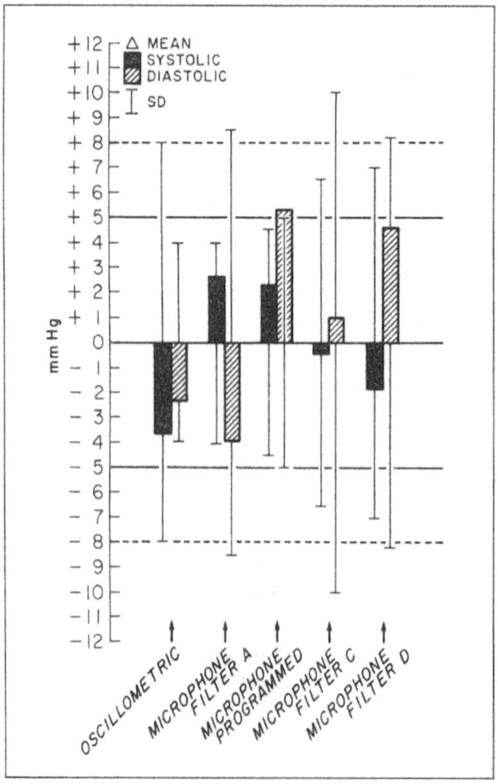

Fig. 7. When comparsions were made between the five selected instruments and auscultatory pressures, the mean differences and standard deviations of all five devices conformed, or nearly conformed, to the AAMI standards.

The analyses of variance for systolic pressure revealed that accuracy was marginally greater for males than females at a P value of 0.05. For diastolic pressure, somewhat greater accuracy was obtained on patients less than 55 years of age than in patients older than 55 years.

In conclusion, the data obtained in this investigation reveal that sphygmomanometers designed for home use, even under the best circumstance, cannot be relied upon to accurately measure diastolic blood pressure. Their performance is better in the measurement of systolic blood pressure. But the performance of any device is a function, to a variable extent, of the skill displayed in its use.

In a limited population sampling, the results showed that variables such as age, sex, and arm circumference had only negligible effects on measurement of blood pressure.

Studies with five selected electronic sphygmomanometers, screened from 65 devices, showed that none of the instruments tested against direct blood pressure fully satisfied the proposed AAMI standards with respect to both systole and diastole.

When the performance of the five selected electronic devices was evaluated against auscultatory blood pressure measurements, all five instruments either fully, or nearly fully, met these standards.

Automatic oscillometric noninvasive blood pressure: theory and practice

M. Ramsey III

Critikon Inc., Tampa, Florida, USA

Introduction to blood pressure measurement

Although the subject of this paper is largely concerned with the automatic oscillometric noninvasive measurement of blood pressure, it is instructive to briefly trace the history of the measurement of blood pressure from its origins. In 1733 Stephen Hales reported that he measured directly the blood pressure of several horses by inserting a brass tube into various arteries and then connecting this brass tube to a short segment of goose windpipe which in turn was connected to a 12 foot glass tube. He observed that in all three animals the blood rose to a height of over 9 feet in height which demonstrated that the mean blood pressure of the horse was approximately 220 mmHg. Almost 100 years later, in 1828, Jean Louis Marie Poiseuille repeated essentially Hales' experiment but this time in the dog, and he used the much more convenient mercury manometer instead of a glass tube filled with blood. These early efforts at measuring blood pressure were all concerned with the invasive measurement and made no attempt at noninvasive measurement. The first practical experiments and devices for noninvasively measuring the blood pressure were those of von Bash and Marey in 1876. Von Bash used a pressure indicating device which indicated the amount of pressure required to occlude a superficial artery by direct pressure. Marey used an occluding device which encompassed the entire hand and forearm and essentially introduced the oscillometric method of blood pressure measurements. However, Marey's device and many later devices were cumbersome because the occluding apparatus required that hands, fingers or even whole arms to be inserted within their pressure cavity. The cumbersomeness of these early indirect measurements was greatly reduced by Riva-Rocci in Italy and Hill and Barnard in England in the late 1890's when they almost simultaneously introduced the use of air-inflated arm occluding cuffs. Although the discovery of the use of the arm occluding cuff to allow the measurement of the systolic pressure by the palpatory method was a great convenience, both the cuffs of Riva-Rocci and Hill and Barnard were considerably too narrow. In 1901 von Recklinghausen investigated the cuff width versus arm size question more thoroughly and showed that a cuff 10—12 cm wide gave accurate results in an adult having an arm circumference of 24 cm. Interestingly, the 12-cm-wide cuff is the one which is today called the standard adult blood pressure cuff. Using this cuff, the oscillometric method was reintroduced and meticulously described by Erlanger in 1903. Using his oscillometric device he showed that the systolic and diastolic pressures could be measured by choosing as systolic the point on the smoked drum recording where the amplitude of oscillations in cuff pressure increased dramatically and he utilized the lowest cuff pressure with maximum oscillations as the diastolic pressure. Although the oscillometric method achieved some degree of popularity, the more convenient auscultatory method introduced by Korotkoff in 1905 largely supplanted the oscillometric method for manual blood pressure determinations. The reason for the auscultatory method's superiority as a manual method for noninvasive blood pressure determination were that (1) the systolic and diastolic endpoints could be judged more accurately by simply listening for the onset and cessation of sounds over the brachial artery just distal to the occluding cuff, and hence not requiring the aid of a smoked drum recording, and (2) the only apparatus required was the previously known arm occluding cuff and the stethoscope.

Thus by 1905 all of the methods in common use today (other than the ultrasonic method which is really a variant of the auscultatory method) were known and being practiced: the flush method (based on return of color in the distal limb during deflation of the cuff), the palpatory method, the oscillometric method and the auscultatory method. The reader is referred to the excellent history by L.A. Geddes (1) from which these preceding facts were taken.

Since the discovery and development of the various methods of indirect blood pressure measurement, many indications for blood pressure have developed. The most common reason for measuring blood pressure is for the detection of hypertension and the monitoring of its therapy. Similarly, it is routine practice that all patients in the hospital have their blood pressure measured at least once a day and most patients will have it measured more often. In both of these applications, the auscultatory method is the one generally utilized and because the patients are generally not in circulatory extremis, the method functions quite successfully in the low normal to modestly elevated range of blood pressure, assuming good technique is used. However, the measurement of blood pressure in the critically ill patient, such as in an intensive care unit or during surgery, requires that not only the measurement be made more frequently than several times per day but also that it be measured in patients who may well be in circulatory shock or extremely hypertensive. This need for measuring blood pressure noninvasively, often, and accurately even in patients with abnormal circulatory status has led to the development of automated noninvasive blood pressure devices based on auscultatory, ultrasonic, and oscillometric principles. Devices based on these methods as well as some variants of the auscultatory method are in routine clinical use today, with the automatic oscillometric devices by the far the most widely used, and in this author's view, the most robust, reliable, and accurate.

Theory of operation

Almost all current blood pressure measuring devices involve the inflation of an occluding cuff to a pressure somewhat above the systolic pressure and the slow deflation of that cuff to a pressure below diastolic pressure. During this deflation of the cuff the device attempts to determine the systolic, diastolic, and mean arterial pressures.

The manually operated devices as well as the automatically operated devices can all be broken down into six major components. These six major components will be referred to as the six building blocks of noninvasive blood pressure measurement and will be briefly described.

1. The pneumatic compression cuff is an essential component of all of the currently used noninvasive blood pressure measurement systems. They vary widely in their size, the material of construction, and the number of inflating and monitoring tubes to the cuff bladder.

2. A cuff inflation means is always present, whether it be a manually operated squeeze-bulb, an electrically operated small pump, or in some cases, a reservoir of compressed gas.
3. A cuff deflation means is likewise always required and this takes the form of the simple hand-operated bleed valve, an automatically operated linear deflate valve or an automatically operated step deflation valve.
4. A pressure sensor and indicator is required and for the manual method is generally an aneroid capsule with attached indicator, or a column of mercury. In the case of automated and semi-automated devices a pressure transducer with digital display is generally used.
5. A signal sensor and endpoint detector are required to determine when the cuff pressure is passing through one of the desired pressures, such as the systolic or diastolic. This endpoint detector is generally a stethoscope in the auscultatory method, an ultrasonic transmitter and receiver in the ultrasonic method, a finger on the radial pulse for the palpatory method and the human eye detecting the change in color of the limb for the flush method. The oscillometric method utilizes the pressure sensing device to judge the amplitude of pressure oscillations at each cuff pressure.
6. All of the previously mentioned apparatuses are utilized in concert towards the goal of measuring the blood pressure noninvasively. It is the overall determination strategy and the algorithms which implement that strategy which provide, the intelligence and coordination that commands the various other component parts to do their work. This determination strategy and the algorithms which implement it may be imbedded in the human mind or in the memory of a microprocessor.

Since the automatic oscillometric method is the automatic method in most common use for the measurement of blood pressure in the critically ill, this paper will henceforth focus primarily on its theory and practice of operation. The hardware required to implement an automatic oscillometric noninvasive blood pressure device consists of an arm occluding cuff which is inflated by an electric pump to the desired initial cuff pressure. This initial inflation pressure is selected by either the user or by the microprocessor itself. Once at the desired upper pressure level, the cuff is deflated either incrementally in steps or continuously with a linear bleed to a pressure below diastolic pressure. During this deflation process, the amplitude of small oscillations which occur in the cuff pressure in response to the increase in arterial pressure at each heartbeat are measured and stored in association with their corresponding cuff pressures. The cuff pressure at which these oscillations increase dramatically is selected as the systolic pressure, the lowest cuff pressure at which they are a maximum is selected as mean arterial pressure, and the cuff pressure at which they decrease rapidly from this maximum is selected as diastolic. (Incidentally, these are very close to the same endpoints which were utilized in the manual oscillometric method by Erlanger and others, and have been shown to give good results.) The difficulty, however, arises in those cases in which the endpoints are not distinct which has given rise to the use of certain ratios of the amplitude of a given oscillation to that of the maximum oscillation amplitude as a means of picking the systolic and diastolic endpoints. How these systolic and diastolic endpoints are judged and tested for validity constitute some of the algorithms which implement the overall strategy of oscillometric blood pressure determination. Other crucial algorithms are those associated with measuring the onset of each oscillation, its peak, the inflation of the cuff to the appropriate pressure and the orderly deflation of the cuff pressure to below the diastolic level.

When these pieces of hardware and the strategies and algorithms which mold them together into a functioning blood pressure unit are rigorously constructed and exhaustively tested and improved, the accuracy of the measurement done automatically is very good when compared to simultaneously measured intra-arterial pressures. When conducted according to the AAMI Standard for automatic noninvasive blood pressure devices, the DINAMAP™ Monitor Model 1846 and over a wide range of patients when compared to simultaneously measured invasive arterial pressure, has a mean difference of less than 3 mmHg and a standard deviation of less than 6 mmHg. (The AAMI Standard requires that the difference be no greater than 5 ± 8 mmHg.)

The robustness of these measurements, that is the device's ability to deliver acceptable accuracy in spite of a modest amount of motion artifact or blood pressure variability, is one of the most important factors in the clinical acceptability of an automatic noninvasive blood pressure device. However, to date no generally acceptable robustness index has been established and thus it is necessary to describe this very important characteristic of a blood pressure device in general terms only. The robustness of the measurements of the DINAMAP™ Monitor Model 1846 are in general very good, meaning that motion artifact, even of an extreme degree, will not adversely affect the readings in most instances unless it is protracted or unless it is at a frequency which mimics that of the human heart. Another way to describe it would be to say that in its use in surgery during an average case of an average patient, the device would be fooled by artifact into displaying erroneous information only rarely, if at all. The speed of the device in its fastest mode of operation will allow up to two and one-half determinations per minute. Since in this mode of operation two systolic pressures are given for each full determination this yields four to five systolic pressures each minute of operation.

The factors which limit the accuracy and robustness of these devices in clinical use can be divided into factors which are constant for each individual patient and those which are variable within that patient. The cuff size versus the arm size is probably the most important constant factor for each patient in determining the accuracy of the readings obtained. It has been shown that if the width of the cuff is 40% of the circumference of the arm, the cuff sizing is optimum. Any deviation from this 40% ratio should be towards making the cuff somewhat larger, since the error introduced as the cuff becomes larger than the 40% of the arm circumference is less than if it is allowed to decrease to a ratio of less than 40% of the arm circumference. Another factor which can influence the accuracy of the readings is the arm shape, i. e., whether it be cylindrical or conical (as well as its consistency), since these factors can influence the effective transfer of cuff pressure to the underlying arm and artery. Obviously without an even and effective transmission of cuff pressure to the underlying arm the accuracy will be degraded. Similarly, if the patient has arterial rigidity of whatever cause, the pressure required to occlude the artery will be higher than would otherwise be the case, resulting in falsely elevated readings.

Factors which can be variable within each subject are related to motion artifact and rapid changes in the blood pressure itself. Motion artifact can be divided into intrinsic and extrinsic motion artifact. Intrinsic motion artifact is caused by voluntary or involuntary patient movement during flexing or moving the arm or another portion of the body intentionally, or during unintentional movement such as caused by a seizure of shivering. Extrinsic motion artifact can be caused by any external pressure on the cuff or by external movement of the patient. For instance, during surgery the surgeon may bump against

the blood pressure cuff causing motion artifact, or the patient himself may be rhythmically disturbed such as during prepping or positioning during surgery.
Rapid changes in the patient's blood pressure during the time of determination by the automatic noninvasive device can cause spurious readings because of the change in the amplitude of the oscillations produced within the time of a single determination. These rapid changes in blood pressure may be due to cardiac dysrhythmia, respiratory variation, dramatic blood loss, or intrinsic or extrinsic arterial compression. These dramatic changes in blood pressure not only make it difficult for the automatic device to make an accurate determination of blood pressure, but likewise make it difficult to specify uniquely the patient's blood pressure even when measured invasively, until the rapid variation ceases. This difficulty in specifying a subject's blood pressure, whether invasively or noninvasively determined during extreme variation of that pressure is not a major problem until the magnitude of variation approaches the 30% level within a 10 to 20 second period. Changes which are slower than this can be faithfully followed since they are occurring more slowly than the measurement being made.

Practice: utilization and interpretation

Adult, child and neonate (lower limit approximately 650 grams) are all suitable subjects for use with automatic noninvasive blood pressure devices of the oscillometric type. As previously discussed, there is a requirement that the patients not be in uninterrupted motion while their pressures are being determined, since this would cause constant motion artifact, thus not allowing the device to function properly. On a given subject, all of the limbs are potential sites for oscillometric blood pressure monitoring and in general the upper arm is the preferred location. However, should an alternative site be needed, it is best to choose one which is basically cylindrical and not greatly tapered as, for example, some thighs are. In general, as an alternative site the ankle works quite well and is very comfortable for the subject. Another factor to be considered, however, is that the location of the blood pressure cuff should be at the same horizontal height as the heart itself, since otherwise there will be a hydrostatic offset resulting in higher readings if the cuff is below the heart level and lower readings if the heart is above the heart level. The magnitude of the hydrostatic offset is approximately 2 mmHg per inch of horizontal difference between the cuff location and the heart itself. In selecting the site for blood pressure cuff placement it is best if it is not placed proximal to a site being used for intravenous infusion (or any vascular access or pathology).

As previously described, the cuff size selected should be of a width approximately 40% of the limb circumference. However, if a cuff of different size than this optimum must be utilized, it is important that it be slightly too large rather than too small, since the errors introduced from utilizing a cuff slightly too large are in general much less than those in utilizing one too small. Before applying the appropriately sized cuff to the selected limb, care must be taken that all air be expelled from the cuff so that when it is applied it can be wrapped quite snugly and contain no residual air before the device is put into operation. If numerous measurements are to be made over a protracted period of time, it is advisable to protect the skin of the arm by first applying a knit stocking over which the cuff ist then snuggly. This stocking material is generally useful, but is particularly desirable in those patients with loose, thin, or fragile skin regardless of the cause.

In most patients, selection of the automatic (that is the automatically repeating) mode in appropriate. The cycle time should be set short enough to provide early warning of blood pressure variation, but with sufficient interim periods of cuff deflation to allow sufficient circulation to the distal limb and skin beneath the cuff. The utility of the automatic oscillometric device can be increased by utilizing appropriately set limit alarms to provide a vigilance assist in case of distraction of the operator.

The accuracy and reliability of the measurements will be enhanced if the extrinsic and intrinsic motion artifact can be reduced or eliminated. This translates generally into keeping the subject quiet and still and shielding the cuff from inadvertent bumping by the surgeon or other healthcare personnel. In the case of readings which are suspect, it is important to always immediately obtain a new reading for verification. Multiple readings with similar values give the best assurance of accuracy. In some instances it is necessary to account for the previously described hydrostatic pressure difference between the heart and the site of the blood pressure cuff. This is particularly true when patients in surgery have their position changed, which results in a relative shift of the level of the cuff and the heart.

During use, it is important to periodically inspect the cuff and arm for any unsuspected problem such as the cuff becoming detached or its position having shifted so that it no longer is snugly and evenly positioned on the arm. Similarly it is important to periodically verify by visual inspection and by feel that the cuff is being inflated and deflated at the appropriate times.

Although not generally practical during the actual utilization of an automatic oscillometric blood pressure device on a patient, if the operation of such device is suspect, a rough indication of its proper function can be obtained by making measurements on people whose approximate level of blood pressure is known, and by measuring the pressure at various sites on the body such as the ankle and the wrist while the arm is held overhead. These checks should indicate whether the device is able to measure pressure over a broad range of values. By comparing the measured pressure with the hydrostatically corrected pressure measured in the arm at heart level should indicate if the device is generally giving the appropriate answer. Similarly the sensitivity of the device can be verified by intentionally loosely wrapping the cuff and determining if proper function can occur in spite of an inappropriately increased cuff volume. These simple user conducted tests can often be utilized to determine the general level of performance of device, but are not a substitute for an appropriate investigation by an authorized and trained electronics technician utilizing the appropriate tools. Similarly the calibration of the instrument should be checked regularly using a mercury manometer as described in the users manual. These devices are extremely reliable, but these tests and precautions are good indirect assurance that an obvious or occult failure is unlikely to have occured.

Conclusion

Today's automatic noninvasive blood pressure device is an extremely useful tool for the monitoring of critical care patients in surgery and intensive care (2). It is the result of the application of electronics technology to the implementation and refinement of methods developed for manual use in the early 1900's. Like those early devices, it utilizes the six fundamental building blocks of noninvasive blood prassure, but in enhanced ways, to achieve accuracy and speed suitable for routine clinical use. Although the automatic oscillometric device is quite simple to use, good results do require a user who is knowledgeable in the basics of its operation, its appropriate application to suitable patients, and the interpretation of the data generated.

Reference

1. Geddes LA (1970) The direct and indirect measurement of blood pressure
2. Frucht U (1989) How reliable are indirect blood pressure measurement devices in the intensive care unit (ICU)? In Meyer-Sabellek W, Anlauf M, Gotzen R, Steinfeld L (eds.): Blood pressure measurements. New techniques in automatic indirect monitoring. p. 61—80, Steinkopff/Springer, Darmstadt/New York

Plethysmographic (volume-oscillometric) method of non-invasive monitoring ambulatory blood pressure

K.-L. Schulte, W. Meyer-Sabellek

Medizinische Klinik und Poliklinik, Klinikum Steglitz, Freie Universität Berlin, Berlin, FRG

Introduction

The value of long-term monitoring of ambulatory blood pressure for the diagnosis of arterial hypertension, as well as for epidemiological, physiological, and pharmacological studies in hypertensive patients has been widely demonstrated (1—4).
A device to monitor intra-arterial pressure was developed in Oxford, England, which has produced the most reliable blood pressure readings and useful data (5). However, as an invasive method with possible severe side effects and complications it is not practical for daily and repetitive measurements in patients.
Therefore, non-invasive automatic or semi-automatic blood pressure recorders based on the Korotkoff sound technique or cuff-oscillometric method using conventional arm-cuffs have been developed (6). As this equipment is relatively noisy and intermittent cuff inflations cause discomfort to patients and frequently disturb sleep, some investigators have been looking for other methods of non-invasive and ambulatory long-term blood pressure monitoring.

Method of plethysmography

One method is based on venous occlusion plethysmography. Venous occlusion plethysmography or volume-oscillometry is a method to measure arterial blood flow or venous capacity in the extremity (7, 8). With water- or mercury-in-silastic strain gauge, or photo plethysmography, volume changes in the arm, leg, or digit are derived from changes in circumference of the extremity detected by changes in water volume, resistance of the applied gauge, or light extinction (9, 10). In Fig. 1a mercury-in-silastic strain gauge finger plethysmograph (Periquant 3500, Gutmann LPM, Eurasburg, FRG) is shown. Total blood flow to an extremity can be derived plethysmographically from the increase in volume of the extremity during the first heart beats immediately after subdiastolic venous occlusion. Venous occlusion is produced by a cuff applied proximal to the measuring site. With such cuff pressure the arterial inflow is not disturbed while the venous outflow is blocked. After the first heart beats the arterial inflow can no longer be determined because of venous congestion, although the devices of digital blood flow and pressure determination are different from the Riva-Rocci method in measurement of the brachial blood pressure.

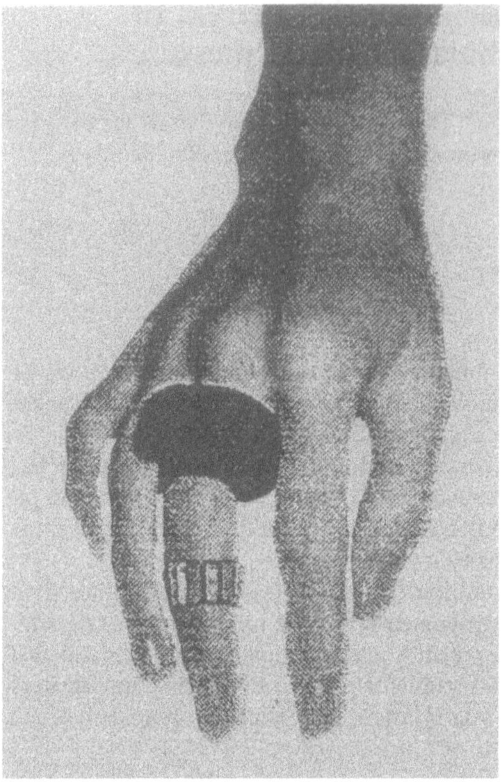

Fig. 1. Mercury-in-silastic strain gauge plethysmograph.

Plethysmographic blood pressure measurement

The basic volume-oscillometric finger discontinous blood pressure measurement device comprises the following components: a digital sensor to detect pulsation, an electrical capacitor converting the sensed pulse into visual indication, a proximal occluding cuff, an air- or fluid-pump to provide inflation or filling and an aeroid manometer for measuring the pressure exerted in the cuff. The cuff obturates the digital artery, and after progressive pressure increases and decreases the pulse sensor downstream from the cuff detects a pulse. Pressure indicated by the manometer represents systolic pressure. The pulse sensor acts as a volumetric transducer, detecting a change in the volume of the finger distal to the cuff when the systolic pressure exceeds cuff pressure. A mercury-in-silastic strain gauge for volume detection or photoplethysmographic probe on the pulp of the digit can be used as a sensor. The available photocell plethysmographs for blood pressure registration consist of an infrared emitting diode as optical source and a photocell detector as appropriate detector, and are based on the large difference between the extinction coefficient of blood and body tissues. The finger cuff is pressurized by a pump and deflated with a constant rate. Via a pressure transducer and after preamplification has taken place, the photo-plethysmographic pulses and cuff-pressure are simultaneously presented to a recorder. In ambulatory devices the signals are led to a recorder for later evaluation (11, 12).

Clinical availability

The main methodological problem of plethysmographic blood pressure is the difficulty of measuring or determining diastolic blood pressure; as described, after progressively increasing and decreasing pressure in the cuff the pulse sensor downstream detects a pulse. Pressure indicated by the manometer represents systolic pressure. Diastolic blood pressure, however, has to be calculated.

Yamakoshi et al. (13, 14), who designed a device for volume-oscillometric ambulatory blood pressure recording, found that the cuff pressure values corresponding to the systolic end-point and to the maximum amplitude of photo-plethysmographic pulsations are in good agreement with systolic blood pressure (SBP) and mean blood pressure (MBP) in the arterial segment concerned. The diastolic blood pressure (DBP) is calculated tentatively according to the conventional formula: DBP = (3 x MBP — SBP)/2. Systolic blood pressure by volume-oscillometry correlates with direct (Oxford system) and conventional arm-cuff methods' measured values, whereas diastolic blood pressure values are tentative and approximate. The absolute blood pressure is different from that measured simultaneously using a conventional arm cuff, which is probably due to the difference in the measuring sites, i. e., arm vs finger and right side vs left side. The reproducibility of systolic and diastolic blood pressure values is high (11).

Another sophisticated method of plethysmographic ambulatory blood pressure measurement is the volume clamp method (12) used in Finapres and further developed by Wesseling (see p. 161). It is possible to record systolic as well as diastolic blood pressure continously using this equipment of plethysmographic blood pressure measurement and registered data are in good correlation with intra-arterial pressure registered in the brachial artery.

Volume-oscillometric devices successfully register, (discontinously, not be beat-to-beat recording) blood pressure during exercise, i. e., sports activities. This is in contrast to conventional arm cuff methods of ambulatory blood pressure readings (11).

The portable volume-oscillometric device developed by Yamakoshi et al. (13, 14) weighs 800 g and causes fewer side effects than any conventional fully-automatic portable recorder. It produces minimal noise, causes less discomfort and minimal sleep disturbance. These factors could facilitate the patients compliance during long-term monitoring and repeatedly allow measurements (11).

Three major problems may occur in outpatients: First, devices with cuff inflation can induce swelling and/or ischemia of the finger in patients with peripheral circulatory disease (i. e., arterio-venous shunt for extracorporal circulation of artificial kidney), occlusive disease (i. e., diabetic macroangiopathy), and vasospastic disease (i. e., Morbus Raynaud) and are not acceptable for these patients. Second, in patients with cardiac arrhythmias, vasospastic, and occlusive arterial diseases, the evaluation of volume-oscillometric recorded blood pressure values is especially difficult. Third, the peripheral vascular tree of the finger reacts more sensibly than the lower and upper arm when there is ischemia or hyperemia induced by changes of outside temperatures. This implicates a restricted ambulatory application.

Conclusion

The plethysmographic (volume-oscillometric) fully-automatic portable finger device allows 24-h monitoring of ambulatory blood pressure with fewer side effects and less disturbance of sleep than the conventional non-invasive equipment; this facilitates blood pressure registrations during daily routine as well as during physical activity. However, only systolic blood pressure can be recorded exactly. With the exception of the volume clamp device diastolic blood pressure has to be tentatively calculated. Furthermore, digital blood pressure measurement by plethysmographic devices is disturbed by ischemia or hyperemia induced by changes in temperature or vascular diseases.

References

1. Sokolow M, Werdegar D, Kain HK, Hinman AT (1966) Relationship between level of blood pressure measured casually and by portable records and severity of complications in essential hypertension. Circulation 34: 279—298
2. Floras JS, Hassan MO, Sever PS, Jones JV, Osikowska B, Sleight P (1981) Cuff and ambulatory blood pressure in subjects with essential hypertension. Lancet II: 107—109
3. Perloff D, Sokoloff M, Cowan R (1983) The prognostic value of ambulatory blood pressure. JAMA 249: 2792—2798
4. Pickering TG, Harshfield GA, Devereux RB, Laragh JH (1985) What is the role of ambulatory blood pressure monitoring in the management of hypertensive patients? Hypertension 7: 171—177
5. Littler WA, Honour AJ, Sleight P (1974) Direct arterial pressure, pulse rate, and electrocardiogram during micturation and defaecation in unrestricted man. Am Heart J 88: 205—210
6. Meyer-Sabellek W, Schulte K-L, Distler A, Gotzen R (1987) Technische Aspekte der ambulanten, automatischen, nichtinvasiven 24-h-Blutdruckmessung. Schweiz Rundschau Med (Praxis) 76: 443—449
7. Brodie TG, Russell AE (1905) On the determination of the rate of blood flow through an organ. J Physiol 32: 47—49
8. Hewlett AE, van Zwaluwenburg JG (1909) The rate of blood flow in the arm. Heart 1: 87—97
9. Schulte K-L, Braun J, Meyer-Sabellek W, Wegscheider K, Gotzen R, Distler A (1988) Functional versus structural changes of forearm vascular resistance in hypertension. Hypertension 10: 220—225
10. Close A, Hamilton G, Muriss S (1986) Finger systolic pressure: its use in screening for hypertension and monitoring. Brit Med J 293: 775—778
11. Imai Y, Nihei M, Abe K, Sasaki S, Minami N, Munakata M, Yumita S, Onoda Y, Sekino H, Yamakoshi K, Yoshinaga K (1987) A finger volume-oscillometric device for monitoring ambulatory blood pressure: laboratory and clinical evaluations. Clin Exp Hypertens A9 (12): 2001—2005
12. Wesseling KH, Penáz J (1986) Indirect blood pressure measurement in the finger: Physiological background of a recent development. Scripta Medica 59: 203—205
13. Yamakoshi K, Shimizu H, Shibata M, Kamiya A (1982) New oscillometric method for indirect measurement of systolic and mean arterial pressure in the human finger. Part 1: model experiment. Med Biol Eng Comput 20: 307—313
14. Yamakoshi K, Shimizu H, Shibata M, Kamiya A (1982) New oscillometric method for indirect measurement of systolic and mean arterial pressure in the human finger. Part 2: correlation study. Med Biol Eng Comput 20: 314—318

The use of piezofilms for noninvasive measurements of blood pressure

W. Nitsche

Institut für Luft- und Raumfahrt, Technische Universität Berlin,
Berlin, FRG

Introduction

Measuring time-dependent blood pressure in the human vascular system creates numerous possibilities for a quantitative and qualitative diagnosis of the functional state of the overall cardiovascular system (4). By examining the time course of blood pressure — shown in Fig. 1a for a typical pulse wave in the left ventricle and the aorta (6) — it is possible to determine the diastolic (p_1) and systolic pressure (p_2) and also to derive information about the state of the pulse for diagnostic purposes. This includes, for instance, information about the elasticity of the vessels, the peripheral resistance of the

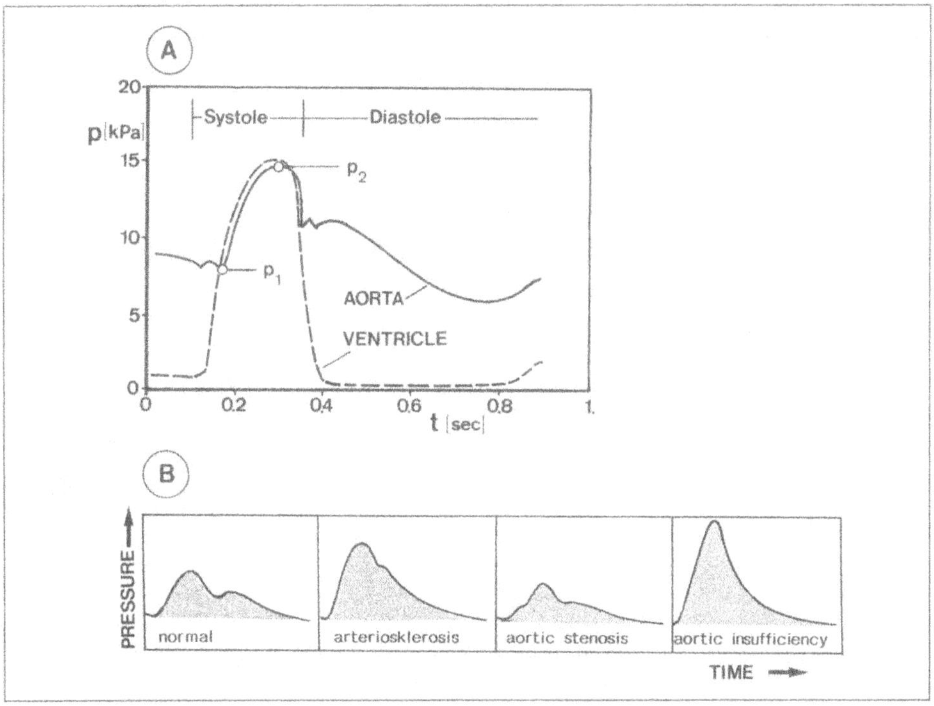

Fig. 1. Time-dependent blood pressure in blood vessels. (A) Static pressure of ventricle and aorta versus time (according to Sommer). (B) Changes in the pressure waveform in the radial artery (according to Schmidt/Thews).

arterial system, the stroke volume, and pulse rate. An example of such diagnostic possibilities can be found in Fig. 1b, which shows changes of the pulse rate in the case of arteriosclerosis, aortic stenosis, and aortic insufficiency based on measurements in the radial artery. Besides their usefulness in form analyses, pulse wave can, together with an electrocardiogram and a phonocardiogram, be taken for a time analysis, which can provide very detailed information about the overall hemodynamics (5).
Systolic and diastolic pressure are still determined chiefly with indirect methods (Riva-Rocci); these have proved very reliable but are not without objections from the point of view of fluid dynamics. In contrast, the time-dependent course of blood pressure, as outlined in Fig. 1, and longterm measurements of systolic and diastolic blood pressure are mainly performed with direct methods (intravascular measurement with cannulas or catheters). These methods naturally pose a burden on the patient as they require a surgical intervention. Moreover, errors of measurement cannot be excluded, since the use of tip catheters, i.e., miniature pressure sensors in the tip of the catheter, can lead to blockages of up to 30% of the cross section of the vessel, e.g., in the upper arm, which naturally lead to considerable signal errors. When using cannulas in connection with external transmitters, this problem can be reduced by selecting very thin probes, yet the basically nonlinear transmission mode of the necessary measurement tubes leads to new problems as regards accuracy.
In view of the above situation it appears appropriate to look for new ways of measuring blood pressure. The following investigations into the use of a novel piezoelectric film for recording the time-dependent arterial blood pressure are a first step in this direction and summarize the current stage in the development of this new technique.

Pulse pressure measurements with piezoelectric films

The extraordinarily high efficiency of the cardiovascular system is chiefly due to the fact that the pumping energy provided by the myocardium is not converted immediately into kinetic energy (flow velocity of blood) but is, during the ejection phase, partially stored as potential energy in the vascular walls. This procedure, known as the windkessel effect, reduces the velocity-proportional frictional losses of the blood circulation. This effect is of decisive importance to the technique under investigation in so far as the energy uptake of the blood vessel walls are associated with considerable radial deformations, which in turn are proportionate to the internal pressure of the vessel. This connection between deformation and vascular pressure can be described by the so-called kessel formula:

$$\sigma = p_i \frac{r}{s}; \quad r \gg s \tag{1}$$

where σ is circumferential tension, p_i, internal pressure; r, vessel radius; s, wall thickness.
This states that the circumferential tension in the wall of a vessel under internal pressure is proportional to the internal pressure multiplied by the ratio of the radius to the wall thickness. According to Hooke's law:

$$\sigma = E \cdot \epsilon \tag{2}$$

where E is elastic modulus; ϵ, strain, the circumferential tension, closely associated with the elastic modulus of the wall material, is also directly proportional to the strain, so that with the Equations (1) and (2) it is possible to relate internal pressure directly to strain. The present task of carrying out a time-dependent measurement of blood pressure thus becomes a problem of recording deformations of the arteries.
As measurements of blood pressure should ideally be noninvasive, arteries close to the surface, such as the radial artery, are the most suitable. Figure 2 shows how a piezoelectric film can be used to measure pulse pressure: the film is completely elastic and therefore adjusts to the surface geometry. As the pressure increases from p_1 to p_2 the film sensor is mechanically shaped in accordance with the deformation of the surface artery, which is converted into a measurable electric signal via the piezoelectric effects of the film material (polyvinylidene fluoride with thermoelectric polarization). With this setup, the time-dependent blood pressure can be documented in the form of a proportional electric signal (see Fig. 2). The results can be used for a direct analysis of form, and, to-

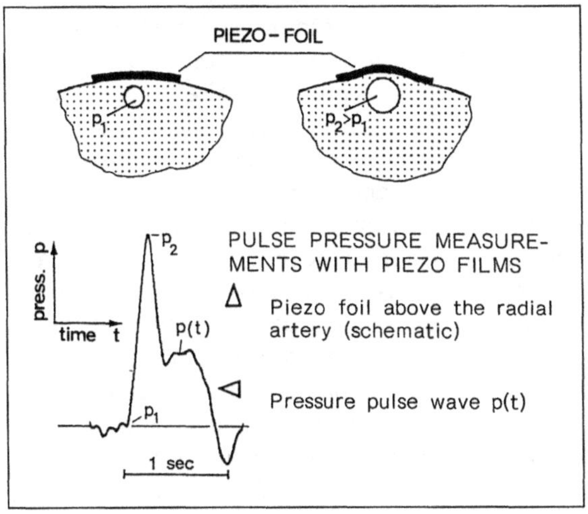

Fig. 2. Pulse pressure measurements by means of piezoelectric films.

gether with electro- and phonocardiograms, of a time analysis of the pulse wave. However, the device must be calibrated for a measurement of the absolute pressure contour (2, 3). This comprises a (basically unproblematic) calibration of the actual sensor, e.g., by applying pressure of a given amplitude to the piezofilm, as well as the individual calibration, taking into account the anatomic boundary conditions of the patient.

Practical application

The above-described technique was first tested under laboratory conditions with very elaborate measuring instruments and process computers to examine the practical applications of the new sensor material for the measurements in question. The investigations also looked into the optimal setup of the piezoelectric measurement process, as illustrated by the comparative measurement of pulse waves in Fig. 3. The piezofilm is an active

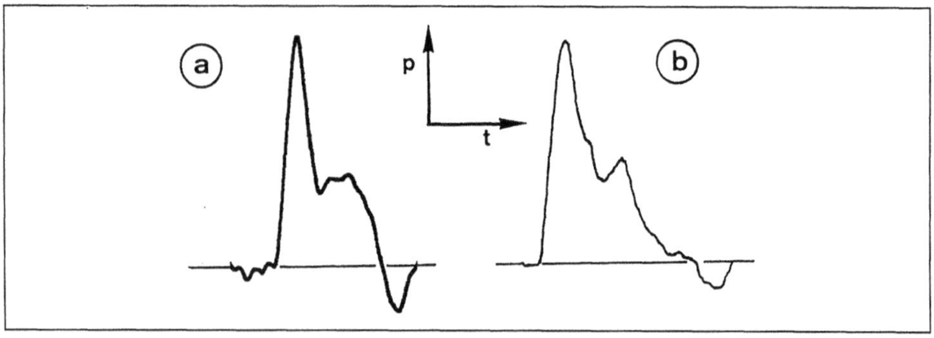

Fig. 3. Comparative pulse wave measurements on the radial artery. (a) Standard wide-band amplifier and numerical integration; (b) Charge amplifier.

sensor, i. e., the film produces a pressure-dependent signal without needing an external power supply for the sensor. Yet the signal indicates changes in the surface charge which have to be picked up by the thin metal coat of the sensor. Since these surface charges are very small, the piezoelectric system is relatively susceptible to noise voltage. Moreover, for the results to be truly proportionate to the applied pressure, specially adjusted amplifier systems (charge amplifiers) have to be incorporated. The first measurements were therefore performed with a standard wide band amplifier with on-line integration of a process control computer to allow simultaneous compensation of signal distortions (2). The basic suitability of the technique can be seen from the results in Fig. 3 a — again illustrated by a pulse wave in the radial artery. Yet this type of processing proved to be too complex for practical applications, and the next stage of development was focused on testing problem-oriented amplifiers that would need no mathematic-numeric signal processing beyond the frequency range relevant to the blood pressure measurements (0.4—4 Hz). Figure 3 b shows such a "direct" measurement; the blood pressure curve is very similar to that in Fig. 3 a and, considering that the measurements are much less complicated, this direct measurement can be seen as the method of choice.

In addition to the technical side of the electronic measurements, there was obviously also the problem of designing a practical probe suitable for the setup shown in Fig. 2. The main priority was to develop a robust pickup that is simple and practical to use. The result is shown in Fig. 4: the probe consists of a metal case (diameter ca. 20 mm) in which an elastic foam base is covered by the film sensor. The probe is placed lightly on the skin above the surface-near artery and can also be fixed with a mechanical cuff. The outer surface of the film forms, together with the case, the electronic shielding, and the signal picked up on the inside of the film is passed on to the amplifier via a shielded cable. Figure 5 shows some practical results with different surface-near arteries obtained with the probe shown in Fig. 4. The curve amplitudes were normalized and the measurement was not calibrated.

To take this piezoelectric method beyond the laboratory stage, a self-contained measuring system was developed (piezo pulse meter), which can also be used as a portable device for external measurements. Figure 6 shows a block diagram of this system: The signal from the piezofilm is first conditioned in an analog amplifying stage and then digitalized with an A—D converter (8 bit) with variable sensitivity. Planned is a multiplex operation with up to eight sensors. The signal is transferred from the A—D converter to a

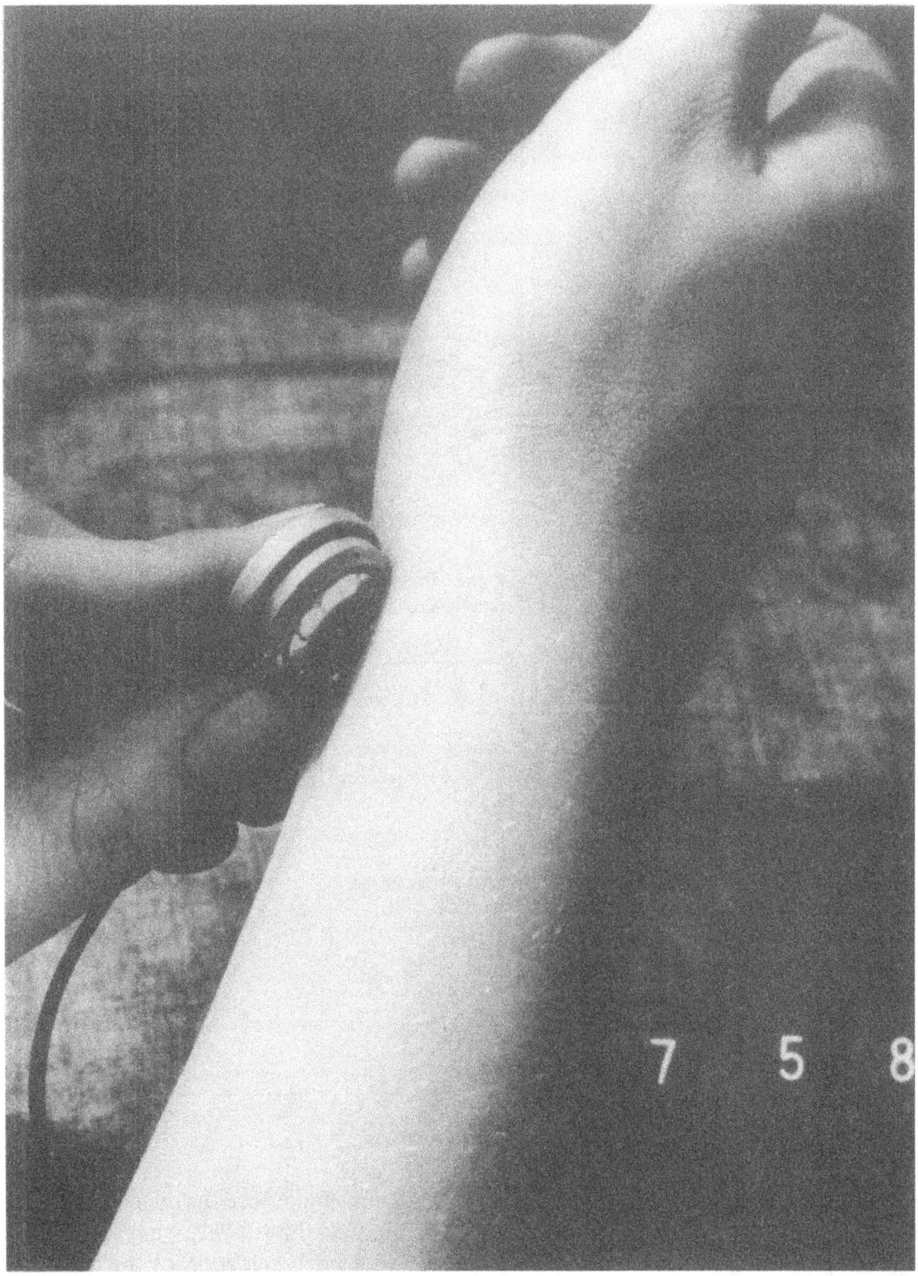

Fig. 4. Piezofoil sensor above the radial artery.

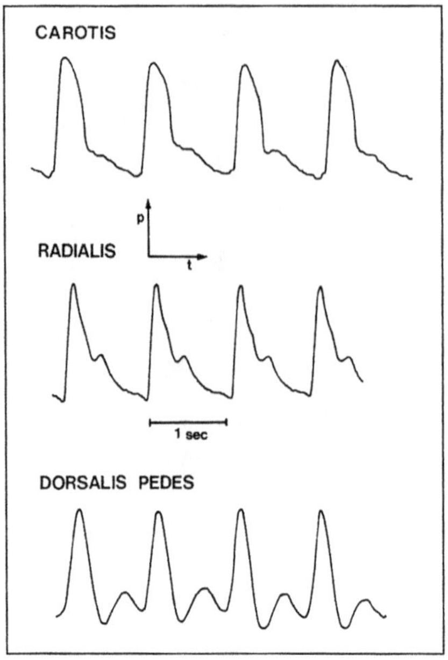

Fig. 5. Pressure waveforms of surface arteries obtained from piezo foil measurements.

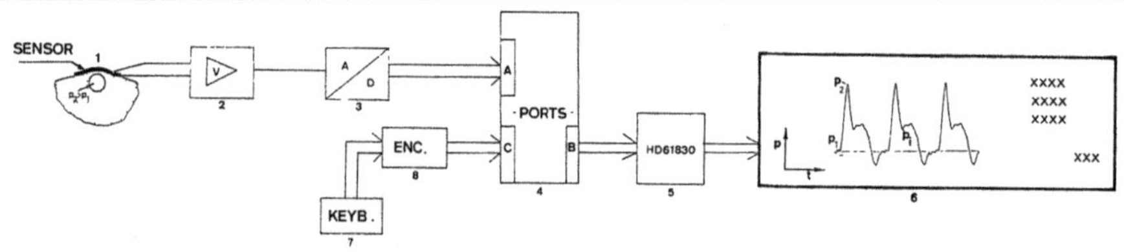

BLOCK DIAGRAM OF THE PIEZO PULSE METER

1 Piezo foil sensor
2 Amplifier
3 A/D-converter
4 Microcomputer miniCON-52
5 Controller (LCD-screen)
6 Screen
7 Keyboard
8 Encoder

Fig. 6. Block diagram of the piezo pulse meter.

miniCon-52 single chip computer equipped with a parallel interface for three input/output ports necessary for communication with additional hardware. The signal conditioning and processing is performed by the computer, e.g., determination of the absolute maxima and minima as well as the secondary minimum, determination of the pulse rate, and conversion of the measurement signal — through the input of calibration factors — into a pressure signal. The computer functions are controlled by a 16-key keyboard. The signals are plotted in 5-s phases on the integrated LCD screen, while the current measurement parameters are continuously displayed. The device has a standard analog output for documentation of the measurement signals. Flexibility was a prime consideration when developing the device, i. e., by making full use of the digital measurement technique the evaluation algorithms of the piezo pulse meter can easily be altered or extended without having to change the system hardware.

Conclusions

The development and testing of the piezoelectric pulse meter has reached a provisional conclusion: the basic laboratory investigations into how the technique functions have now been successfully completed and a device for practical implementation has been developed.

The efficiency of the piezo pulse meter has been shown in long-term test series, and the very principle of measuring pulse pressure with piezoelectric films has been confirmed by another investigation (1). The next stages will concentrate on its clinical applications and further development. Alongside its use in time analyses of hemodynamic investigations, the main priority will be to calibrate the system reliably. One objective is to apply the technique in long-term monitoring examinations, for instance in industrial medicine, thus giving it a broad range of potential applications.

References

1. Karr SG, Karwoski T, Jacobs JE, Mockros LF (1985) Transducer System for the Noninvasive Recording of Arterial Pressure Contours. Annals Biomed Eng 13
2. Nitsche W (1984) Anwendungen des piezoelektrischen Effekts zur Messung des zeitabhängigen Arteriendruckes (Pulsdruck-Messung). Proc "Piezo- und Pyroelektrische Folien aus PVDF", Düsseldorf

2a. Nitsche W, Thünker R, (1987) Application of the Piezo-Electric Effect in Measuring the Arterial Pressure Pulse. Ferroelectrics 75

3. Nitsche W, Thünker R, Weiser N (1985) Piezo-Folien als Sensor für instationäre Drücke am Beispiel von Wanddruck- und Pulsdruckmessung. Proc Sensor 85, 1
4. Schmidt F, Thews G (Hrsg) (1983) Physiologie des Menschen. Springer, Berlin New York Tokyo. 21 Aufl
5. Siegenthaler W, (Hrsg) (1976) Klinische Pathophysiologie. Thieme, Stuttgart, 3 Aufl
6. Sommer K (1983) Der Mensch-Anatomie, Physiologie, Ontogenie. Volk und Wissen, Berlin

Automatic registration of Korotkoff sounds: clinical experiences with automatic blood pressure measurement devices as compared to the auscultatory method

M. Anlauf and F. Weber

Medizinische Klinik und Poliklinik der Universität Essen (GHS), Essen, F.R.G.

Introduction

To a technician it often is hardly comprehensible why quality testing of physically well-defined devices should be performed on biological systems, taking into account their instabilities and variabilities. On the other hand, chemicals are also well-defined, and no one would dare to apply them on a greater number of patients without knowledge of clinical tests which have been built up stocastically. In particular this holds true in the field of preventive medicine. Right from the start of their development, the so-called electronic blood pressure measuring devices were looked upon with great scepticism, which was confirmed by initial clinical experiences 10 years ago. In the Federal Republic of Germany it was to the credit of "Stiftung Warentest" that they realized the need for an extensive technical and clinical testing programme. In 1980 and 1983 we took over work on the clinical aspects of the programme (4, 6). What follows represents the most important results in an abridged form.

Methodological Remarks

In principle there are four possibilities of comparative blood pressure measurement using different devices (2). They may be done simultaneously or non-simultaneously on one or on both arms. We decided in favor of simultaneous measuring on one arm, aware as we were of the following advantages and disadvantages: The test results may be influenced — except with fixed-display equipment — by differences between necessarily different testers. These differences can be avoided to some extent by providing special training for testers and adequate statistical design. As a microphone or a stethoscope is usually built into the cuff, the registration of Korotkoff sounds has to result from simultaneous comparative measurements at two different locations, over the brachial artery and over the cubital artery. The advantage of the above procedure is the independence of differences in blood pressure on both arms and changes of blood pressure with time. In simultaneous measurements, the dimensions of the single cuff used, as well as the deflation rate, influence test and control measurements equally. Thus they have no influence on measured differences and should be rated separately.
In 1980 we had to test 19, and in 1983, 21, different electronic devices available on the German market at that time. Each of the devices was tested on 24 probands, 12 men and 12 women, half of them were young and the other half were elderly patients.

Results

Accuracy of measurement

The ordinate of Fig. 1a und b gives the systolic differences of comparative measurements, i.e., the result of the tested instrument minus the result of the standard method of measuring. Thus a negative value means that blood pressure values measured by the robot were lower than values of simultaneous standard measurements. Each column represents one instrument. In 1980, the weakest (No. 33) had a medium systolic deviation of 11 mmHg with a standard deviation of ±12 mmHg, the best (No. 22) corresponded on average exactly with the simultaneous measurement with a standard deviation of ±3 mmHg.

Three years later the assortment of instruments had almost completely changed. Only a few instruments had the same shape as in 1980.

In general, apart from a lack of positive differences, the medium systolic differences between test and standard values now were as high as in 1980, but the standard deviations had lessened to values of between ±2 and ±9 mmHg.

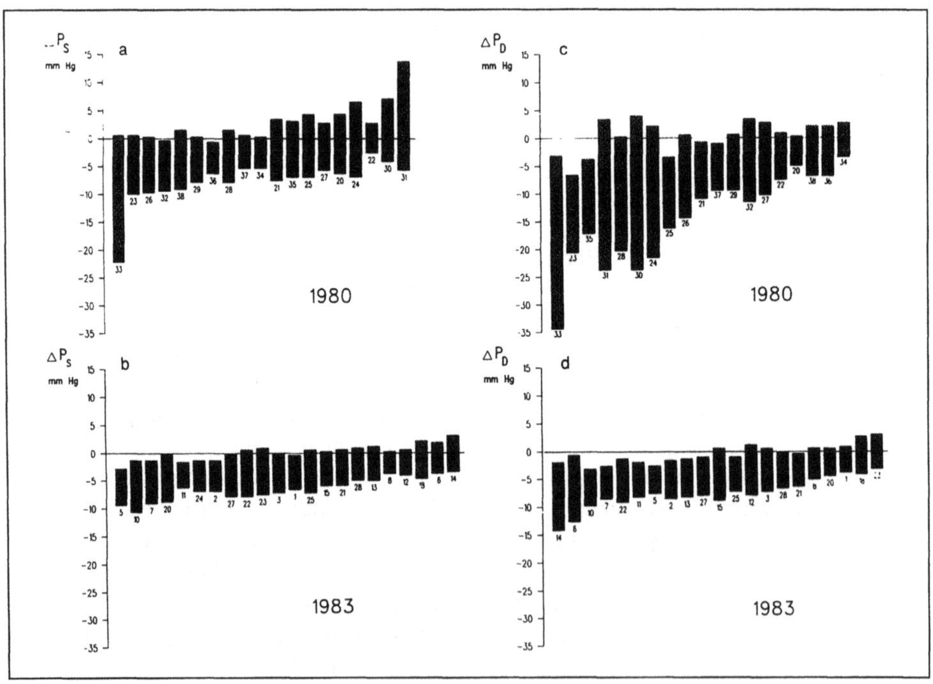

Fig. 1. Systolic and diastolic differences of blood pressure values (ΔP_s; ΔP_d, device to be tested minus control) of all devices (abscissa = number of device) tested in 1980 (a and c) and in 1983 (b and d). ● mean ± standard deviation of patients' averages.

More alarming than the systolic test results were the diastolic (Fig. 1c and d). In 1980 the weakest instrument measured diastolic pressure at about 19 mmHg lower than the standard method, with a standard deviation of ±16 mmHg. The mean differences of four instruments were about —10 mmHg, with standard deviations of ±10 mmHg. Only a few instruments showed tolerable results.

The repetition of the test in 1983 showed a fundamental improvement. The mean differences were found to be between —8 and 0 mmHg, with standard deviations between ±3 and ±6 mmHg.

Without doubt the increasing quality of blood pressure measuring devices between 1980 and 1983 was due to the fact that administrative regulations had been issued in the meantime (3). On the basis of the test results from 1980, the Physikalisch-Technische Bundesanstalt, the authority responsible for the approval of new devices brought onto the market, established the following limits for the blood pressure differences in the abovementioned method of clinical testing: The mean systolic difference must not exceed ±8 mmHg with a maximum standard deviation of ±6 mmHg. For physiological reasons to be discussed later the minor diastolic differences of ±6 mmHg were fixed symmetrically around —2 mmHg. Thus they range between +4 to —8 mmHg, with a standard deviation of ±6 mmHg, as with systolic pressure.

Influences indicated by individual characteristics of patients

The homogeneous testing of a large number of instruments on very similar groups of patients differing in age, sex and height of blood pressure enables one to make general observations concerning the influences of the above characteristics on test results.

A step-by-step analysis of the variance of data for the diastolic pressure in 1983 clearly showed that on average the readings differed more in young probands, and male and hypertensive patients than in elder probands, and female and normotensive patients. This means that in young hypertensive men, in particular, the self-measurement of blood pressure with electronic devices may lead to falsely low diastolic blood pressure values.

Influences of the location of auscultation

The differences in measured values between automatic recording and the auscultation of Korotkoff sounds are dependant on, among other things, the arterial place at which sounds are recorded or heard. Simultaneous comparative auscultation on the same arm with identical stethoscopes over the brachial artery and over the cubital artery leads to diastolic blood pressure differences which correlate closely with the age of the probands, regardless of height of the absolute blood pressure. Auscultations over the brachial artery in young probands in particular yielded lower diastolic values than auscultations over the cubital artery (Fig. 2). These results were not only detected by nursing staff, who may be able to hear even the last fainting Korotkoff sound of phase 5, but also by people like patients who are less experienced in auscultation.

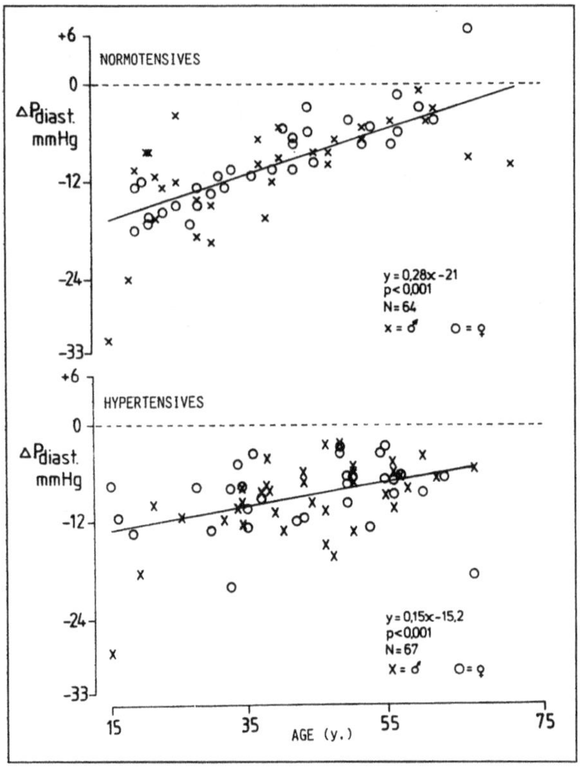

Fig. 2. Diastolic differences of blood pressure values for normotensive and hypertensive probands from simultaneously auscultated Korotkoff sounds at cubital artery and brachial artery of the same arm.
Δ brachial minus cubital.

Dislocation of the cuff

Additional errors may be expected from incorrect use of the instruments. Often the microphone in the cuff is not placed exactly over the brachial artery. One possibility may be the circular ventral dislocation of the microphone, if the patient has not learnt to find his own brachial artery. We investigated the consequences of this error in 19 stethoscope and 19 electronic devices designed for self-measurement of blood pressure. In these a stethoscope and a microphone, respectively, were built into the cuff. In a randomized test arrangement the cuff was placed exactly or ventrally displaced by about 2 patient's fingers' width (Fig. 3). Whereas the systolic differences with stethoscope devices as compared to correct placement did not appear significantly enlarged and the diastolic differences were not significantly reduced, the changes with electronic instruments were larger and statistically significant. This means that electronic devices have a higher sensitivity for dislocation than stethoscopic devices.

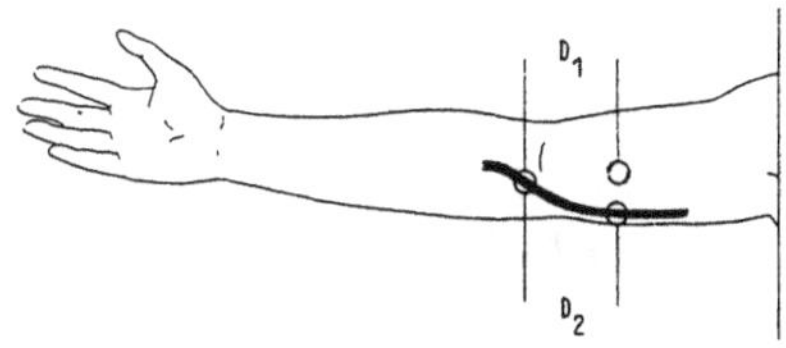

	stethoscope devices		microphone devices		
	D2	D1	D2		D1
syst.	-0,1±2,5	-0.9±3.5	-2,5±5,6	**	-5.1±5.8
diast.	-5,1±2,7	-4,5±2,8	-6,6±8	*	-4,6±8,7

Fig. 3. Differences of blood pressure values (brachial minus cubital artery) with correct (D_2) and incorrect (D_1) position of stethoscope or microphone. 19 different divices were used in each trial. ** $p < 0.01$; * $p < 0.05$.

Deflation rate

In the chosen test arrangement the deflation rate of the cuff does not influence the test results, provided that both manometers used show the same coefficient of inertia. If the deflation rate exceeds the recommended 2 to 3 mmHg/s, falsely low systolic and falsely high diastolic pressure values may be measured as a consequence, especially with low heart rates.

In the 1983 test, the automated deflation rate of nine electronic devices was checked by strain gauge measurements. Only one instrument covered the recommended rate of 2 to 3 mmHg/s in all pressure ranges, whereas the other instruments in the range of high, i. e. normally systolic, blood pressure deflated too fast, but correct, sometimes too low in the range of low, i. e. mainly diastolic, blood pressure range. These difficulties have been overcome in some of the recently developed instruments by means of a simple valve.

Constancy of device quality

A further question to be answered is whether the results of clinical tests on medical instruments prove true for all specimens of the same product, as should normally be the case with pharmaceutical compounds, or whether the manufacture of these sometimes very complicated instruments leads to greater differences between individual products, so that instruments are put on the market which measure differently. We only have some general impressions in this respect because there is no representative choice of instruments, and we rarely obtained reliable test results owing to the small, inhomogeneous groups of patients. In 1980, 6 out of 19 different instruments showed diastolic differences between identical specimens exceeding 5 mmHg. In 1983 all differences between the specimens available were below this limit.

Conclusion

To summarize our experiences with electronic devices developed for the self-measurement of blood pressure, a decisive improvement in measuring accuracy has been achieved in the course of the last few years. Nonetheless there still are diagnostically relevant errors in measurement with different types of instruments.

Our own experience and communications in the literature (1) show that this also applies true for technically more complicated instruments which were developed for clinical use.

A statistical analysis of all the results of measurements shows a relation between the accuracy of measurement and the characteristics of probands, such as age, sex and height of blood pressure. This relation may differ in intensity with each individual instrument.

The sensitivity for dislocation of the microphone is a very important fact to be considered as a characteristic of an instrument. This ought to be tested additionally.

Differences between individual specimens of the same product should be tested and the recommended deflation rate of the cuff should be checked by technical, not clinical means.

Taking into account the experiences with automatic blood pressure measurement devices, there should be comparative standard measurements on each patient for whom an electronic device is to be used. This must be possible before purchase of a self-measurement device. The information manual should refer to the documentation of clinical test results and thereby help the patient to choose the appropriate instrument.

In any case clinical tests of automatic blood pressure devices are indispensable for the time being. This was also proposed by the American Association for the Advancement of Medical Instrumentation (AAMI) in February 1986.

References

1. Adorjani C, Siegenthaler W, Vetter W (1979) Eignen sich automatische Geräte zur Blutdruckmessung? Schweiz, Med, Wschr, 109: 1225
2. Anlauf M (1980) Physiologische und technische Gesichtspunkte bei unblutigen Vergleichsmessungen. In: Deutsche Liga zur Bekämpfung des hohen Blutdruckes e. V.: Klinische Prüfung von Blutdruckmeßgeräten. 4. Tagung der wissenschaftlichen Sektion der Deutschen Liga zur Bekämpfung des hohen Blutdruckes, 20.11.1980, Berlin, S. 21—29
3. Physikalisch-Technische Bundesanstalt Berlin (1982) Vorläufige Richtlinien für klinische Eignungsuntersuchungen im Rahmen der Bauartzulassungsprüfungen von nichtinvasiven Blutdruckmeßgeräten. Berlin
4. Weber F, Hirche H, Simonides R, Anlauf M (1981) Vergleichende klinische Untersuchungen zur Meßgenauigkeit konventioneller und elektronischer Blutdruck-Selbstmeßgeräte. Z Kardiol, 70: 700
5. Weber F, Anlauf M, H Hirche (1983) Indirekte Blutdruckmessung: Simultane Vergleichsmessungen über der Arteria brachialis am Oberarm und in der Ellenbeuge bei normotonen und hypertonen Probanden. Verh Dtsch Ges Inn Med 89: 1129
6. Weber, F, Hirche H, Simonides R, Anlauf M (1985) Vergleich der Meßgenauigkeit elektronischer Blutdruckselbstmeßgeräte 1980—1983. Z Kardiol, 74: 610

Direct and indirect blood pressure measurement — rheologic and pathophysiologic considerations

T. Kenner

Physiological Institute of the University of Graz, Graz, Austria

Introduction

The measurement of blood pressure is still one of the procedures which are most often performed on human individuals. On one hand this fact is due to the diagnostic and prognostic importance of blood pressure. On the other hand, the usual noninvasive techniques are so simple and safe that nearly no limitation to the frequency of application is necessary. Several recent reviews on the theory and application of direct and indirect blood pressure measurement from our group (13) as well as from other authors (1, 3, 15) have summarized historical viewpoints and new developments.

In this paper I intend to present and discuss some general views about pressure and about the measurement of pressure and its assessment in biology and medicine. Among others I will attempt to answer the following questions:

What is pressure?

How is pressure generated?

What are the main effects of pressure?

How can pressure be measured?

Finally I will present some thoughts about the question of assessment:

What do we really want to know if we measure pressure?

What is pressure?

From the viewpoint of physical classification, pressure is a so-called intensive magnitude because its value does not depend on the extension — i. e., the amount or volume — of the medium. Pressure is defined as force per area, or as momentum (impulse) per area and time, or as energy per unit volume (i. e., energy density).

This study will be restricted to the discussion of arterial blood pressure. In order to extend this discussion to the measurement of pressure in gases we would have to include questions of compressibility. Since — in the range of biological pressure values — blood is incompressible, the measurement of blood pressure can only be performed by observing the deformation or reaction of some test system.

How is pressure generated?

If, in a fluid, viscous friction can be neglected, the relation between pressure and fluid be described by the so called Euler's equation. This equation includes three terms (5):

i. A term expressing inertial force,
ii. A term expressing a pressure gradient,
iii. A term expressing an external force.

In a somewhat symbolic form, Euler's equation can be written:

$$(i) + (ii) = (iii) \qquad (1)$$

The inertial force describes the effect of accelerations on the mass of the fluid. This effect of acceleration generates a pressure gradient, or vice versa. Both (i) and (ii) can be effected by external forces. Euler's equation can be called an equation of motion, since it relates forces to motion. For the description of pulsatile pressure and flow in large arteries Euler's equation can be used because the influence of viscous friction under this condition is relatively small.

For the particular condition of stationary nonpulsatile flow the solution of Euler's equation leads to the so called Bernoulli equation:

$$H = p + 1/2\, \varrho\, v^2 + \varrho\, g\, h \qquad (2)$$

This equation leads us into the center of problems concerning the measurement of pressure. H is the total pressure head which can be measured with a catheter with the opening directed against the direction of flow. p is the pressure or the lateral pressure which can be measured with a catheter with the opening directed parallel to the direction of flow. $1/2\, \varrho\, v^2$ is the dynamic pressure, whereas $\varrho\, gh$ is the hydrostatic pressure generated by the gravitational acceleration g in a fluid of density ϱ and depth h.

If fluid is flowing through a stenosis, the pressure p within the stenosis is lower by about $1/2\, \varrho\, v^2$ compared with the pressure in the wide tube or the ventricle before the stenosis. This effect of lowering the pressure within a narrow part of the stenosis, which can be observed during catheterization, has been called "Venturi-effect". Due to energy loss in the jet behind the stenosis, the pressure — regain p_r from narrow (n) to wide (w) is less than the fall of pressure by the Venturi-effect:

$$p_r = \varrho\, v_w(v_n - v_w) \qquad (3)$$

Coming back to the general description of the equation of motion, we now have to discuss the effects of viscosity. Whenever the viscosity of the fluid plays a marked role in determining the flow of a fluid, a term describing the effect of the viscous force has to be added to the equation of motion as a fourth term. The resulting equation is called Navier-Stokes equation and is the most general form of describing the pressure flow relation in a fluid (5, 20). In symbolic form the Navier-Stokes equation can be written in the following way:

$$(i) + (\text{viscous force}) + (ii) = (iii) \qquad (4)$$

The description of fluid movement in all models of the arterial system somehow is derived by simplification from the Navier-Stokes equation.

In order to summarize the two main phenomena in the arterial system we can firstly mention Poiseuilles law as the description of the pressure — flow relation during viscous flow in a circular tube (Eq. [5]) and secondly the relation between pressure- and flow-amplitude in an elastic tube (Eq. [6]). Poiseuille's equation is a special solution of the Navier-Stokes equation. The effect of the viscous flow through the so called resistance vessels in the circulation gives rise to the relation between peripheral resistance R, mean arterial pressure p and cardiac output q:

$$p = q\,R \tag{5}$$

Whereas Eq. (5) is mainly governed by the effects of viscous friction, the relation between pressure amplitude Δp and flow amplitude Δq in an elastic tube primarily depends on inertial and elastic forces:

$$\Delta p = \Delta q\,Z \tag{6}$$

Z is the so-called characteristic impedance of the tube (e.g., the aorta) and depends on pulse wave velocity c, the density of the blood ϱ and the cross-sectional area of the tube A:

$$Z = c\,\varrho/A \tag{7}$$

c is the pulse wave velocity which depends on the elastic properties, the dimensions of the tube and on the density of the fluid ϱ:

$$c = [ED/(2r\varrho)]^{1/2} \tag{8}$$

Equation (8) is the so called Moens-Korteweg equation. E is Youngs modulus of the arterial wall, r is the wall radius and D is the thickness of the wall.
Equation (5) and (7) describe in a somewhat approximated form the most important relations between pressure and flow in the arterial system which lead to the actual values of mean pressure and pressure amplitude.

What are the effects of pressure?

The three most obvious effects are (20):

1. Driving the blood through the peripheral parts of the vascular system
2. Distension of the arteries
3. Determining the amount of work the heart has to perform in order to eject a certain stroke volume

The effects of pressure are, on one hand, related to the movement caused by the pressure gradients. On the other hand, the effects depend on biomechanical phenomena like the stress generated in the wall of an artery or in the wall of the left ventricle. In approximation this force per cross-sectional area of stressed wall material in circumferential direction is equal to

$$\sigma = pr/D \tag{9}$$

r/D is the relation of arterial radius to the thickness of the wall. It is obvious that with equal pressure the material of a thick walled artery has to carry less load per cross-sectional area than a thin walled vessel. It is for this reason that the term hypertension actually distracts the attention from the more fundamentally important role of wall stress, at least as long as hypertension implies increased pressure and not increased wall stress.
Similar arguments are valid for the heart and the forces in the ventricular wall. The arterial pressure is generated by the left ventricle and is therefore the result of an interaction between ventricle and arterial system. The work of the left ventricle depends on the stroke volume and on the arterial pressure. In a somewhat approximated form the stroke work can be calculated by the following equation:

$$W = V_s p \tag{10}$$

Here, p is the mean arterial pressure during systole. The actual load on the heart muscles during contraction can be expressed by the wall stress similar to Eq. (8).

Why has the arterial pressure the value it actually has?

All mammals have, independent of their size, nearly the same blood pressure (5). If we consider Eq. (8) we can argue that equal pressures are related to equal wall stress values if there is a certain constant relation between arterial radius and wall thickness. Therefore, the problem of equal pressure in animals of different size can be reduced to a problem of stress-strain behavior and dimension of vascular wall material. The question of size dependence of cardiovascular variables is governed by the laws or rules of biological similarity (16).
It is important to note that the composition of blood is quite similar in different mammals: the electrolyte composition, the protein concentration, (the colloid osmotic pressure and also the number and size of erythrocytes (at least within certain limits) are similar. It seems that the colloid osmotic pressure plays a particularly important role in determining the fundamental magnitude of all pressure values in the cardiovascular system.

What is the fundamental principle of pressure measurement?

Pressure can be measured by observation of the compression or the displacement of some internal or external device. The number of possible techniques applicable for such a measurement in an incompressible fluid is limited. The historical development proves this statement. Since the first development of blood pressure measurement (Steven Hales, 1733, invasively, and Riva-Rocci 1896 and Korotkoff, 1905, noninvasively) the principles — manometry, occlusion method using a cuff, tonometry — have been continuously improved over the years of application, but no fundamentally new way has been invented.
During the process of measurement the measured variable is always subjected to filtering and transformation, which includes a loss of information. This process may even lead to a distortion of the recorded signal, e.g., by resonance phenomena.

The filtering process performed during an invasive measurement of blood pressure with a manometer connected to a catheter can be described by the equation of motion of the fluid in the catheter. The displacement x of the membrane of the manometer depends on the elasticity E of the membrane, the effective inertia M of the fluid in the catheter and the friction R of the fluid in the catheter (15).

$$E\,x + R\,dx/dt + M\,d^2x/dt = p\,(t) \tag{11}$$

The displacement x is the transformation or the projection of the arterial pressure p (t) and yields a more or less distorted reproduction of the "true function". This distortion can be minimized by shortening the catheter. The best results can be obtained by placing the manometer to the tip of the catheter.

How can the quality of a measurement technique be described?

In order to characterize a measurement technique we can describe it in terms of accuracy, precision and resolution (9). Accuracy means how well estimates of the value of interest represent the true value. Precision describes the reproducibility of an estimate — precision may be high even in the presence of a constant bias. Resolution describes this smallest possible variation of the variable which can be observed with a certain technique. For blood pressure measurement, it seems that usually accuracy is the most important of these properties of a technique.

Which phenomena are related to the pressure measurement by a cuff occlusion method?

A. Proximal to the occlusion

In most descriptions of the noninvasive cuff methods, the phenomena at the proximal site of the compressed arterial segment are completely neglected. Actually, it seems that these proximal events play quite an important role because they determine the entering of the volume pulse into the compressed arterial segment, and also the conditions which determine the first transition of a pulse wave through the compressed segment (6, 8). The pulse wave consists of orthograde and reflected wave components. If Δp is the pressure amplitude of such a wave component, it is related to the corresponding amplitude of the flow velocity Δv (as can be measured by Doppler ultrasound technique) by the so called waterhammer equation:

$$\Delta p = \varrho\, c\, \Delta v \tag{12}$$

Actually, this equation is just another form of writing Eq. (6). However, from the historical point of view, it is the more "classical" notation (20).
The wave pattern in a side branch of the aorta, like the brachial artery, depends on the pressure pattern at the location of the branching. Any obstacle in an arterial tube, like

a stenosis or an obstruction by an inflated cuff, leads to wave reflection. This reflection distorts the pressure wave proximal to the location of the cuff (6, 8). However, the closer towards the point of branching of the artery from the aorta this location is positioned, the less the pressure wave will be distorted.

B. The arterial segment in the cuff area

In the cuff area, the artery is collapsed whenever the cuff pressure exceeds the arterial pressure. The length of the collapsed segment depends on the radius of the extremity. The arterial pressure pulse contains a certain amount of energy which is used to open the collapsed segment. Therefore, as the cuff pressure decreases, the collapsed segment is opened and filled successively deeper, which each pulse as the available energy increases. Only the energy in the part of the pressure pulse above the value of the cuff pressure is available to be converted into the work which can be used for shifting fluid volume into the collapsed segment.

At the same time, and for the very same reason, the effects of the reflection of a part of the pulse wave can be observed proximally to the occlusion, as explained above. The phenomenon of wave reflection is governed by the laws of conservation of energy and of momentum.

As soon as the cuff pressure is decreased below a certain value which, in the correct setting, should correspond to the systolic arterial pressure, the first pulse appears distally to the occluded segment.

As long as the cuff pressure is within the systolic and the diastolic value of the arterial pressure, the arterial segment collapses during each diastolic pressure fall after each complete systolic opening. During this phase, the cuff area acts as a valve: it permits arterial pressure and volume pulses to pass through the collapsed area under the cuff as long as the pulse pressure is higher than the cuff pressure, and inhibits backflow as soon as the peripheral pressure falls below the cuff pressure (8).

C. Peripheral to the cuff

For the reasons explained in the preceeding section, the diastolic pressure in the arteries distal to the cuff may become markedly higher than in the aorta and in the proximal part of the artery, due to the valve function of the cuff pressure.

On the other hand, variations of the peripheral resistance in the extremity may, in the absence of an occluding cuff, lead to corresponding variations of the local arterial pressure amplitude, due to variations of the reflection factor. However, since the phenomena which lead to the opening of the collapsed segment are not influenced by whatever happens peripherally to this location, the values of the observed blood pressure, as measured with the application of an occluding cuff, are independent thereof (8).

D. The criteria

Besides the classical criteria — palpatory, auscultatory, oscillometric — the observation of arterial pulsations by ultrasound or by impedance plethysmography can be used. The origin of the Korotkoff sounds is not yet explained unanimously. Drzewiecki, Melbin and Noordergraaf ((2); personal communication) present a list of the following possibilities:

Pressure origin:
- dispersion in finite amplitude waves
- arterial wall instability

Flow origin:
- water hammer
- disturbed flow
- jet noises
- periodic wakes
- self excited oscillations in a collapsible tube

According to these authors, it can be assumed that their results support the pressure origin theory and indicate that the Korotkoff sound arises from oscillations resulting from distortion of the arterial pulse under the cuff, due to nonlinear pressure- flow relations in the collapsed segment of the artery. They conclude that, although not yet categorically established, the theory appears to embody experimentally observed features and predicts the genesis of sound from the arterial pulse.

The oscillatory criterion can be explained by the distension of the collapsed arterial segment by the pulse wave. This pulsatile distension leads to pressure oscillations in the cuff which appear to have a maximum amplitude at a cuff pressure which corresponds to the mean arterial pressure.

The arterial unloading technique

The technique of the so-called arterial unloading in its current form was invented by Peñaz (10) and was further developed by Peñaz et al. (11) and Wesseling et al. (9). It is interesting to note that the basic idea of arterial unloading is as old as any other principles of blood pressure measurement. Staub (17) in an extensive review on blood pressure measurement, mentions experiments which Marey performed in as early as 1876 with arterial unloading.

The technique used by Peñaz is based on the possibility of inflating a cuff around a finger to exactly the pressure p_c (t), which equals the arterial pressure p (t), such that the transmural pressure becomes zero at all times t:

$$p(t) - p_c(t) = 0 \qquad (13)$$

This goal can be achieved by a feedback system. The sensor of this system is a photo diode which receives the light transmitted trough the tissue of the finger. The feedback system actually keeps constant the amount of transmitted light: since the transmitted amount of light depends on the volume of blood in the arteries, which depends on the transmural pressure and on the compliance of the arteries, the condition of Eq. (10) is fulfilled by such a feedback system — at least as long as the compliance of the arteries does not change. The compliance C is related to the transmural pressure p and the volume V of an arterial segment by:

$$V = C\,p \tag{14}$$

Most of the electronic additions had to be made because of a certain physiologic variability of arterial compliance, in order to guarantee proper calibration and thus to improve the quality of the measurement. Since the invention of the feedback system by Peñaz, several other similar systems have been developed, e.g. by Yamakoshi (21), which use the same principle of arterial unloading with a slightly different setup.

Tonometry

Many attempts have been made to measure blood pressure noninvasively by application of a technique which uses the indentation or deformation of an artery by a local device for the estimation of arterial pressure. Actually, this approach is older than the cuff method. One technique of this type was constructed by S. von Basch in Vienna in 1876. It is, of course, possible to apply the principle of the arterial unloading technique locally with a tonometric device. It may be possible to apply modern methods of ultrasound echo in order to localize the artery and to estimate the degree of unloading. A recent review of tonometry was published by Drzewiecki et al. (1).

Wave velocity and blood pressure

It has been well known for many years that the pulse wave velocity in any artery depends on the transmural pressure, because with increasing pressure and wall stress (see Eq. [9]) the modulus of elasticity E of the arterial wall material increases. According to the Moens-Korteweg equation (Eq. [8]) the pulse wave velocity is proportional to the square root of the modulus of elasticity (5, 20). Besides this interrelation, however, there are individual differences due to activation of the arterial smooth muscles and differences which depend on age, and/or on pathological changes. It should be noted, furthermore, that the wave velocity is frequency dependent (20), and also depends on the steepness of the wave front. Nevertheless, the noninvasive recording of the wave velocity for observation of the trend in arterial pressure variations seems to be an interesting approach.

Automated devices

Automated sensing and data handling permits the construction of more or less automated blood pressure measuring devices. These devices use the same principles as the non-automated machines. However, the possibility of electronic data analysis permits the use of certain algorithms in order to handle more complex sets of criteria. One of these devices, which uses the oscillatory criterion, was examined in detail by Pessenhofer (12) who compared the pressure readings with the results of the Korotkoff method. The conclusion of this study was that although the oscillometric method exhibited a trend towards higher systolic and lower diastolic values compared to the auscultatory method, both methods are well comparable and the differences are below the level of physiological and clinical significance. An interesting fact which may lead to problems in the future is that the manufacturer does not usually explain the algorithms used in the program of the microcomputer in detail.

What do we really want to know if we measure pressure?

A. The Count Bobby effect

Count Bobby is a "famous" old Austrian joke figure. It is told that one late evening he was observed somewhat drunk after coming out of a Viennese wine bar. He was looking for something on the ground in the close surrounding of the next street lamp. When asked what he was looking for, he said that he had lost his key somewhere back in the dark when he stepped out of the wine bar. However — said he — since it is clearly easier to search and find a lost key in the light of a street lamp, he had decided to look around in this spot.

This little story is intended to demonstrate the problem that, if a method is available — like the street lamp — it is tempting to use this method, irrespective of usefulness or deeper sense (7). If we measure blood pressure and if we even derive a name for a disease like hypertension from measuring pressure, we should be aware of the fact that, as was explained above, not arterial pressure, but arterial wall stress and ventricular wall stress are the important variables. Wall stress, however, is not always simply proportional to blood pressure. The wall stress is — given a certain arterial pressure — relatively higher in thin walled arteries (see Eq. [9]).

B. Sensitivity and Specificity

Sensitivity is the conditional probability that if a certain sign (e. g. a blood pressure reading above a certain limit) is present, the "disease" is also present (18).

Specificity is the conditional probability that if the diagnostic sign is not observed, the person is healthy, i. e. the "disease" is not present.

Usually one can say that a method or technique is better, the higher sensitivity and specificity are. The problem in the case of blood pressure is that the "disease" is defined by the blood pressure reading, so that — if we accept this definition — both these statistical measures may always be close to 1.0.

C. The fuzzy diagnosis

As modern techniques for invasive as well as for noninvasive blood pressure measurement are improved and, particularly, as modern numerical displays permit an increase in the actual, as well as the apparent, accuracy of the reading, we are faced with an interesting problem. This has been discussed with respect to a slightly different cardiological question by Kalmanson and Stegall (4), and is related to the question which will be posed in the next section.

Using advanced technology we now seem to be able to determine blood pressure with an absolute accuracy of much less than a tenth of a mmHg. Every physician knows that, due to the physiologic variation of the blood pressure reading with an accuracy of better than $\pm$ 5 mmHg. If the only conclusion drawn by the physician from a highly accurate pressure reading is simply to label the person as either a "normotensive" or a "hypertensive" patient, then the question arises of why we need such a high accuracy of pressure recording at all. This question will not be answered here, since it certainly not only includes technical or medical but also ethical viewpoints. One viewpoint is presented in the following section.

D. "The mysterious viability of the false"

With respect to the assessment of the observed values of arterial pressure, Sir G. Pickering (14) wrote, under the title mentioned above: "There is no agreement as to what is the dividing line between so called normotension and so called hypertension, although WHO, that great propagator of science by committee, has made a recommendation. The dividing line that an authority chooses is based not on fact but on a whim."

This admonition interestingly summarizes not only the viewpoint of a responsible physician, but also the viewpoint of fundamental physics. Blood pressure is an individual magnitude, not only in terms of its actual value in a certain person, but also with respect to its effect on the cardiovascular system. As explained above, it is not the pressure but the wall stress which describes the load on the artery. Considering the variability of anatomical and histological configurations, it seems clear that the limit between normal and pathological blood pressure must be rather fuzzy.

Conclusion

Pressure is an intensive magnitude which does not depend on the extension of the medium. Pressure has static and dynamic components and in the arterial system is composed of a mean value, which depends on cardiac output and peripheral resistance, and of a pressure amplitude which depends on the flow amplitude and on the characteristic impedance of the artery. The measurement of arterial pressure can be done either invasively or by one of the following noninvasive methods: occlusive cuff method, vascular unloading, arterial tonometry, measurement of pulse wave velocity. Once the blood pressure has been measured in a person, the problem of the assessment has to be considered. According to the decision of the WHO, certain limits are defined which distinguish normotension from hypertension. The actual procedure used by each physician has to take into account the fact that these limits are subject to individual variations in each case.

Acknowledgement

This study has been supported by the Austrian Heart Fund.

References

1. Drzewiecki GM, Melbin J, Noordergraaf A (1983) Arterial tonometry: review and analysis. J Biochem 16: 141—152
2. Drzewiecki GM, Melbin J, Noordergraaf A. The noninvasive measurement of blood pressure and the origin of the Korotkoff sound. In: Skalak R, Chien S (eds) Handbook of Bioengineering. McGraw-Hill (1987)
3. Grashuis JL (1984), Arterial blood pressure measurement. ESA Report 5464/83/NL/HP, Paris
4. Kalmanson D, Stegall HF (1975) Cardiovascular investigations and fuzzy sets theory. Am J Cardiol 35: 80—84
5. Kenner T Flow and pressure in the arteries. In: Fung YC, Perrone N, Anliker M (eds.): Biomechanics: its foundations and objectives. Prentice Hall, New Jersey (1972)
6. Kenner T Pulse wave reflection at the collapsed segment of an artery in Riva-Roccis method. Pflügers Arch. 363, 263—265 (1976)
7. Kenner T Einspieler Ch, Holzer A. Risk, cost-effectiveness and profit: problems in cardiovascular research and practice. Theoret Med 7, 283—297 (1986)
8. Kenner T Gauer OH. Untersuchungen zur Theorie der auskultatorischen Blutdruckmessung. Pflügers Arch 275, 23—45 (1962)
9. Murphy EA The logic of medicine. The Johns Hopkins Univ. Press. Baltimore — London, 1976
10. Penaz J Czech Patent 133205, Prague, 1969
11. Penaz J, Voigt A, Teichmann W Beitrag zur fortlaufenden indirekten Blutdruckmessung. Z. Gesamte Inn. Med. Grenzgeb.j 31, 1030—1033 (1976)
12. Pessenhofer H Single cuff comparison of two methods for indirect measurement of arterial blood pressure: standard auscultatory method versus automatic oscillometric method. Basic Res. Cardiol. 81, 711—720 (1986)
13. Pessenhofer H, Kenner T (1983) Neue Entwicklungen auf dem Gebiet der nichtinvasiven Blutdruckmessung. In: Bergmann H, Gilly H, Kenner T, Schuy St, Steibereithner K (Hrsg) Monitoring in der Anaesthesiologie und Intensivmedizin. Verlag W. Maudrich, Wien — München — Berlin, S 145—161
14. Pickering G (1978) Normotension and hypertension: the mysterious viability of the false. Am J Med 65: 561—563
15. Schabert A, Bauer RD (1982) Methoden zur Messung von Druck, Durchmesser und Strömung im Kreislauf. In: Busse R (Hrsg), Kreislaufphysiologie, Georg Thieme Verlag Stuttgart — New York, S 219—256
16. Schmidt-Nielsen K Scaling. Why is animal size so important? Cambridge University Press, Cambridge, 1985
17. Straub H Bestimmung des Blutdruckes. In: Abderhalden E (Hrsg): Handbuch der biologischen Arbeitsmethode, Abt. V, Teil 4, I. S 134—266, Urban & Schwarzenberg, Berlin, Wien 1923
18. Taube A Sensitivity, specificity and predictive values: a graphical approach, Statistics in Medicine 5, 585—591 (1986)
19. Wesseling KH, de Wit B, Settels JJ, Klewer WH On the indirect registration of finger blood pressure after Penaz. Funkt. Biol. Med 1, 245—250 (1982)
20. Wetterer E, Kenner T. Dynamik des Arterienpulses. Springer Verlag, Berlin — Heidelberg — New York, 1968
21. Yamakoshi K, Kamiya A, Shimazu H, Ito H, Togawa T Noninvasive automatic monitoring of instantaneous arterial blood pressure using the vascular unloading technique. Med. Biol. Eng. Comp. 21, 557—565 (1983)

Ambulatory blood pressure monitoring: use in clinical practice and in research

J. Conway

Department of Cardiovascular Medicine, John Radcliffe Hospital, Headington, Oxford, UK

Introduction

Home blood pressure measurement was introduced some 40 years ago after the first effective anti-hypertensive medications became available (1, 15, 32). The problem at that time was to avoid the serious side effects, mostly postural hypotension, produced by the agents then available. Tremendous advances have been made since in the control of blood pressure. Malignant hypertension is now rarely seen and the level of diastolic blood pressure at which treatment is recommended has fallen progressively to levels just above those which are regarded as "normal". The problem today is to determine whether hypertension is present or not. In the absence of symptoms and signs of secondary organ involvement, reliance has to be placed exclusively on the blood pressure level. Yet this varies considerably throughout the day (3, 6, 13, 29) (Fig. 1) and, to add to this, the level rises considerably when a patient presents himself to the physician (1, 5, 20, 30). The magnitude of this change is not generally recognised but it has recently been shown to vary from 4—75 mmHg systolic and 1—36 mmHg diastolic (23). This alerting response

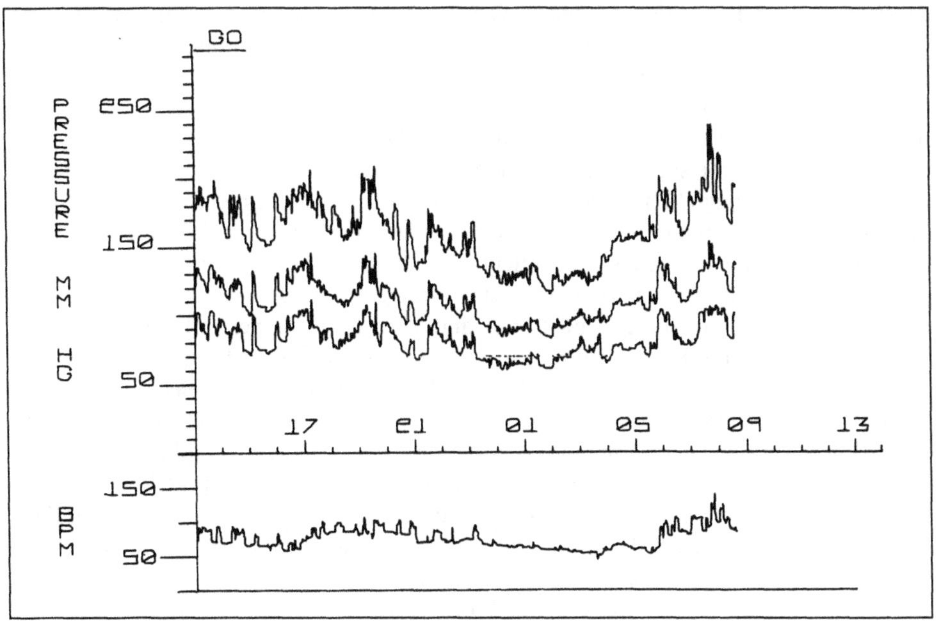

Fig. 1. Blood pressure and heart rate recorded directly from the brachial artery. Note the variability in blood pressure throughout the day. Both blood pressure and its variability decline with sleep.

generally, but not always, declines with time. The most important need in the management of hypertension today, then, is the accurate measurement of the true level of blood pressure.

Home blood pressure devices have long been used to obtain reliable readings but they suffer from several disadvantages. First their use requires a continuing commitment on the part of the patient to the proper use of the apparatus. Secondly the patient records the reading and has a recurring reminder of their illness. This is undesirable.

Ambulatory blood pressure devices

Over the last few years several devices have been developed for the automatic recording of blood pressure throughout the day. These are portable machines generally using the Korotkoff sounds (2, 4, 8, 11, 14, 16, 17, 21, 24). They have proved to be reasonably accurate when compared with the random-zero sphygmomanometer but it has to be said that they are untested in "field" use. Their accuracy with the patient standing and during exercise has not been extensively assessed. Some devices use the oscillometric method, largely as a back-up when the Korotkoff sounds are not readily audible. This method is untested and algorithm used by individual devices to indicate systolic and diastolic pressure is not provided. This method is of doubtful value.

Ambulatory devices then are convenient and, within limits, accurate enough for clinical purposes. Although the devices are adequate, the details of their use needs some clarification. The first decision is on posture. Blood pressure changes as the subject moves from the recumbent to the sitting and standing positions (35). Obviously then, the proportion of readings taken in each position will affect the daily average. This must either be standardized or a single position adopted. We have settled for the sitting position with the arm supported (7, 8) (Fig. 2). This has the added advantage of minimizing the number of unsatisfactory readings. There is some debate in the literature (8, 18, 27) as to the conditions under which blood pressure should be read. The level rises progressively as one passes from sleeping to wakefulness to mental activity and working (6, 27, 34). A case has been made for the superiority of blood pressure readings at work in the prediction of target organ damage (27). This needs to be more firmly established since the problems involved in taking pressure readings at work have not been adequately addressed. With direct intra-arterial recordings the patient may move around freely and every blood pressure reading is measured. With indirect recording the word "ambulatory" is a bit of a misnomer, since the subject must stop and keep the arm perfectly still while the measurement is made. Furthermore, it is not always socially convenient for subjects to take readings during working hours. Practically all the devices use electric pumps to inflate the blood pressure cuff and these are noisy. Consequently, the act of measurement attracts attention. There are also many occupations (e. g., teachers, assembly line workers, etc.) in whom "work-time" blood pressure recordings are clearly impractical. Ambient noise may also make it impossible to take recordings (e. g., in an automobile). Recordings at night also disturb sleep. Accepting therefore that some information is inevitably lost we use readings taken in the sitting position on a "rest" day. The subjects are nevertheless encouraged to be active around the house and with recreational activities (Fig. 2). With our own device a signal alerts the subject some 30 s before each reading to enable the subject to prepare for the activation of the device (8). The output from such

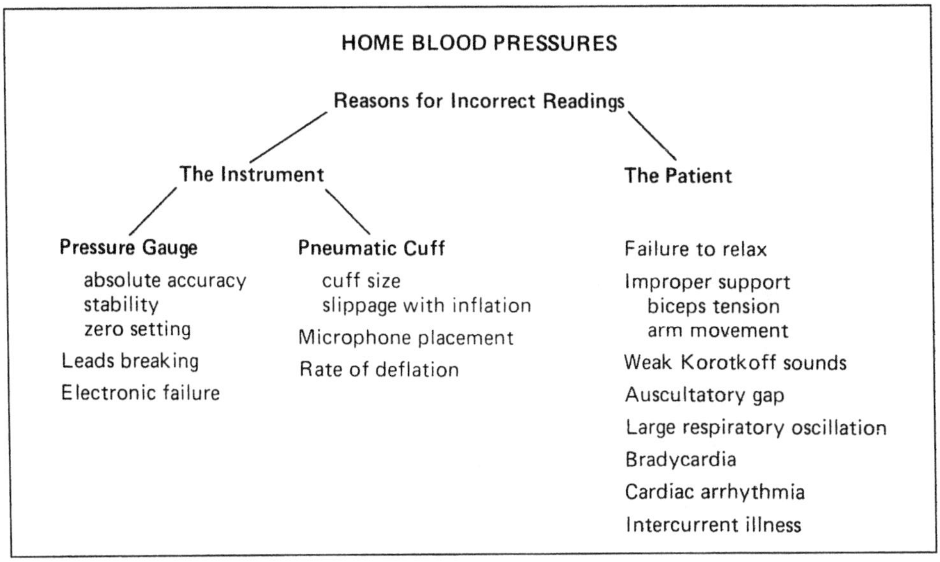

Fig. 2. Home blood pressure monitoring technique with suggestions for accurate recording (From ref. (7) with permission).

a device is shown in Fig. 3. The analogue output, of each recording is given along with the mean of the day's readings.

The frequency of readings and the duration over which they should be carried out has to be considered (10, 11, 13). Ambulatory recordings are a method of obtaining a sample of measurements throughout the day of a variable parameter. Obviously the best estimate

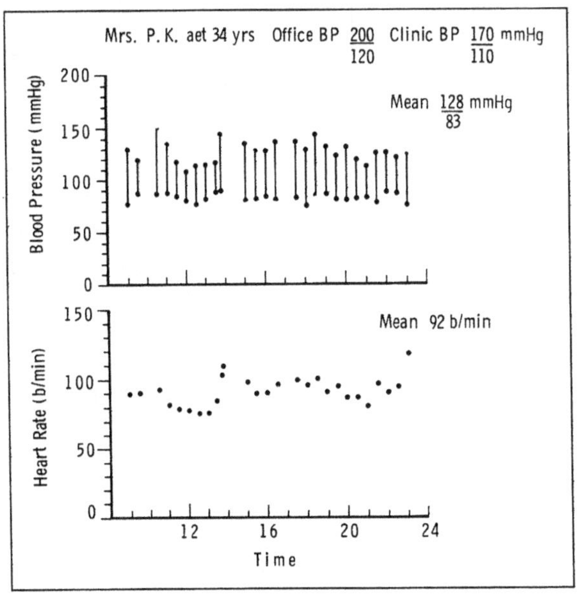

Fig. 3. Blood pressure and heart rate measured at 30-min intervals over the daytime hours. Note: The patient had very high blood pressure in the doctor's office and in the hospital clinic yet the average ambulatory record was clearly normal.

would be provided by the greatest number of readings but this must be balanced against the interruption of activity for the 2 min required to achieve the recording. Repeated inflations of the cuff ultimately cause some discomfort in the arm. For various reasons therefore we have settled for half-hourly-readings. Thus 20—30 readings are made throughout the waking day. We have shown that fewer measurements than this seriously affects the accuracy of blood pressure estimates (7, 8) (Fig. 4).

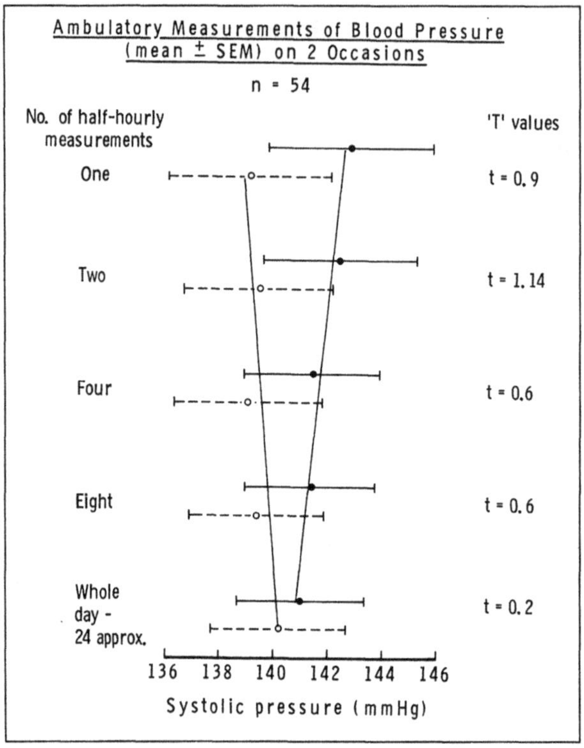

Fig. 4. Blood pressure readings taken in a group of 40 subjects on two separate occasions showing the mean levels and standard errors of the readings while they were on a placebo medication when 1, 2, 4, 8 and 20+ readings are used to estimate blood pressure level. It can be seen that the difference between the two means and the variability declines progressively as the number of readings taken during the day increases. If only one or two readings are taken, the difference between two measurements approaches significance (t = 0.9 and 1.14) and this declines as the number of readings increases (t = 0.2) to approximately 24.

Disadvantages

The use of the ambulatory apparatus obviously interferes with the patient's daily life and its use during work is difficult. The patient has to be prepared to spend time on blood pressure recordings. Compliance is, however, less of a problem than it is with multiple home recordings. Nevertheless, some subjects find the use of the apparatus quite distressing. Others find it difficult to remain stationary enough for the device to record blood pressure without artifacts. Fortunately these subjects are few if trained personel properly instruct the patient on the use of the apparatus. The importance of this aspect of ambulatory monitoring connot be overstressed.

Artifacts inevitably occur and there is no general advice available as to how these should be handled. We have taken as a rule of thumb that if the pulse pressure of a single reading is less than half of the daily average it is rejected (8). This would appear to be justified from the intra-arterial recordings (Fig. 1).

The chief handicap to the wider use of ambulatory blood pressure monitoring is cost. We have therefore constructed our own device for $ 500 and we are pressing for this to be the aim of commercial manufacturers (7).

Clinical application

Diagnosis of the presence of hypertension is clearly the most important application of the ambulatory technique. It is well known that clinic readings are almost always higher than ambulatory recordings. In patients referred to the hospital with mild hypertension we have found the average difference between clinic and ambulatory recordings was 20/10 mmHg (8). Approximately one third of patients who are referred to us do not have hypertension when an ambulatory recording is taken into account (1, 8, 33). It could be argued that as clinic readings have been used in epidemiological surveys to assess prognosis (22) then ambulatory recordings should not be used as a guide to treatment. This, however, is an over-simplification of the problem. It is an altogether different psychological situation when blood pressure is measured in a "survey" as against one made when the patient presents himself to a physician. Strangely, no attempt has been made to compare clinic readings with those obtained during epidemiological surveys. The normal distribution in the population of blood pressure taken by ambulatory devices would be desirable, as would the value of prognosis determined on the basis of ambulatory recordings. These are formidable and largely impractical tasks.

As a clinical guide, then, one has to rely on the as yet imperfect information available. Perloff and others in a large retrospective survey have shown that ambulatory blood pressure recordings will more clearly reflect mortality and morbidity of hypertension than clinic readings (25, 31). Their findings have generally been supported by others (5, 9, 12, 26). Obviously further work is needed in this area. For the present, an ambulatory blood pressure level of 90 mmHg diastolic is used to consider the patient as hypertensive and to recommend treatment, though not necessarily the use of drugs.

The accurate estimate of blood pressure provided by ambulatory recordings is a clear advantage in monitoring anti-hypertensive treatment and in achieving a target blood pressure (11, 13, 19, 28, 30). This confidence makes it possible to reduce the number of clinic visits and to prevent side effects which might result from excessive reductions in blood pressure. These advantages alone justify the technique.

Research applications

The ability to measure blood pressure with reasonable accuracy has a wide variety of research applications in physiological and pharmacological research.

It should be possible to monitor trends in blood pressure with time and with environmental changes. It might be thought that studies of blood pressure variability could be made with the use of ambulatory recordings. When one considers that half-hourly readings provide but two estimates of the 4.000 beats which occur each hour it will be appreciated that the sample is too small to reliably reflect variability. This is not to say that research into the response to induced stress would not be of value. It is well known that some subjects respond to psychological and physical stresses with much higher blood pressure rise than others. Whether this is good or bad has not yet been determined. Research in this area is underway with the European co-operative study of ambulatory recordings being organized by Professor Clement in Belgium.

Response to antihypertensive agents

The use of ambulatory recordings will find its greatest use in clinical pharmacology. Repeatability of ambulatory recordings has been shown to be reasonable (4, 8, 13, 20, 24). In our experience, when blood pressure was measured on two occasions 1 month apart with the patient on a placebo, the average difference in systolic pressure was 1.8 mmHg systolic with a standard deviation of the difference of 8.1 mmHg and for diastolic pressure the difference was —0.3 and a standard deviation of the difference was 5.6 mmHg (8). The difference between one occasion and another can be further reduced by making a repeat estimate on 2 different days. It has already been found that the well known "placebo" effect does not occur with ambulatory recordings (8, 11, 16, 28, 34). It is therefore possible to obtain an accurate estimate of blood pressure from a single session and study interventions from that base line.
It should be possible to make reasonable estimates of the dose-response curves to antihypertensive agents on relatively small samples of subjects and to make comparisons between two drugs (19).

Conclusion

Ambulatory blood pressure monitoring provides a reasonably accurate estimate of the level of blood pressure throughout the day. There are several devices available on the market. Although accurate and convenient to use, these are inordinately expensive and the true potential of this method will not be realized until manufacturers can be persuaded to produce devices at a reasonable cost.
The technique makes it possible to separate true hypertensives from "clinic reactors" and thereby avoid unnecessary and possibly harmful treatment. It improves the confidence in the assessment of therapy. The improved accuracy of blood pressure measurement makes it possible to compare different agents and to assess dose-effect relationships on small numbers of subjects.
Much remains to be done however. To mention only two problems; we must know whether subjects who are "clinic" reactors have an increased tendency to a rise in pressure with time. We must also know the level of ambulatory pressure at which medical treatment is recommended.

References

1. Ayman D, Goldshine AD (1970) Blood pressures determinations by patients with essential hypertension: I. The difference between clinic and home readings before treatment. Am J Med Sci 200: 465—474

2. Bassein L, Borghi C, Costa FV, Strocchi E, Mussi A, Ambrosioni E (1985) Comparison of two automatic devices and the standard mercury sphygmomanometer in hypertensive patients. Clin Exper Hypertension A 7: 387—390
3. Bristow JD, Honour AJ, Pickering GW, Sleight P. (1969) Cardiovascular and respiratory changes during sleep in normal and hypertensive subjects. Cardiovasc Res 3, 476—485
4. Brunner HR, Combes BJ, Waeber B and Porchet M. (1983) Accuracy and reproducibility of ambulatory blood pressure recordings obtained with the Remler system. J Hypertension 1 (suppl 2), 291—292
5. Brunner HR Waeber B and Nussberger J. (1985) Blood pressure recording in the ambulatory patient and evaluation of cardiovascular risk. Clin Sci 68, 485—488
6. Conway J, Boon N, Vann Jones J and Sleight P. (1985) Mechanisms concerned with blood pressure variability throughout the day. Clin Exper Hypertension A 7, 153—157
7. Conway J (1986) Home blood pressure recording. Clin Exper Hypertension A 8: 1267—1294
8. Conway J, Johnston J, Coats A, Somers V, Sleight P. (1988) The use of ambulatory blood pressure monitoring to improve the accuracy and reduce the numbers of subjects in clinical trials of antihypertensive agents. J Hypertension 6, 111—116
9. Devereux RB, Pickering TG, Harshfield GA, Kleinart HD, Denby L, Clark L, Pregibon D, Jason M, Kleiner B, Borer JS, Laragh JH (1983) Left ventricular hypertrophy in patients with hypertension: importance of blood pressure response to regularly recurring stress. Circulation 68: 470—476
10. Di Rienzo M, Grassi G, Pedotti A, Mancia G. (1983) Continuous versus intermittent blood pressure measurement in estimating 24-hour average blood pressure. Hypertension 5: 264—269
11. Drayer JIM, Weber MA, DeYoung JL, Brewer DD. Long-term BP monitoring in the evaluation of antihypertensive therapy. Arch Intern Med 1983; 143: 898—901
12. Drayer JIM, Weber MA, DeYoung JL (1983) BP as a determinant of cardiac left ventricular muscle mass. Arch Intern Med 143: 90—92
13. Drayer JIM, Weber MA, DeYoung JL (1983) The use of short-term ambulatory blood pressure monitoring in differing forms of hypertension. Clin Exper Hypertension A 5: 1597—1610
14. Fitzgerald DJ, O'Callaghan WG, O'Malley K, O'Brien ET (1981) Accuracy of the London School of Hygiene and Remler M 2000 sphygmomanometers. Clin Sci 61(s): 399—401
15. Freis ED (1954) The discrepancy between home and office recordings of blood pressure in patients under treatment with pentopyrolidinium. Importance of home readings in adjusting dosage. Med Ann DC 23: 363—367
16. Gould BA, Kieso HA, Hornung R, Altman DG, Cashman PMM, Raftery EB (1982) Assessment of the accuracy and role of self-recorded blood pressures in the management of hypertension. Br Med J 285: 1691—1692
17. Harshfield GA, Pickering TG and Laragh JH (1979) A validation study of the Del Mar Avionics ambulatory blood pressure system. Ambulat Electrocardiol 4: 7—12
18. Harshfield GA, Pickering TG, Kleinert HD, Blank S and Laragh JH (1982) Situational variations of blood pressure in ambulatory hypertensive patients. Psychosomatic Med 44: 237—245
19. Jacot Des Combes B, Brunner HR, Waeber B, Porchet M, Biollaz J (1984) Blood pressure variability in ambulatory hypertensive patients: effect of beta-blocking agents and/or diuretics. J Cardiovasc Pharmacol 6: 263—266
20. Jacot Des Combes B, Porchet M, Waeber B, Brunner HR (1987) Ambulatory blood pressure recordings. Reproducibility and unpredictability. Hypertension 6: 110—114
21. Kain HK, Hinman AT, Sokolow M (1964) Arterial blood pressure measurements with a portable recorder in hypertensive patients. Circulation 30: 882—892
22. Kannel WB (1974) The role of blood pressure in cardiovascular morbidity and mortality. Prog Cardiovasc Disc 17: 5—23
23. Mancia G, Bertinieri G, Grassi G, Parati G, Pomidossi G, Ferrari A, Gregorini L, Zanchetti A. (1983) Effects of blood pressure measurement by the doctor on patient's blood pressure and heart rate. Lancet ii: 695—697
24. Palatini P, Sperti G, Cordone L, Mormino P, Di Marco A, Bastanzetti M, Pessina AC (1985) Reliability of indirect blood pressure monitoring for the evaluation of hypertension. Clin Exper Hypertension A7: 437—443
25. Perloff D, Sokolow M and Cowan R (1988) The prognostic value of ambulatory blood pressure. I An Med Ass 249: 2792—2798

26. Pessina AC, Palatini P, Sperti G, Cordone L, Libardone M, Mos L, Mormino P, Di Marco A, Dal Palu C (1985) Evaluation of hypertension and related target organ damage by average day-time blood pressure. Clin and Exper Hypertension A7: 267—278
27. Pickering TG, Harshfield GA, Kleinart HD, Blank S, Laragh JH (1982) Blood pressure during normal daily activities, sleep and exercise. Comparison of values in normal and hypertensive subjects. I AM Med Ass 247: 992—996
28. Pomidossi G, Parati G, Casadei R, Mancia G (1985) Absence of alarm reactions with use of non-invasive blood pressure monitoring devices. Clin Exper Hypertension A7: 429—436
29. Richardson DW, Honour AJ, Fenton GW, Stott FH, Pickering GW (1964) Variation in arterial pressure throughout the day and night. Clin Sci 26: 445—460
30. Rion F, Weber B, Graf HJ, Jaussi A, Porchet M, Brunner HR (1985) Blood pressure response to antihypertensive therapy: Ambulatory versus office blood pressure readings. J Hypertension 3: 139—143
31. Sokolow M, Werdegar D, Kain HK, Hinman AT (1966) Relationship between level of blood pressure meansured casually and by portable recorders and severity of complications in essential hypertension. Circulation 34: 279—298
32. Taylor RD, Corcoran AC, Dustan HP, Page IH (1954) Further evaluation of hydralazine in treatment of hypertensive diseases. Arch Int Med 93: 705—712
33. Waeber B, Jacot Des Combes B, Porchet M, Biollaz M, Schaller D, Brunner HR (1987) Ambulatory blood pressure recording to identify hypertensive patients who truly need therapy. J Chron Dis 37: 55—57
34. Weber MA, Drayer JIM, Wyle FA, DeYoung JL (1982) Reproducibility of the whole-day blood pressure pattern in essential hypertension. Clin Exper Hypertension A4: 1377—1390
35. Webster J, Newnham D, Petrie JC, Lovell HG (1984) Influence of arm position on measurement of blood pressure. Br Med J 288: 1574—1576

How reliable are indirect blood pressure measurement devices in the intensive care unit (ICU)?

U. Frucht[1], G. Papadopoulus[1], L. Richter[1], S. Mieke[2]

[1]Klinik für Anaesthesiologie und operative Intensivmedizin, Klinikum Steglitz, Freie Universität Berlin, Berlin
[2]Physikalisch-Technische Bundesanstalt, Berlin

Introduction

Indirect blood pressure measurement has been used for more than 100 years to determine arterial blood pressure in clinical routine. The extensive literature on the different methods (auscultatory and oscillometric) and their use is confusing, because the reports are contradictory in their assessment of the comparability of indirect and direct methods for blood pressure measurement (2, 3, 5—8, 11, 15, 16, 19, 20, 24, 27).
These problems have not been overcome by the development and clinical use of automated indirect blood pressure monitors. Difficulties arise when the different methods and/or devices for blood pressure measurement are used simultaneously in one patient. The observed differences apparently contradict not only the precision and accuracy of the individual devices, but also the plausibility of the results from measurement to measurement. The user derives this plausibility from the observation of the clinical symptoms whose relation to the measured blood pressure values is always evident. When confronted with these problems, the manufacturers of blood pressure recorders refer to clinical trials that have proven the usefulness of their devices and to the fact that, in the Federal Republic of Germany, blood pressure monitors can only be used in clinical practice after having been approved by a Federal institute. The stethoscope technique according to RIVA-ROCCI/KOROTKOFF is used as a reference method for this approval.

Aims of our study

The studies performed by Bruner (5) mainly contributed to disclosing the problems involved in the comparison of direct and indirect measurements and to developing the theoretical concepts for possible solutions. On the one hand, he stated the necessity to describe the method used for direct blood pressure measurement, in a comparison of direct and indirect measurements, by indicating the resonance frequency and the damping coefficient. On the other hand, he introduced the new concept according to which differences between directly and indirectly measured values should not be attributed to a disturbance or measurement error alone. Instead, it should be considered that changes in the quality and temporary relation between pressure pulse and blood flow also influence these methods (4, 23).

Efficiency of noninvasive measurement

Technically complex, noninvasive blood pressure monitors analyze parameters which the classical stethoscope method does not yield. This is achieved by electronic components which use mathematical procedures for the calculation of blood pressure values by analyzing special parameters, such as the oscillation of the cuff pressure or frequency changes of the Korotkoff sounds. The concept of automated blood pressure measurement necessarily requires additional technical sophistication for the recognition and suppression of artifacts. These techniques are designed to imitate an experienced examiner. However, human beings process information much more efficiently than do technical procedures (10). Our selective hearing and sight or our ability to analyze shapes make it easy for us to distinguish between important und unimportant information. Automated blood pressure monitors therefore have to be assessed with regard to their efficiency in signal processing.

Error analysis in relation to CO (each for p/sys, p/mean, and p/dia)

On the assumption that an increase in CO (cardiac output) likewise increases the blood flow under the blood pressure cuff, i.e., at the site of indirect blood pressure measurement, we analyzed the measurement error of the devices in relation to CO (4, 26). Furthermore, the examinations were repeated in 23 patients (see Section 3.7) at different COs in order to study the intraindividual influence of CO on the error.

Methods and technical devices

One direct and four indirect blood pressure monitors were used in our study.

a. Direct measurement:
   HP 78342 A patient monitor, Hewlett-Packard, West Germany.
b. Indirect measurement:
   Auscultatory measurement by three physicians
   BOSO BS 40, Bosch und Sohn, West Germany
   DINAMAP 845, Criticon, USA
   ACCUTORR2, Datascope, USA
   INFRASONDE D 4000, Puritan Bennet, USA.

Direct measurement

The direct measurement was carried out using a HP 78342 A monitor, a HP 1290 A quartz transducer, a 15-cm catheter (Sorensen Res) and a cannula of 32 x 0.6 mm ID (Abbocath-T 20G*32 mm). The frequency response of the whole system (3, 4, 13, 14, 21, 28) is presented in Fig. 1. It shows the influence of the two main factors, the electronic and hydrodynamic frequency response. The bandwidth (—3dB) of the whole system reached a maximum of 16 Hz due to the fact that there was a resonance at 35 Hz in the catheter system, and the bandwidth of the HP 78342 A monitor was 12 Hz (4, 14). The damping coefficient of the whole system was 0.21.

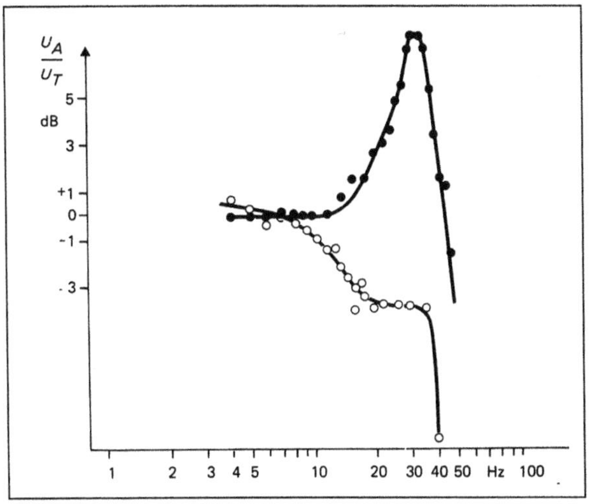

Fig. 1. Frequency response of the measurement system for direct blood pressure measurement. (●) Resonance of the system at 35 Hz; (○) same signals modified by a 12 Hz filter of a HP 78342 A patient monitor.

Auscultatory measurement by physicians

The auscultatory measurements were done by three physicians according to the recommendations of the AHA (1). In contrast to these recommendations, however, all diastolic values were determined in phase 5 to make them comparable to those obtained by automated sphygmomanometers, although most patients showed a hyperdynamic hemodynamic status. Standard stethoscopes were used.

DINAMAP 845

The DINAMAP 845 is one of the two representatives of automated sphygmomanometers operating with the oscillometric method. Criticon was the first manufacturer to develop an algorithm for the calculation of systolic and diastolic blood pressure values from the shape of the collected oscillations. They also set up special routines to minimize the influence of artifacts.

ACCUTORR 2

The ACCUTORR 2 is the other representative of automated sphygmomanometers based on the oscillometric method. It likewise uses oscillations stored in the microcomputer for the calculation of systolic and diastolic blood pressure. But the algorithm is totally different from that used by the DINAMAP 845. Another obvious difference is the continuous deflation compared to the stepwise deflation of the DINAMAP 845.

INFRASONDE D 4000

The INFRASONDE D 4000 is an auscultatory device that records Korotkoff sounds in the range of 10—50 Hz via a microphone and processes them via a static band pass filter (this device has not been approved in the Federal Republic of Germany). Due to the fact that the number of measurements is comparatively small and that the instrument was not available all the time, not all the analyses could be done for this monitor.

BOSO BC 40

The BOSO BC 40 blood pressure monitor likewise uses the auscultatory method. The Korotkoff sounds are recorded by a microphone and filtered by a digital filter with the possibility of changing the frequency band during the measurement (minimum frequency: 2.2 Hz, maximum frequency: 300 Hz).

Patients

We analyzed 59 measurement series of a total of 36 patients (Table 1) from the Surgical Intensive Care Unit of the Steglitz Medical Center of the Free University of Berlin. 17% of the patients were less than 31 years old, 36% were aged between 31 and 60 years, and 47% were over 60 years old. About 2/3 of the patients were men. Repeated measurements (measurement series) under markedly changed circulatory conditions were performed in 23 patients (twice in 15 patients, three times in 5 patients and four times in 3 patients). For medical reasons, all patients were artificially ventilated, sedated, and had an indwelling balloon-tipped pulmonary artery catheter (Swan-Ganz type) at the time of measurement. Twelve patients received dopamine (dosage: 2.5—5 μg/kg/min), 20 patients received dopamine + dobutamine, 22 patients received dopamine + dobutamine + noradrenalin, and five patients did not receive catecholamines.

Study design

Since it was not possible to perform direct and indirect blood pressure measurements at the same arm, we determined possible differences between the two arms prior to the measurement. This was done by simultaneously performing auscultatory blood pressure measurements at both arms. Patients in whom the side difference did not exceed respiratory blood pressure variations (2nd order blood pressure changes (17, 18)) were the study. Before and after each measurement series (45 min), CO was determined according to the usual guidelines (12, 25, 29). The mean value of both measurements is given in Table 1.

Table 1. Patient datas

Series No.	Patient No.	code	age/sex	Diagnosis	Site of direct measurement	Catecholamines DOP $\mu g/kg$ min	DOBUT	ARTE 1/min	Hemodynamic profile CO	CI 1/min m^2	SVR dyn*s*cm^{-5}
DINAMAP 845											
1	1	M.R.	25 m	1A, 2, 3	b	2.9	5.0		9.8	5.19	742
2	2	L.H.	60 f	1, 4, 5	f	2.8	19.0	0.40	10.0	5.80	632
3	3	J.M.	22 m	2, 6	b	5.0			16.0	7.50	290
4	4	H.S.	66 f	2, 2A, 4A	f	7.2	22.0	0.40	3.7	2.31	691
5	5	R.L.	50 m	1, 5, 6	f	2.4	10.0	0.29	10.5	5.06	680
6	6	E.S.	85 m	2A	b	2.3	19.0		6.6	3.65	630
7	6	E.S.	85 m	2A	b	2.3	19.0	0.2	12.0	6.44	460
8	7	K.H.	79 f	2, 2A, 5	b	3.3	23.0		6.9	4.50	660
9	8	G.S.	50 m	1, 2, 7	b	2.8	14.0	1.50	12.5	6.70	352
10	9	A.Z.	18 m	3, 3A	b	2.5	8.0		14.0	7.60	513
11	10	L.P.	74 f	1, 2	b	2.8	12.0	0.08	9.5	5.12	627
12	11	E.R.	61 f	1, 2, 3B,	5f	3.1	20.0	0.76	7.4	4.30	562
13	10	L.P.	74 w	1, 2	b	3.1	20.0	0.06	8.0	4.30	560
14	12	H.S.	85 f	1, 4A, 6A	b	2.6	20.0		12.9	7.40	359
15	13	A.V.	82 f	2, 2A, 4A	b	3.1	10.0	0.15	8.4	5.23	698
16	14	W.S.	60 f	1, 2	f	3.0	22.0		5.6	3.22	850
17	15	W.B.	50 m	1, 2	b	2.8	12.0	0.12	14.0	7.55	485
18	15	W.B.	50 m	1, 2	b	2.8	12.0	0.12	16.5	8.90	378
19	14	W.S.	60 f	2	f	3.0	22.0		11.0	5.98	350
20	16	W.K.	68 m	4B	r				6.0	3.03	666
ACCUTORR 2											
21	17	H.L.	70 w	1, 4A, 5	f	2.8	19.0	0.4	10.0	5.80	632
22	5	R.L.	50 m	1, 5, 6	f	2.4	10.0	0.29	9.4	4.59	731
23	3	J.M.	22 m	2, 6	b	3.0			16.0	8.30	397
24	18	H.S.	68 f	2, 2A, 4A	f	7.2	22.0	0.40	4.1	2.50	884
25	19	J.S.	20 m	2, 3	b	3.0			11.0	5.50	627
26	6	E.S.	85 m	2A	b	2.3	19.0	0.20	12.0	6.30	480
27	6	E.S.	85 m	2A	b	2.3	19.0		6.2	3.70	639
28	20	K.H.	72 f	2, 2A, 5	b	3.3	23.0		6.9	4.60	660
29	12	H.S.	85 f	1, 4A, 6A	b	2.6	2.0		12.9	7.40	359
30	10	L.P.	74 f	1, 2	b	3.1	20.0	0.06	8.0	4.30	560
31	16	W.K.	68 m	4B	r				5.2	2.63	753
32	21	H.K.	55 m	2, 2A	b	3.0	19.0		15.0	7.88	437
33	16	W.K.	68 m	4B	r				7.5	3.70	512
34	22	H.L.	71 m	1	b	3.0			6.5	4.40	849

Series No.	Patient No.	code	age/sex	Diagnosis	Site of direct measurement	Catecholamines DOP	DOBUT	ARTE	Hemodynamic profile CO	CI	SVR
						µg/kg min		1/min	1/min	m^2	dyn*s*cm^{-5}
INFRASONDE D 4000											
35	23	K.E.	58 m	1, 6	b	3.0			8.4	5.45	746
36	23	K.E.	58 m	1, 6	b	3.0			10.0	5.70	803
37	24	W.P.	72 f	9	b	3.0			8.1	4.53	814
38	25	F.D.	16 f	1	b	2.5	9.6		7.5	5.36	664
39	26	A.M.	46 m	2, 6	f	2.5	9.6	0.6	11.4	6.50	531
40	27	B.F.	71 m	8	r				6.2	3.9	873
41	28	R.E.	46 m	1, 2	r				8.8	5.25	596
42	29	K.T.	74 m	2	r	2.5	16.0		10.8	6.00	726
43	30	W.S.	48 m	2, 2A	f	2.5	20.0	0.8	11.1	5.10	656
BOSO BC 40											
44	24	L.P.	74 f	1, 2	b	2.8	13.0	0.08	9.6	5.20	692
45	15	W.B.	50 m	1, 2, 2A	b	2.8	12.0	0.12	14.0	7.50	486
46	15	W.B.	50 m	1, 2, 2A	b	2.8	12.0	0.12	16.5	8.90	378
47	14	W.S.	60 f	1, 2	f	3.0	22.0		4.9	2.80	881
48	11	E.R.	61 f	1, 2, 3B, 5	f	3.1	20.0	0.76	7.4	4.30	562
49	25	H.K.	55 m	2, 2A	b	3.0	19.0		15.0	7.88	437
50	16	W.K.	68 m	4B	r	3.0			8.2	4.10	487
51	22	H.L.	71 m	1	b	3.0			6.5	4.40	849
52	21	H.K.	55 m	2, 2A	b	3.0	19.0		12.2	6.40	505
53	31	R.E.	40 m	3B	b	2.5			6.5	3.50	886
54	32	H.N.	72 m	2A	b	2.9	12.0		11.0	5.50	604
55	33	A.S.	20 m	3A, 3B	b	2.5			8.5	4.20	922
56	34	E.V.	45 m	1A	r	2.5			11.3	5.70	396
57	35	M.G.	56 f	3B	b	13.2	9.0		4.9	3.13	1551
58	35	M.G.	56 f	3B	b	3.6	6.1		7.3	4.70	1096
59	36	M.B.	65 f	6A	b	2.5	8.0		6.0	4.40	730

Each measurement series and each patient was numbered consecutively. The following key indicates the most important diagnoses in the patients:

Diagnosis:

ARDS	1	pneumonia	1A		
sepsis	2	peritonitis	2A		
brain trauma	3	brain death	3A	intracranial bleeding	3B
cardiac infarction	4	cardiac insufficiency	4A	cardiac arrhythmia	4B
renal insufficiency	5				
poly trauma	6	hip endoprothesis	6A		
pancreatitis	7				
bypass aorta	8				
gastrectomie	9				

Site of direct arterial measurement: r = arteria radialis;
b = arteria brachialis
f = arteria femoralis

Mathematical methods

The following mathematical procedures were used (31):

1. Correlation analysis: correlation coefficient (r) and coefficient of determination ($B = r^2$) as percentages
2. Determination of linear regression (a, b)
3. Histograms of the errors of measurement ΔP (class interval of 2 mmHg).

Results

Figures 2a to 5c show the results of the comparative measurements for the different methods and instruments; the results of the mathematical assessment of these figures are summarized in Table. 2.

Table 2. Results of regression — and correlation analysis

Method/device	n	a mmHg	b	r	$r^2 = B$ %
Systolic					
Stethoscope	849	9	0.89	0.82	67
DINAMAP 845	299	35	0.77	0.78	61
ACCUTORR 2	210	43	0.63	0.79	62
INFRASONDE	129	62	0.69	0.56	31
BOSO BC 40	240	2	0.91	0.84	71
Mean					
Stethoscope	849	⁒	⁒	⁒	⁒
DINAMAP 845	299	29	0.68	0.71	50
ACCUTORR 2	210	38	0.67	0.76	58
INFRASONDE	129	⁒	⁒	⁒	⁒
BOSO BC 40	240	21	0.78	0.88	77
Diastolic					
Stethoscope	849	21	0.69	0.69	48
DINAMAP 845	299	28	0.62	0.70	49
ACCUTORR 2	210	43	0.52	0.56	31
INFRASONDE	129	−3	1.02	0.74	55
BOSO BC 40	240	26	0.65	0.68	46

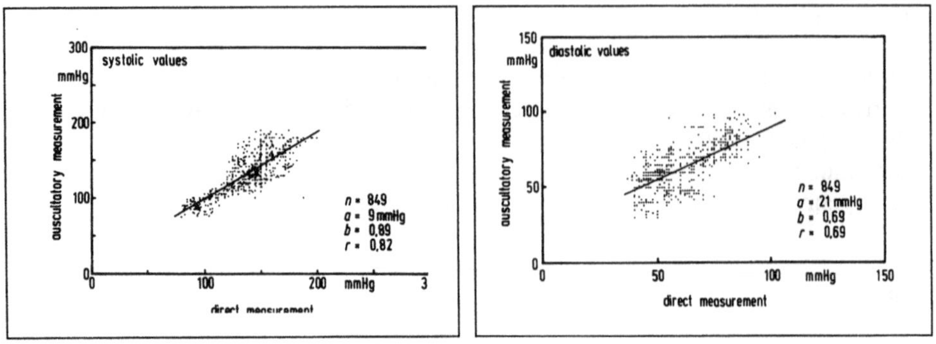

Fig. 2 a—b. Relationship between direct and indirect stethoscope measurements of systolic and diastolic pressure.

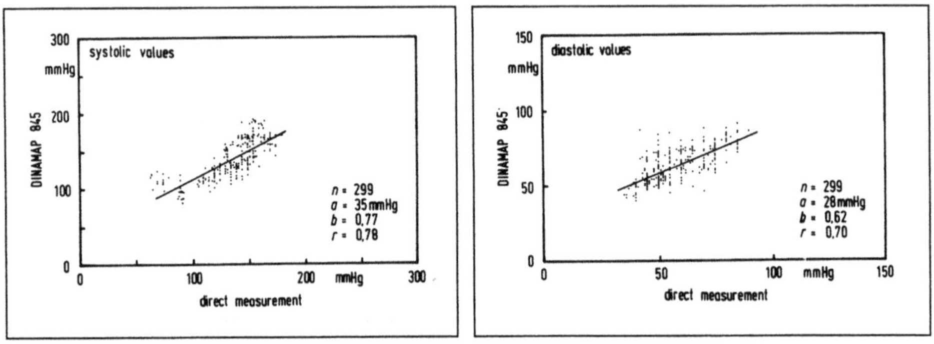

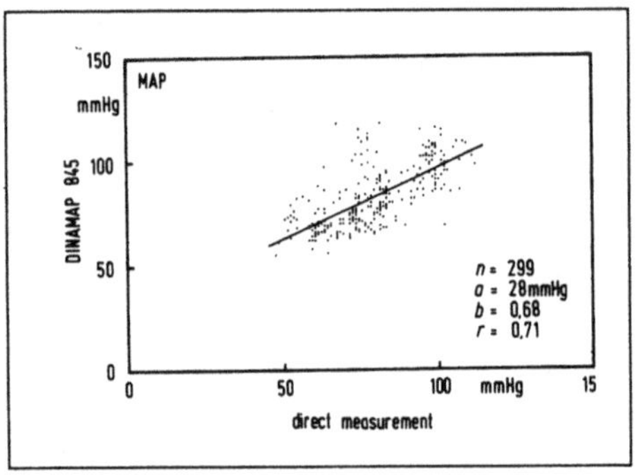

Fig. 3 a—c. Relationship between direct and indirect (DINAMAP 845) measurements of systolic, mean and diastolic pressure.

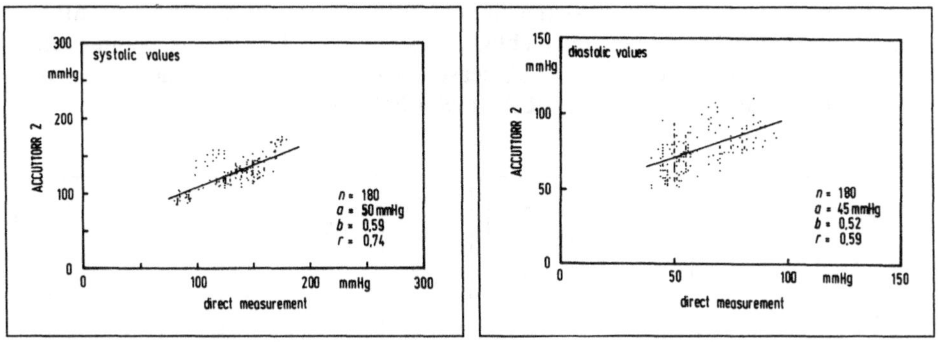

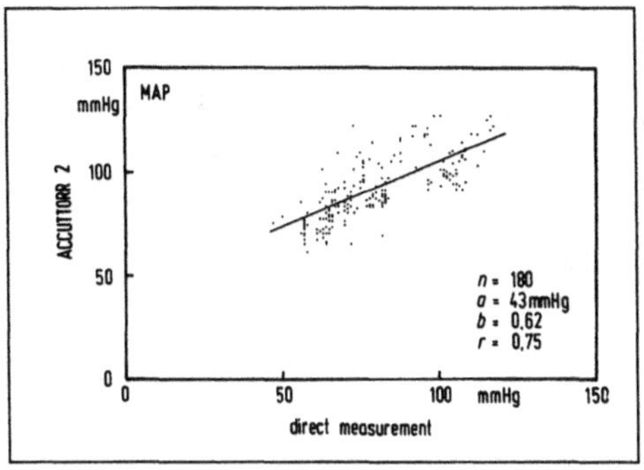

Fig. 4 a—c. Relationship between direct and indirect (ACCUTORR 2) measurements of systolic, mean and diastolic pressure.

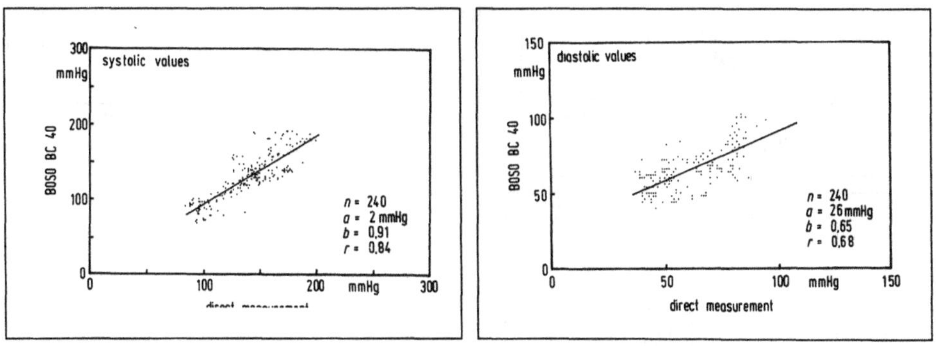

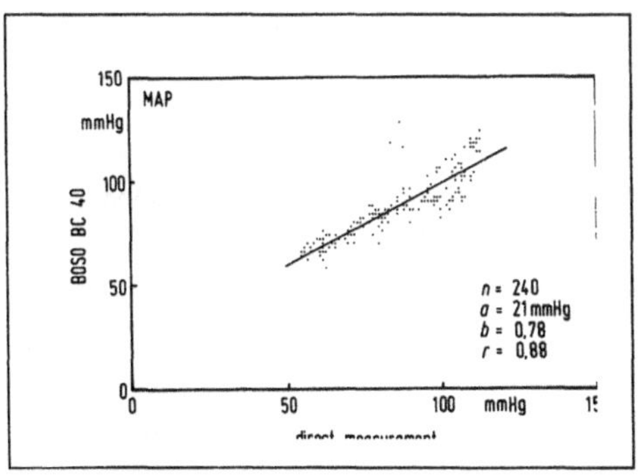

Fig. 5 a—c. Relationship between direct and indirect (BOSO BC 40) measurements of systolic, mean and diastolic pressure.

The histograms (Figs. 6a—9c) show the differences in the error of measurement ΔP between directly and indirectly determined blood pressure levels. Figures 17a, b and c summarize the representations of the errors of measurement ΔP for the three most important devices (DINAMAP 845, ACCUTORR 2, BOSO BC 40).

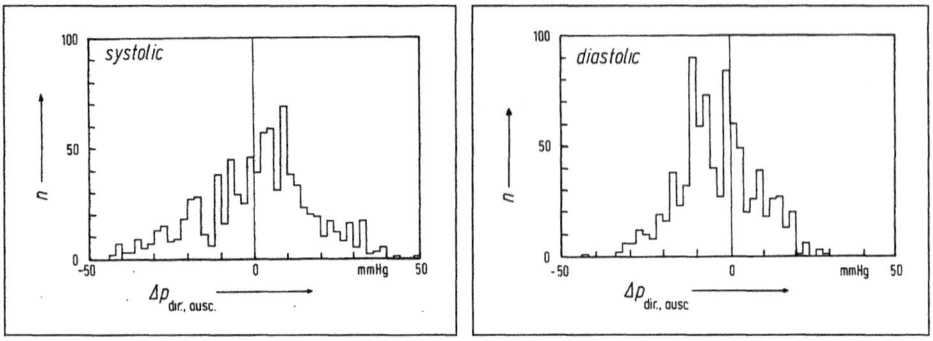

Fig. 6 a—b. Histograms direct vs stethescope (systolic, diastolic).

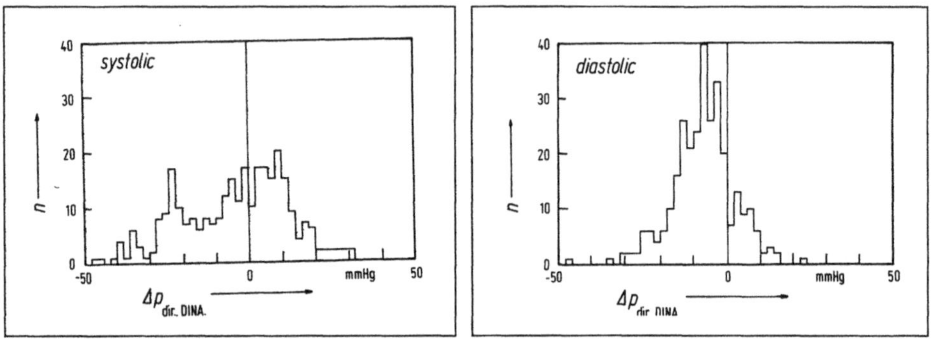

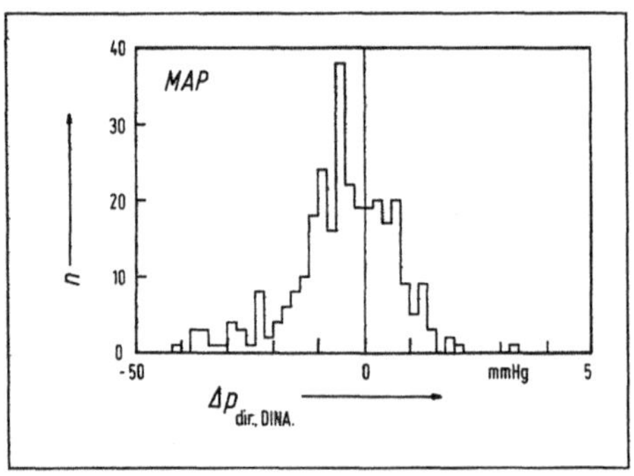

Fig. 7 a—c. Histograms direct vs DINAMAP 845 (systolic, diastolic, mean).

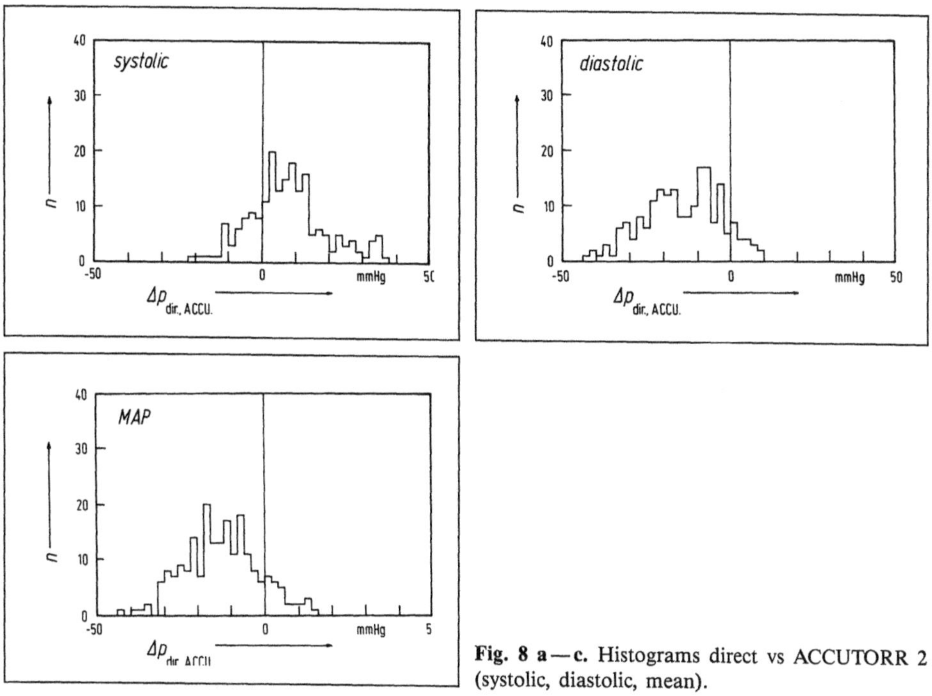

Fig. 8 a—c. Histograms direct vs ACCUTORR 2 (systolic, diastolic, mean).

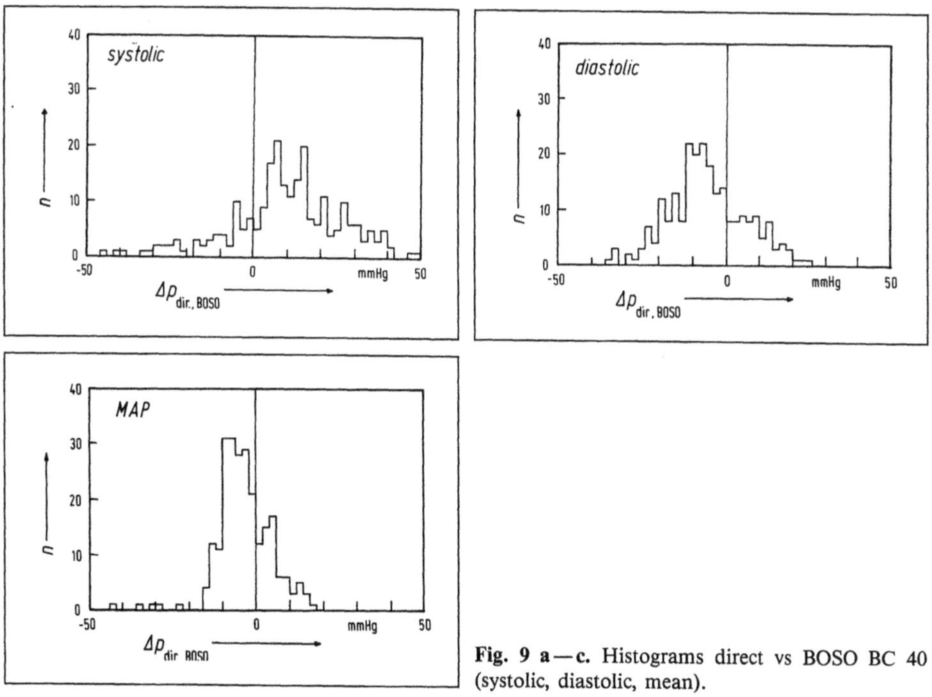

Fig. 9 a—c. Histograms direct vs BOSO BC 40 (systolic, diastolic, mean).

Figures 10—13 show how the error of measurement ΔP is influenced by changes in CO.

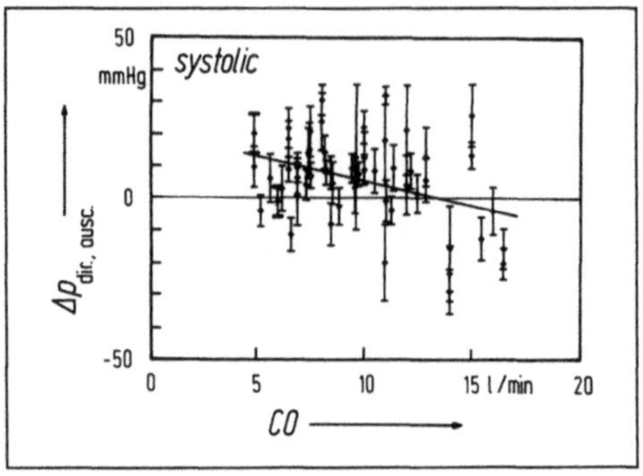

Fig. 10a. Correlation between measurement error (P) and CO (direct vs stethescope, systolic) n = 56, r = —0.37 (sig.: p = 0.01).

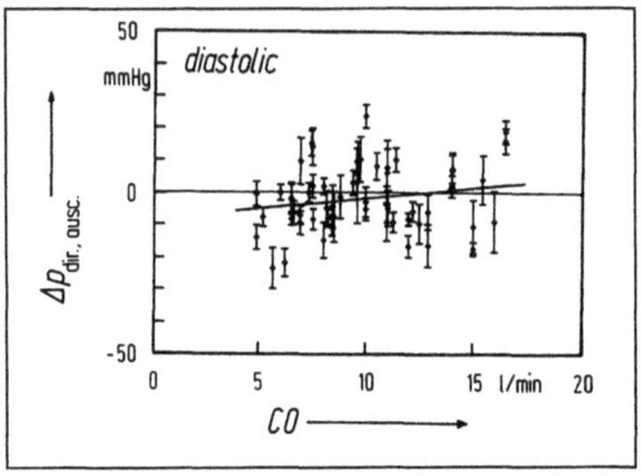

Fig. 10b. Correlation between measurement error (ΔP) and CO (direct vs stethescope, diastolic) n = 56, r = 0,26 (sig.: p = 0.05).

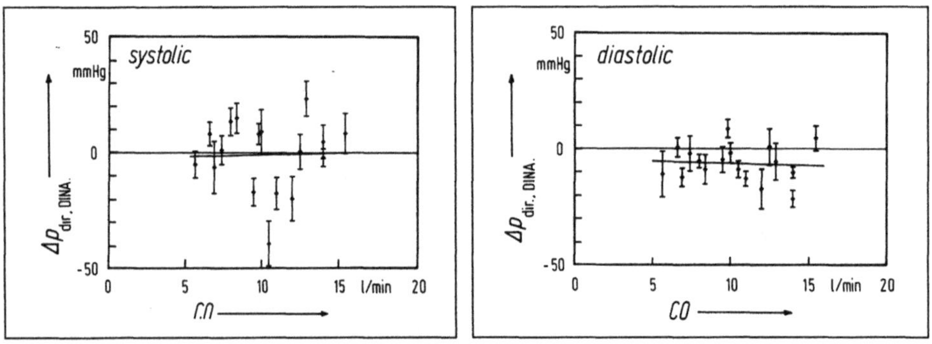

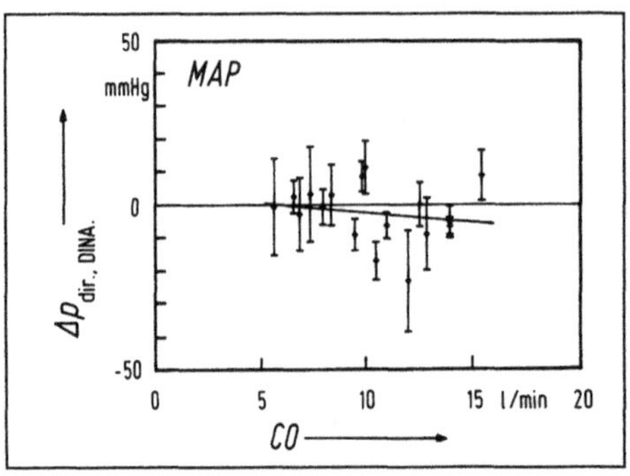

Fig. 11 a—c. Correlation between measurement error (ΔP) and CO (direct vs DINAMAP 845, systolic, diastolic and mean).

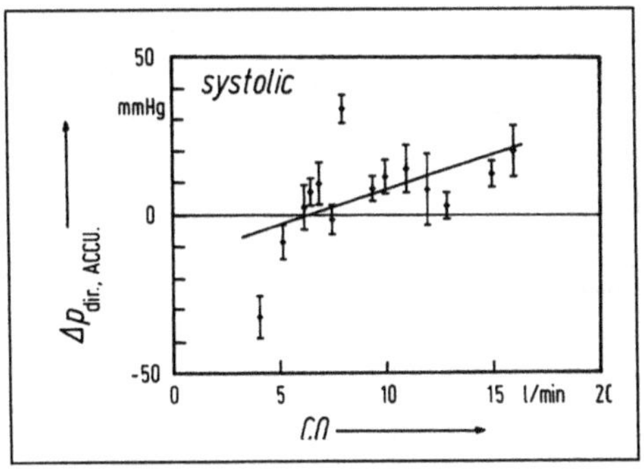

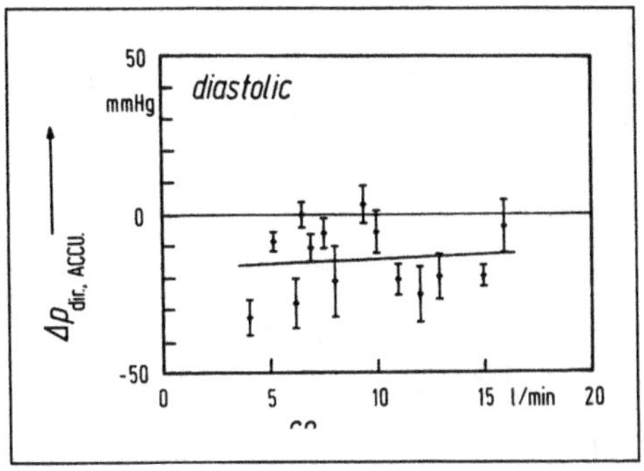

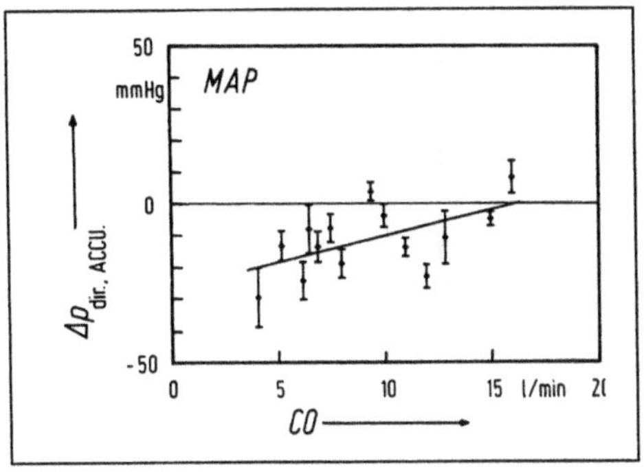

Fig. 12 a—c. Correlation between measurement error (ΔP) and CO (direct vs ACCUTORR 2, systolic, diastolic and mean) n = 14 (systolic r = +0.54 n. s.).

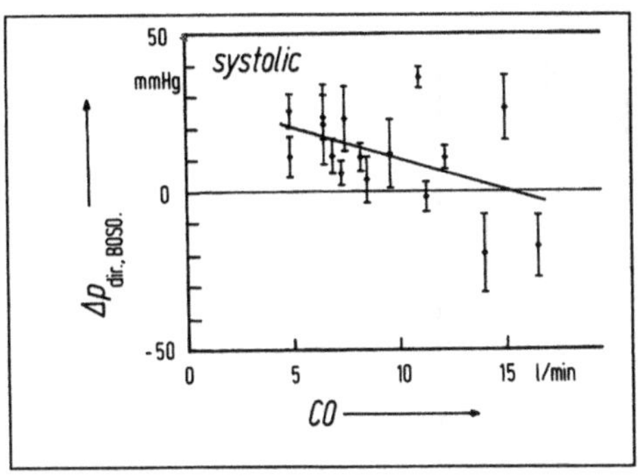

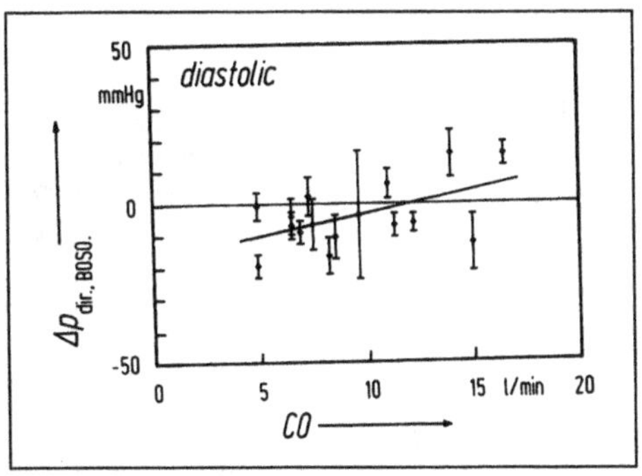

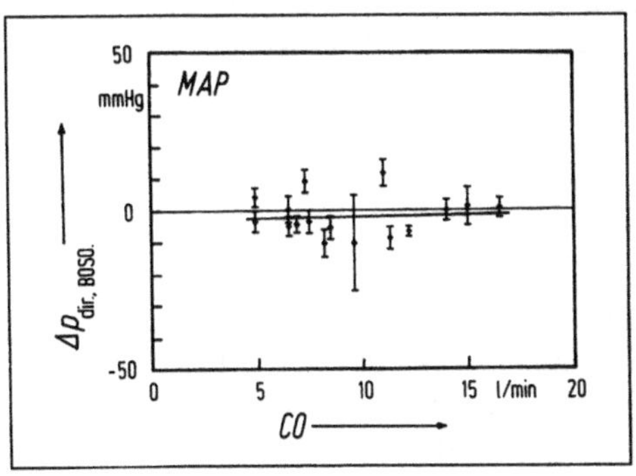

Fig. 13 a—c. Correlation between measurement error (₉₈ΔP) and CO (direct vs BOSO BC 40 systolic, diastolic and mean) n = 16 (systolic r = —0.47, border line n. s.).

The results obtained in patients in whom measurements were repeated under markedly changed circulatory conditions are summarized in Fig. 14. Each point in the figure represents the mean value of the error of one measurement series (ΔP = direct-indirect measurement). The standard deviation of the error in each measurement series is represented as a vertical line.

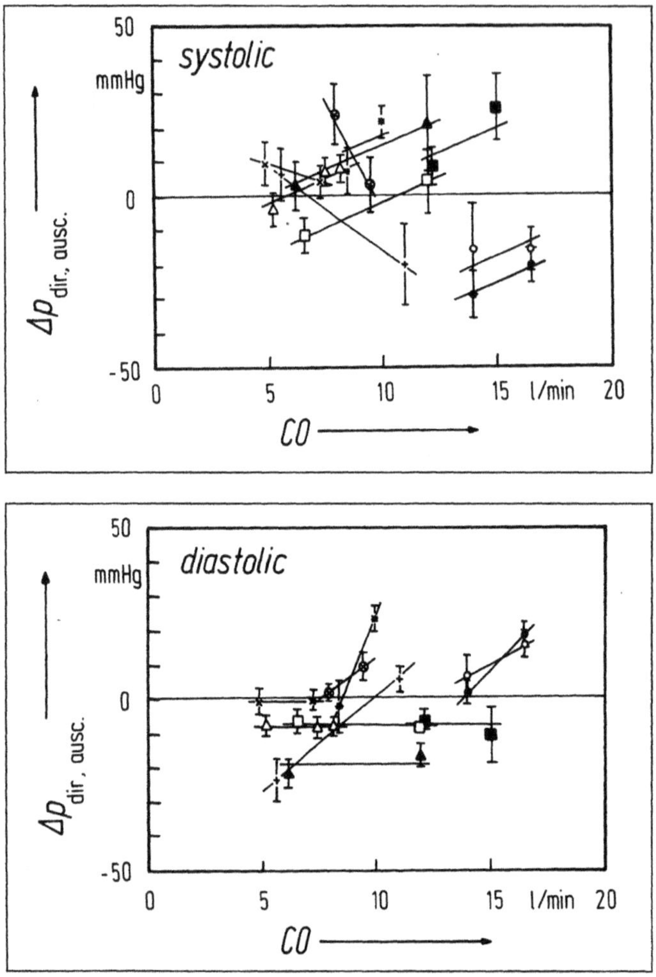

Fig. 14 a—b. Repeated measurements under changed circulatory conditions, direct/stethescope (systolic, diastolic).

Discussion

To assess the results of a measuring technique, it is advisable to differentiate between accuracy and precision. Measured values are accurate if they coincide with those obtained using a reference method; a measuring technique is precise if the results differ only slightly from measurement to measurement (9). This definition also implies that a precise technique does not necessarily have to yield accurate results.

Correlation coefficient and coefficient of determination

The graphic presentation of the comparison between the various indirect methods and the direct technique (Fig. 2—5), as well as the values given in Table 2, indicates that no clear correlation exists between the measuring techniques. The measured values are widely scattered around the averaged straight lines; the correlation coefficients r range between 0.56 and 0.88.
On inspection of Figs. 2 to 5, it is apparent that the measurement results of individual patients are frequently arranged in clusters of points. This means that the error from measurement to measurement in one patient can be relatively small; thus, the precision of the indirect technique is high. Since, however, it is impossible to predict on which side of the bisectors the measured values will lie, i. e. whether the measured values will be too high or too low, and since, in addition, there are strong individual fluctuations in the degree of error, it seems to us senseless in connection with comparative measurements of this type to make statements about the mean error of a technique. Thus the possible precision of techniques for indirect blood pressure measurement deceives the users as to the accuracy of the results. This approach also makes it possible to reconcile two apparently contradictory observations: the "good results" reported by the users and the rather depressing results of comparative measurements (27).
Interpretation of the statistics represents a further problem. The correlation coefficient r derived from correlation analysis of two variables, one of which serves as a reference, is a parameter that is not very expressive. This makes it difficult to deal with and often leads to misinterpretation. It is much more advantageous to use $B = r^2$, the coefficient of determination. This expresses in percentage the extent of the relation between the variables to be tested. For example, in the test of the direct/indirect systolic pressure (Table 2), only 31% of the variability of the indirectly measured blood pressure, at the worst, can be ascribed to the arterial blood pressure. This is nevertheless 67% for the stethoscope method, the standard blood pressure measuring technique.
The correlation coefficients we determined do not differ significantly from results of other authors (4, 6, 8, 11, 16, 19, 20, 24, 27); the differences lie in the assessment. Surprisingly, the highest value of $r = 0.88$ is achieved by BOSO BC 40 for the MAP, although this device calculates the MAP according to the well-known formula:

$$P_{MAP} = P_{diast} + 1/3\,(P_{syst} - P_{diast})$$

The correlations were particularly poor in connection with diastolic blood-pressure measurements. There are probably several reasons for this:

1. Despite hyperdynamic circulatory conditions, it was not the usual criterion (phase IV) that was applied for determination of diastolic blood pressure, but phase V.
2. It is extremely unfavorable to determine the blood pressure at the time the Korotkoff sounds diminish under the conditions of intensive-care medicine and during anesthesia (high external noise level, etc.).
3. The threshold of audibility varies for low frequencies depending on the stethoscope used.
4. The ability to recognize Korotkoff sounds depends on many individual factors, such as spectral sensitivity of the ear, and the amplitudes of Korotkoff sounds vary in the range of the diastolic pressure (22).

Thus, the indirect determination of diastolic pressure continues to represent a considerably greater problem than that of systolic blood pressure.

Slope of the averaged line

The impression that arterial blood pressure can only be inadequately determined by the indirect techniques applied under the conditions of intensive care medicine is strengthened on inspection of slope b of the averaged straight lines. The optimal value, b = 1.0, is not reached in any representation; the values range between 0.52 and 0.91. The values of indirect measurements are too high for low arterial pressures and too low for high ones.

Histograms

The histograms (Figs. 6—9) show, on the one hand, that the values scatter widely and, on the other hand, that the indirect methods frequently yield systolic values that are too low and diastolic values that are too high. The results of the Korotkoff method and oscillometric methods do not differ significantly with regard to this point, although these are fundamentally different methods. This fact might be the result of the effort of the manufacturers to achieve a high degree of conformity with the stethoscopic technique (Fig. 15).

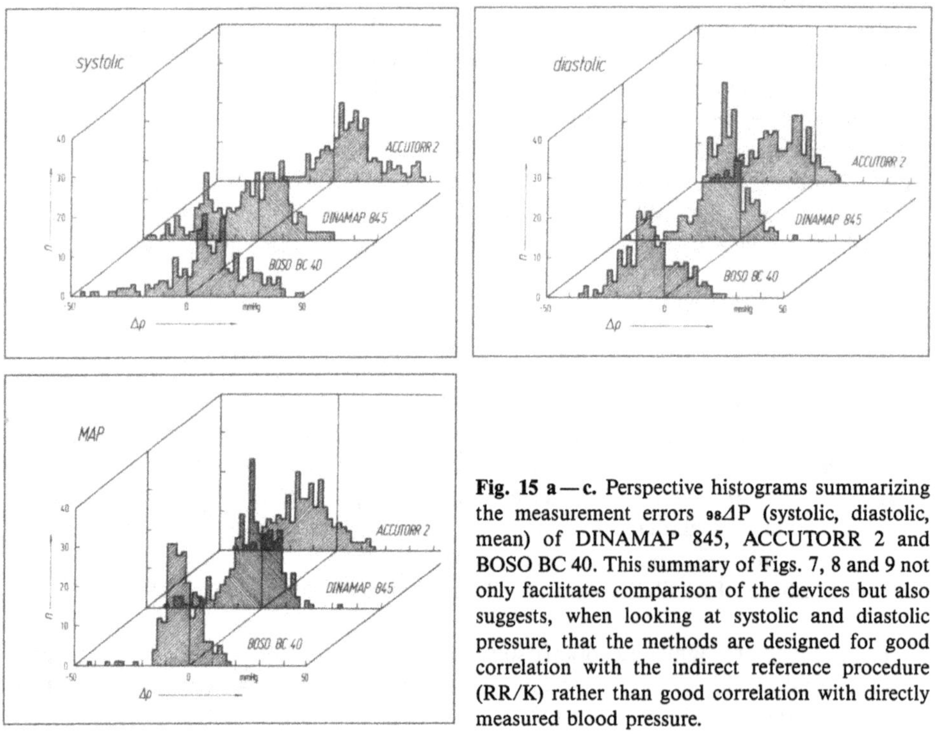

Fig. 15 a—c. Perspective histograms summarizing the measurement errors 98ΔP (systolic, diastolic, mean) of DINAMAP 845, ACCUTORR 2 and BOSO BC 40. This summary of Figs. 7, 8 and 9 not only facilitates comparison of the devices but also suggests, when looking at systolic and diastolic pressure, that the methods are designed for good correlation with the indirect reference procedure (RR/K) rather than good correlation with directly measured blood pressure.

Relation of the measurement error to CO

Discriminating consideration must be given to the question as to the influence exerted by CO on the differences between direct and indirect blood pressure measurements (ΔP). One of the hypotheses for this study was that flow-dependent techniques for blood pressure measurement are subject to flow-dependent errors of accuracy (4, 7, 26, 29). This was believed to be in contrast to techniques that interpret the pressure pulse and are thus pressure-dependent (oscillometric method).

As far as the auscultatory methods (BOSO BC 40, INFRASONDE and the stethoscope technique) are concerned, the result is not uniform and must be more closely elucidated here. The representation of the error of measurement (ΔP) of all auscultatory measurement values (stethoscope technique) shows contrary tendencies with respect to CO in Figs. 10a and 10b. In consideration of the number of observations ($n = 56$), the gradients of the curves in Figs. 10a and b deviate significantly from zero (systolic $n = 56$, $r = -0.37$, sig. $p = 0.01$; diastolic $r = 0.26$, sig. $p = 0.05$) according to the tables of Fisher and Yates (31). The results of the auscultatory blood pressure measurements change with alterations of the CO. Incontestable, however, is the fact that it is not possible, with the number of measurements in the present study, to confirm a relation between CO and the values determined by BOSO BC 40 and INFRASONDE.

The seemingly clear picture changes when consideration is given exclusively to multiple measurements in individual patients under different hemodynamic conditions (Fig. 14). First the systolic values: here the relationship can take a contrary course in individual cases (decrease of systolic measurement values with increasing CO). There have also been single observations of diastolic measurements values in which the error of measurement ΔP is independent of the CO. The concept of multiple measurements was chosen because it was considered to be the only method that eliminated the many individual influences, leaving CO as the only parameter influencing the error of measurement. The shortcoming of this hypothesis might be the fact that increases in CO do *not* necessarily result in increased blood flow in the upper arm artery. Some patients showed signs of peripheral vasoconstriction despite high CO.

In accordance with the theoretical assumption, the auscultatory measuring device BOSO BC 40 is apparently not unaffected by alterations of the CO, although the numbers of cases do not allow this observation to be statistically confirmed (Fig. 13). It was also in accordance with expectations that the error of measurement (ΔP) of DINAMAP 845 and ACCUTORR 2 is statistically independent of the CO (see Figs. 11, 12). The differences in the course of the curve between DINAMAP 845 and ACCUTORR 2 are obvious, however, and can only be explained by the different evaluation algorithms.

Conclusion

The present investigation shows that, in several important points, the number of examinations were not sufficient to confirm the conjectured relationships between the blood flow and the flow-dependent auscultatory techniques (BOSO BC 40, INFRASONDE). This is due to a variety of indeterminable influences which affect auscultatory measurements and interfere with the postulated flow-dependence. The influence of accidental errors coud only be minimized by substantially increasing the number of patients and additional parameters, such as blood flow in the upper arm artery. Repeated measurements in the same patient under different hemodynamic conditions could be helpful but cause new problems (ethical, legal).

Although our study does not allow us to make a final statement as to the causes of the error of measurement ΔP, the extent of the deviations suggests that indirect blood pressure measuring devices cannot serve as a replacement for direct blood pressure measurement in intensive care units and that the differences in price of these devices are not justified by differences in efficiency.

References

1. American Heart Association (1980/81) Recommendations for human blood pressure determinations by sphygmomanometers. News from the AHA
2. van den Broeke JJ, Karliczek G (1979) DINAMAP eine neue automatische Blutdruckmessung, Ergebnisse von Vergleichsmessungen. Prakt Anasth 14: 533—536
3. Broemser Ph (1930) Anwendung mathematischer Methoden auf dem Gebiet der physiologischen Mechanik. In: Abderhalden E (ed) Handbuch der biologischen Arbeitsmethoden. Urban & Schwarzenberg, Berlin, Wien, pp 81—166
4. Bruner JMR (1978) Handbook of Blood Pressure Monitoring. PSG Publishing Co. Inc., Littleton, MA
5. Bruner JMR, Krenis LJ, Kunsman JM and Sherman AP (1981) Comparison of direct and indirect methods of measuring arterial blood pressure. Med Instrum 15/1: 11—21; ibid 2: 97—101; ibid 3: 182—188
6. Chastonay P, Morel D, Forster A, Suter PM (1982) Evaluation of a new monitoring device for arterial blood pressure and heart rate measurement by automatic sphygmomanometry. Anästh Intens Notfall med 17: 348—350
7. Cohn JN (1967) Blood pressure measurement in shock. J Am Med Assoc 199/13: 972—976
8. Colan SD, Fujii A, Borow KM, McPherson D, Sanders SP (1983) Noninvasive determination of systolic, diastolic and end-systolic blood pressure in neonates, infants and young children: Comparison with central aortic pressure measurements. Am J Cardiol 52: 867—870
9. Deutsche Norm DIN 1319 (1983) Grundbegriffe der Meßtechnik, Teil 3
10. Ellis DM 1985 Interpretation of beat-to-beat blood pressure values in the presences of ventilatory changes. J Clin Monit 1: 65—70
11. Finnie KJC, Watts DG, Armstrong PW (1984) Biases in the measurement of arterial pressure. Crit Care Med 12: 965—968
12. Forrester JS, Ganz W, Diamond G, McHugh T, Chonette DW, Swan HJC (1972) Thermodilution cardiac output determination with a single flow-directed catheter. Am Heart J 83/3: 306—311
13. Gauer OH (1972) Messung von Druck, Volumen und Stromstärke im Kreislauf. In: Gauer O, Kramer K, Jung R (eds) Physiologie des Menschen. Bd 3, Urban & Schwarzenberg, München, Berlin, Wien, pp 283—304
14. Gardner RM (1981) Direct blood pressure measurement — dynamic response requirements. Anesthesiology 54: 227—236
15. Geddes LA (1970) The direct and indirect measurement of blood pressure. Year Book Publishers, Chicago
16. Hausmann D, Rommelsheim K (1983) Automatische nichtinvasive Blutdruckmessung — Vergleichsmessungen und Erfahrungen mit dem DINAMAP Vital-Daten-Monitor 845 XT auf der Intensivstation. Anästh Intensivther Notfallmed 18: 93—97
17. Koepchen HP (1962) Die Blutdruckrhythmik. Steinkopff, Darmstadt
18. Koepchen HP (1984) History of studies and concepts of blood pressure waves. In: Miyakawa K et al. (eds) Mechanisms of blood pressure waves. Japan Sci Soc Press, Tokyo/Springer Berlin, pp 3—23
19. Loubser PG (1985) Comparing direct and indirect arterial blood pressure. Anesthesiology 63: 566—567

20. Loubser PG (1985) Accuracy of automated oscillometric pressure measurement devices inhypertensive patients. Anesthesiology [Suppl] 63: A188
21. Bedford RF (1985) Invasive Blood Pressure Monitoring. In: Blitt CD (ed) Monitoring in Anesthesia and Critical Care Medicine. Churchill Livingstone, New York, Edinburgh, London and Melbourne, pp 41—85
22. McCutcheon EP, Rushmer RF (1967) Korotkoff sounds, an experimental critique. Circ Res 20: 149—161
23. Milnor WR (1972) Pulsatile blood flow. Physiology in medicine. N Engl J Med 287: 27—34
24. Nystrom E, KH Reid, R Bennett, L Couture, HL Edmonds (1985) A Comparison of two automated indirect arterial blood pressure meters: With recordings from a radial arterial catheter in anesthetized surgical patients. Anesthesiology 62: 526—530
25. Pace NL (1977) A Critique of flow-directed pulmonary arterial catheterization. Anesthesiology 47: 455—465
26. Rodbard S (1953) The significance of the intermediate Korotkoff Sounds. Circulation 8: 600—604
27. Rutten AJ, Ilsley AH, Skowronski GA and Runciman WB (1986) A comparative study of the measurement of mean arterial blood pressure using automatic oscillometers, arterial cannulation and auscultation. Anaesth Intens Care 14: 58—65
28. Shinozaki T, Deane RS, CHrand B, Mazuzan JE (1980) The dynamic responses of liquid-filled catheter systems for direct measurements of blood pressure. Anesthesiology 53: 498—504
29. Swan HJC, Ganz W, Forrester J, Marcus H, Diamond G and Chonette D (1970) Catherization of the heart in man with use of a flow-directed balloon-tipped catheter. N Engl J Med 283/9: 447—451
30. Ur A, Gordon M (1970) Origin of Korotkoff sounds. Am J Physiol 218/2: 524—529
31. Weber E (1972) Grundriß der biologischen Statistik. Gustav Fischer, Stuttgart

Common clinical problems of measuring arterial pressure in the elderly

F.H. Messerli, E. Grossman, S. Oren

Department of Internal Medicine, Section on Hypertensive Diseases, Ochsner Clinic and Alton Ochsner Medical Foundation, New Orleans, Louisiana, USA

Introduction

Arterial pressure increases with age in westernized populations, and more and more patients reach values considered to be hypertensive. Thus, prevalence of essential hypertension may exceed 50% of the total population in the geriatric age group (1). Despite these impressive numbers, there is nothing benign about hypertension in the elderly (2). A variety of studies have indicated that cardiovascular morbidity and mortality increase in parallel with systolic pressure even more in the geriatric than in the middle-aged population (3—6). However, a variety of facts can interfere with blood pressure measurement in the elderly patient. Among them is the increased variability of arterial pressure commonly present in the elderly patient, the hiatus of the Korotkoff sounds occasionally encountered, as well as pseudohypotension and pseudohypertension due to increased arterial stiffness (7—11).

Increased variability of arterial pressure

Variability of arterial pressure has been found to increase with age (12, 13). This increase parallels the increase in arterial pressure, and it remains unknown whether the two phenomena can be dissociated. Several factors could contribute to the increased variability of arterial pressure in the elderly hypertensive patient: (1) Baroreflexes have been shown to become more sluggish with progressive aging (and also with an increase in arterial pressure) (14, 15); therefore, any change in arterial pressure is less effectively counteracted by the baroreceptors. (2) Intravascular volume declines with aging, making the patient's blood pressure more prone to the effects of volume depletion (14). (3) Arterial (and venous) wall stiffness increases with aging thereby impairing elasticity of resistance and capacitance vessels. Thus, acute volume expansion within the intravascular space will raise pressure, and volume depletion will lower pressure much more dramatically in elderly than in younger patients (16, 17).

The unusual lability and variability of arterial pressure have to be taken into account when blood pressure is measured in the elderly. Depending upon fluid volume status, position, postprandial state, bladder distention, etc., blood pressure may be high on one occasion and normal or even low on another. Many patients who initially meet the blood pressure criteria for hypertension will have normal blood pressure on repeated examinations (18, 19). Thus, repetitive measurements of blood pressure must be taken before a patient is labelled as hypertensive.

Pseudohypertension

In patients with distinct arteriosclerosis, stiffness of the arterial wall can interfere with blood pressure measurement. Clearly, a higher cuff pressure is needed to compress a hardened sclerotic artery than an elastic one. A systematic evaluation of pseudohypertension by Spence et al. indicated that discrepancies of up to 64 mmHg can be demonstrated between cuff and intra-arterial pressures in certain elderly patients (20). We recently evaluated a maneuver that was originally described by Osler for the detection of pseudohypertension in elderly patients (11). Osler's maneuver was performed by inflating the blood pressure cuff above systolic pressure and carefully palpating the radial or brachial artery. When either of these arteries remained clearly palpable (despite being pulseless), the patient was described as being *Osler positive*. In contrast, when the artery collapsed and could not be palpated, the patient was described as being *Osler negative*. We classified 24 elderly hypertensive patients as either Osler positive or Osler negative and subsequently measured their intra-arterial pressure, arterial compliance, and systemic hemodynamics. Our study revealed that patients with pseudohypertension (Osler positive) had falsely elevated blood pressure readings, with a difference of 10 to 54 mmHg between cuff and intra-arterial pressure. At the same time, arterial compliance was distinctly lower in Osler-positive subjects and correlated with the difference between cuff and intra-arterial pressure. This indicates that the stiffer the artery, the more pronounced was the degree of pseudohypertension.

Clinical consequences arising from this spurious elevation of arterial pressure are most important. The Framingham study allows us to calculate that an increase of arterial pressure of 15 mmHg (such as simulated in the Osler-positive subjects) would increase the risk of stroke fourfold, of congestive heart failure threefold, and of myocardial infarction twofold in an elderly population (21, 22). Moreover, subjects misdiagnosed as having essential hypertension could be subjected needlessly to the inconvenience, cost, risk, and adverse effects of the antihypertensive regimen. Elderly patients are particularly susceptible to the adverse effects of antihypertensive therapy, and inappropriate treatment has been shown to lead to transient ischemic episodes as well as to even fatal neurologic events (22—26).

Pseudohypotension

Localized atheromatosis occurring bilaterally in both subclavian or brachial arteries may occasionally lead to a drastic drop in pressure so that blood pressure becomes low or unmeasurable in the upper extremities (27). We recently observed a patient who had peripheral pressures of 80/60 mmHg at the time when aortic root pressure was 220/116 mmHg. At the same time, distinct left ventricular hypertrophy was present by echocardiographic and electrocardiographic criteria, and renal function was impaired. Blood pressure differences between the two arms are common in the elderly population (28). However, bilateral, high-grade occlusion is fortunately quite rare. This entity should be borne in mind in any patient who suffers from excessive target organ disease, i. e., Grade III and IV retinopathy, left ventricular hypertrophy, and renal failure in the presence of normal arterial pressure. Wide differences in the pressure in the two arms is sometimes associated with the subclavian steal syndrome (stenosis of the subclavian or brachiocephalic artery proximal to the origin of the vertebral artery). This syndrome results in a steal of blood flow from the carotid and opposite vertebral artery across the basilar artery flowing backward down the ipsilateral vertebral artery on the obstructed side.

Hiatus of Korotkoff sounds

In patients who have distinct systolic hypertension, occasionally a hiatus occurs when blood pressure is measured and the Korotkoff sounds are assessed (28). When the cuff is progressively deflated, the Kortokoff sounds may be heard from (for example) 220 to 190 mmHg, then disappear and become audible again at 140 mmHg, to disappear completely at the diastolic level of 90 mmHg. Little is known about the exact pathophysiologic mechanism of this hiatus or auscultatory gap. For practical purposes, it is important to remember that in the elderly patient the cuff must be inflated until the arterial pulse disappears (by digital palpation) and should then be deflated very slowly. This is not usually a problem for the thorough examiner but may lead to spuriously low or normal pressure readings with automated equipment.

References

1. Ostfeld AM (1978) Elderly hypertensive patient: epidemiologic review. NY State J Med 78: 1125—1129
2. Kannel WB, Dawber TR, McGee DL (1980) Perspective of systolic hypertension: The Framingham study. Circulation 61: 1179—1182
3. Ostfeld AM, Shekelle RB, Klawans H, Tufo HM (1974) Epidemiology of stroke in an elderly welfare population. Am J Public Health 64: 450—458
4. Shekelle RB, Ostfeld AM, Klawans HL Jr. (1974) Hypertension and risk of stroke in an elderly population. Stroke; 5: 71—75
5. Kannel WB, Dawber TR, Sorlie P, Wolfe PA (1976) Component of blood pressure and risk of atherothrombotic brain infarction: The Framingham study. Stroke; 7: 327—331
6. Amery A, Hansson L, Andren L, Gudbrandsson T, Sivertsson R, Svensson A (1981) Hypertension in the elderly. Acta Med Scand; 210: 221—229
7. O'Callaghan WG, Fitzgerald DJ, O'Malley K, O'Brien E (1983) Accuracy of indirect blood pressure measurement in the elderly. Br Med J; 286: 1545—1546
8. Vardan S, Mookherjee S, Warner R, Smulyan H (1983) Systolic hypertension: direct and indirect BP measurements. Ann Intern Med; 143: 935—938
9. Taguchi JT, Suwangool P (1974) "Pipe-stem" brachial arteries: a cause of pseudohypertension. Am Med Ass; 228: 733
10. Messerli FH, Glade LB, Ventura HO, Dreslenski GR, Suarez DH, MacPhee AA, Aristimuno GG, Cole FE, Frohlich ED (1982) Diurnal variations of cardiac rhythm, arterial pressure and urinary catecholamines in bordeline and established essential hypertension. Am Heart J 104: 109—114
11. Messerli FH, Ventura HO, Amodeo C (1985) Osler's maneuver and pseudohypertension. N Engl J Med 312: 1548—1551
12. Schmeider RE, Lavie CJ, Messerli FH (1987) The variability of arterial pressure: what is the clinical importance? Cardiovasc Rev Reports 8: 65—69
13. Kobrin I, Oigman W, Kumar A, Ventura HO, Messerli FH, Frohlich ED, Dunn FG (1974) Diurnal variation of blood pressure in elderly patients with essential hypertension. J Am Geriatr Soc; 32: 896—899
14. Messerli FH, Ventura HO, Glade LB, Sundgaard-Riise K, Dunn FG, Frohlich ED (1983) Essential hypertension in the elderly: haemodynamics, intravascular volume, plasma renin activity and circulating catecholamine levels. Lancet; II: 983—985

15. Gribbin B, Pickering TG, Sleight P, Peto R (1971) Effect of age and high blood pressure on baroreflex sensitivity in man. Circ Res; 29: 424—431
16. Ventura HO, Messerli FH, Oigman W, Suarez DH, Dreslinski GR, Dunn FG, Reisin E, Frohlich ED (1984) Impaired systemic arterial compliance in borderline hypertension. Am Heart J; 108: 132—136
17. Learoyd BM, Taylor MG (1966) Alterations with age in the viscoelastic properties of human arterial walls. Circ Res; 18: 278—292
18. Colandrea MA, Friedman GD, Nichaman MZ, Lynch CN (1970) Systolic hypertension in the elderly — an epidemiological assessment. Circulation 4: 239—245
19. Hulley SB, Feigal D, Ireland C, Kuller LH, Smith WM (1986) Systolic Hypertension in the Elderly Program (SHEP), the first three months. J Am Geriatr Soc 34: 101—105
20. Spence JD, Sibbald WJ, Cope RD (1978) Pseudohypertension in the elderly. Clin Sci Mol Med; 58 (Suppl 4): 3995—4025
21. Kannel WB, Gordon T (1978) Evaluation of cardiovascular risk in the elderly: the Framingham study. Bull NY Acad Med; 54: 573—591
22. Jackson G, Pierscianowski TA, Mahon W, Condon J (1976) Inappropriate antihypertensive therapy in the elderly. Lancet; II: 1317—1318
23. Traub YM, Aygen MM, Rosenfeld JB (1979) Hazards in treatment of systolic hypertension. Am Heart J; 97: 174—177
24. Jones JV, Graham DI (1978) Hypertension and the cerebral circulation — its relevance to the elderly. Am Heart J; 96: 270—271
25. Hypertension in the elderly. Lancet (Editorial) 1977; 1: 684—685
26. Dangerous antihypertensive treatment. Br Med (Editorial) 1979; 2: 228—229
27. Kirkendall WM, Feinleib M, Freis ED, Mark AL (1980) Recommendations for human blood pressure determination by sphygmomanometers. Subcommittee of the AHA Postgraduate Education Committee. Circulation; 62: 1146A—1155A.
28. Kirkendall WM, Burton AC, Epstein FH, Freis ED (1967) Recommendations for human blood pressure determination by sphygmomanometer. Circulation 36: 980—988

Clinical relevance of casual blood pressure readings versus self-measurement

D. Magometschnigg

Medical University Clinic, Department of Clinical Pharmacology, Vienna, Austria

Introduction

Blood pressure is determined and regulated by multiple influences such as by myocardial, vascular and rheological factors (1). Therefore, a single blood pressure reading does not permit any conclusions to be drawn as to one specific mechanism influencing blood pressure. There is, however, an abundance of epidemiologic evidence that people with blood pressure readings at the upper end of the scale are at higher risk (2—14). We rely on this fact to calculate the rate of adverse, hypertension-related events, especially stroke, cardiovascular failure, coronary heart disease and progressive renal impairment. The belief in the value of casual blood pressure readings to predict an increased risk started with the advent of modern medicine at the beginning of the 20th century (15). Up to now it has been customary to estimate individual risks on the basis of population risks. Strangely enough, we continue judging our patients on the wisdom of mean values in spite of our knowledge of statistics and of the great variations in the epidemiological data which are taken as the scientific basis for our decisions. Generally, we predict individual risks on the basis of the same crude method which, on account of its poor predictive value ought to be used only for judging groups. For all decisions concerning individuals, for diagnosis as well as for the control of treatment, we still use just one informal blood pressure reading, mostly obtained by the Riva-Rocci technique. We do this although drug studies based on this method and performed on large numbers of patients have hardly shown any benefits at all (16—21). It may well be that taking casual blood pressures as a basis for judging hypertension is to a large extent responsible for the difficulty in proving the protective effect of lowering arterial blood pressure.

In addition to the above arguments there are other reasons why the common use of casual blood pressure readings for judging individual hypertensives is open to severe criticism.

Doctor's cuff blood pressure

Another problem associated with casual blood pressure readings is the basic tendency of blood pressure to increase with physical and psychological stress. It is certainly natural for a patient who sees his doctor to be in a state of expectation or even apprehension, or at best anxious to hear the doctor's opinion of his/her health. Therefore it is not surprising to find the doctor's blood pressure readings to be generally higher than those measured by other persons or in different environments. Blood pressures taken by nurses, automated devices or recorded by the patient himself are generally distinctly lower than those recorded by the doctor (22—25). The individual discrepancy between the various

readings cannot be predicted. We can neither assess the degree of anxiety, alertness or nervousness of the patient, nor can we define the extent to which a vascular system reacts to a certain stress. The discrepancies differ widely within normotensive and hypertensive individuals. It is common to find deviations ranging from 0 to 60 mmHg systolic and from 0 to 30 mmHg diastolic. Unless we decide to ignore this effect the only chance of predicting the individual degree of blood pressure elevation caused by the medical doctor is by direct measuring. If we want to take this effect in account we have to compare the different recordings, i. e. the doctor's reading and the self-recorded pressures.
If we further consider the small differences in blood pressure of 10 mmHg diastolic, which are used by the Arterial Hypertension Committee of the WHO (26) as well as by Subcommittee on Definition and Prevalence of 1984 Joint National Committee (27) to differentiate the severity and prognosis of hypertensive groups, the weakness of casual blood pressure readings for judging individuals becomes even more apparent.

Blood pressure variability

Further severe criticism of casual blood pressure readings is based on continuous inter-arterial blood pressure recordings. This data demonstrate clearly that blood pressure is a continuous variable and as such not amenable to simple methods of measurement (23, 28). In normotensives, as well as in hypertensives, blood pressure varies widely during daytime and especially between day and night. Within 24 h differences of 40 mmHg systolic and 25 mmHg diastolic are quite normal. Therefore the casually recorded blood pressure reading depends on the hour and on the individual circadian variability.

Population risk versus individual risk

Casual blood pressure reading by the traditional sphygmomanometer method has proved to be a valid basis to guide our decisions in respect of hypertensive cohorts. Various epidemiological studies (16—21) have demonstrated that up to 20% of the mild to moderate hypertensives are at higher risk. If we assume that about 20% of patients with such a low level of blood pressure elevation are at risk, we can logically conclude that about 80% of them are not at risk. Consequently, in 80% of mild to moderate hypertensives, elevated casual blood pressure readings have no precdictive value. As we base our decisions on these readings we tend to make false judgments in the majority of cases showing slightly elevated blood pressures. Even more problematic is the fact that we base our therapeutic decisions on these measurements. If we decide to medicate all our mildly to moderately hypertensive patients, the conclusions we draw as to the no-risk majority must of necessity be wrong. On the basis of these considerations, casual blood pressures can only be satisfactory for judging cohorts, not individuals.

Casual blood pressure as a guide to treatment

Another feature which is often overlooked is the quality of casual blood pressures as a guide for treatment. As the above considerations have led us to conclude that casual readings cannot judge individual risk in a satisfactory way, the method obviously can not be used as a guide to individual therapy. This is important, as we cannot expect that normal-risk patients will benefit from medication, while we have to take into account the normal rate of side effects of pharmacological treatment. Furthermore, persons who are unnecessarily treated will — unnecessarily — consider themselves to be ill, they will be expected to visit their doctor regularly and will thus at least cause unnecessary health care expenditures.

Even in the 20% of patients for whom the decision to treat is justified, we are not of much help. Quite apart from the grounds for criticism mentioned so far, there are other drug-related variables influencing blood pressure that would have be taken into consideration. Any medication based on a single blood pressure reading ought to take certain pharmacodynamic features of the drug into account. We should at least know the time interval between drug intake and blood pressure recording, as well as the effect a given drug dosage had on blood pressure as a continuous parameter.

Besides, the mean values obtained in drug trials only suggest what might happen in our patient, but they do not tell us anything about the actual effect the drug dosage has on the individual patient we are treating.

24-hour blood pressure recordings

While casual blood pressure recordings give us little base for judging individuals, 24-h blood pressure recordings as well as self-measurements seem to be more useful. There is strong evidence that 24-h blood pressure recordings improve the predictability of risk (29—36). It appears that hypertension-related organ damage can be predicted more reliably on the basis of 24-h blood pressure readings. Also, an analysis of 24-h blood pressure profiles can be used to classify patients with comparable casual blood pressures into at least three groups (37).

In 40% of the patients, blood pressure will be elevated only occasionally. In 20—30% of the patients, blood pressures are elevated only during daytime and hardly ever at night, while in about 20% of hypertensives blood pressures are elevated both day and night. Our analysis of 24-h blood pressure readings has convinced us that the views of Brunner and Mancia (24, 25), who think that we overtreat at least 40% of our patients on the basis of casual blood pressure readings, are entirely correct. A further advantage of 24-h blood pressure readings is that they allow a better assessment of drug effectiveness in the individual patient.

24-h blood pressure profiles give a more realistic picture of blood pressure as a continuous variable rather than reflecting only a momentary situation.

Unfortunately the method still has some imperfections and equipment costs as well as the cost of individual studies are still high, so that general application of the method is not yet possible.

Self-recording

Self-monitoring is another method superior to casual blood pressure readings. Like 24-h blood pressure readings, self-monitored blood pressures tend to be lower than those mea-

sured by the doctor and, at the same time, are a better prognostic tool for predicting hypertension-related risks (30, 38, 39).
Furthermore, values recorded by the patients themselves correlate better with 24-h blood pressure readings than office blood pressures (40). Like the Remler device, selfrecordings may be used by the patient to determine his diurnal blood pressure profiles (Fig. 1). The main difference between this device and other automatic devices, (e. g. Spacelabs) is that we do not obtain any values from the patient while he is asleep.

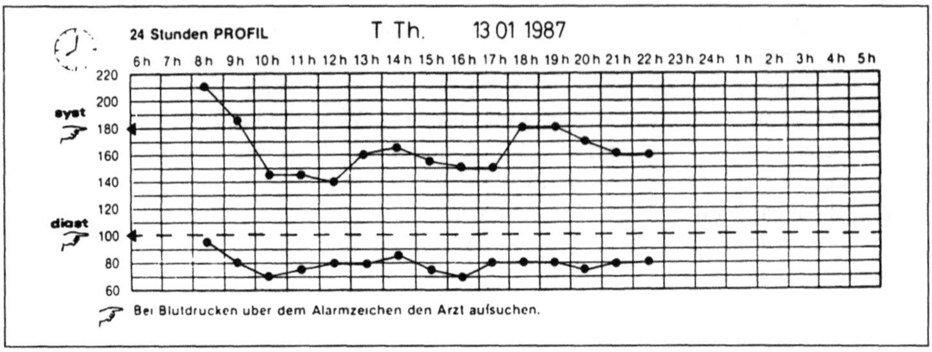

Fig. 1. Self-recorded diurnal blood pressure profile. Blood pressure measurements were taken by the patient himself using his own simple device.

This might be important for all those hypertensives whose blood pressure is elevated during the night, as well as in those cases where it is important not to depress the nocturnal blood pressure too much. To date, there is hardly any information on the influence of drugs on the blood pressure of sleeping patients.

The advantages of self-monitoring over 24-h blood pressure monitoring

Self-monitored blood pressure records are the source of information on long-term blood pressure variability, since they allow us to trace changes in blood pressure taking place over the course of days, weeks or even months (Fig. 2). This means that we are also able to monitor blood pressure changes during periods of increased psychological stress, but also during holidays.
In about 10% of our patients, blood pressure readings vary considerably despite continuous drug therapy, not only from hour to hour but also from day to day, and even from week to week (Fig. 3). In such patients therapy can be successful only if the patient is trained to cooperate actively in the treatment effort and to adapt his medication to the self-monitored blood pressure values.

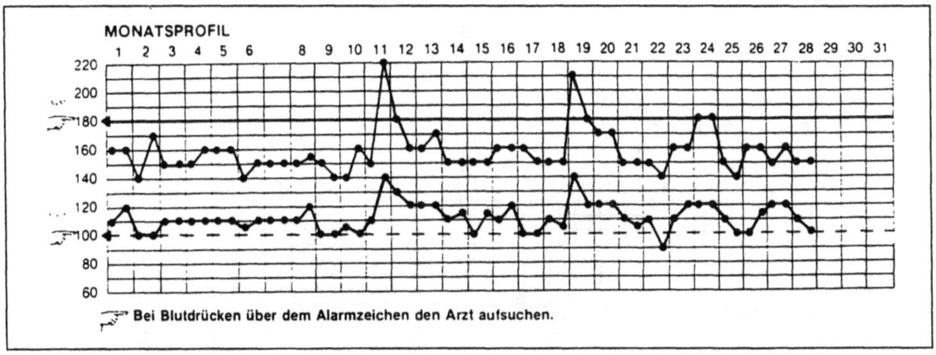

Fig. 2. Self-recorded blood pressure profile over a month. Peak values were caused by increased psychological stress.

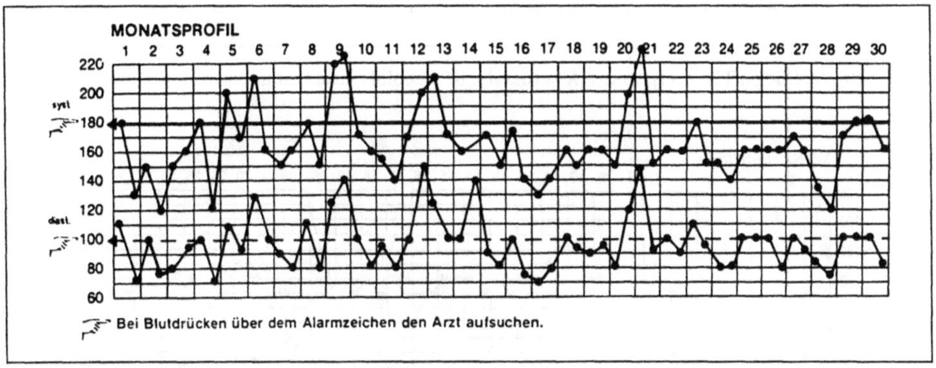

Fig. 3. Self-recorded blood pressure profile over a month. Blood pressure variability takes place in spite of constant drug intake.

Self-monitoring also offers additional advantages which regard to drug therapy:

1. Ever since we started to base our decision of whether or not to institute treatment mainly on blood pressures recorded at home and decided not to treat patients whose blood pressure was elevated only when they where seen in the out-patient department, we have been able to exclude 40% of the patients from therapy. Of course, our decision to treat is not only based on blood pressure, but also on such factors as additional cardiovascular risk and hypertension-related organ damage.
2. Self-monitored blood pressure readings show immediately whether the drug or the dosage prescribed are adequate or not and, regardless of whether the effect is too mild or too strong, remedial action can be taken without delay (Fig. 4).
As a result, the use of this technique makes therapy safer.
3. Patients with unpredictable episodes of high blood pressure can protect themselves immediately by self-medication.
4. Blood pressure self-recording has a positive influence on compliance (41). The self-monitoring records are a good way to keep the patient on an effective therapy, as they instantly get a negative feedback whenever they do not comply with the necessary hypertensive treatment scheme.

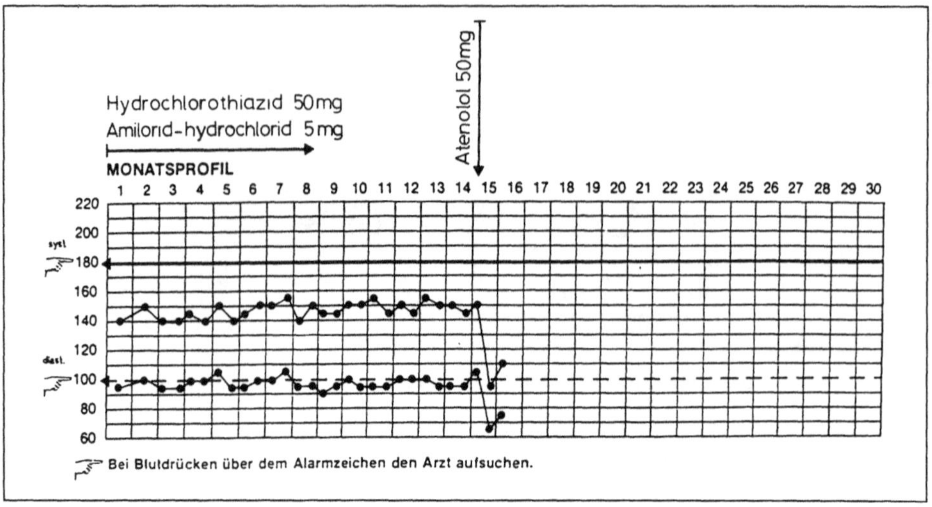

Fig. 4. Self-recordings. The decision to add a diuretic to atenolol caused an intense fall in blood pressure.

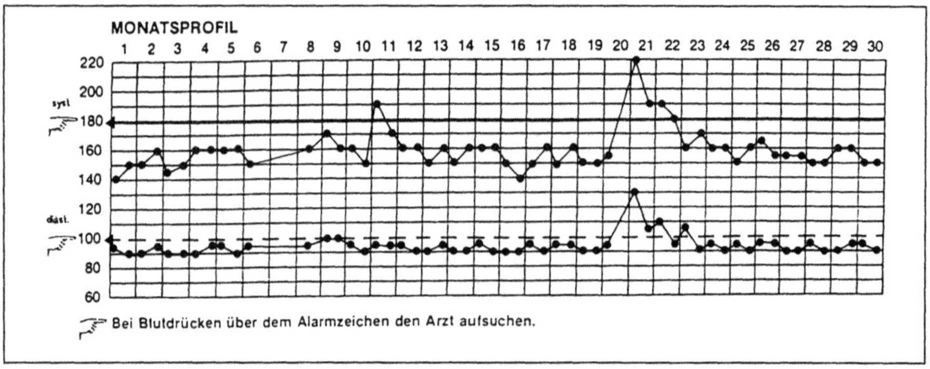

Fig. 5. Self-recorded blood pressures over a month. Peak values could not be attributed to an obvious cause. The elevated pressures were treated by the patient's decision with an additional dose of nifedipine.

A further benefit of blood pressure diaries is that the patient and his doctor learn a great deal about the patient's blood pressure profile. Consequently, it is easy to adapt drug administration to individual needs. At the same time, the patients learn more about their disease and how certain activities influence their blood pressure values.

On the other hand, self-monitoring may also give rise to new problems:

1. In order to obtain accurate blood pressure diaries, the patient must be trained to take his blood pressure properly.

2. In order to obtain accurate records, the patient must be told how to document his blood pressure readings in such a way that they can be easily read and interpreted. We ask our patients to document their blood pressure readings in such a way that they can be easily read and interpreted. We ask our patients to document their blood pressure

readings in the form of graphs (Figs. 1—5). Unlike lines or columns of figures, this technique allows the doctor to review the records of several months at a glance. At the same time, the patient obtains a feedback on his blood pressure status in a summary form.

3. As the patient learns more about his disease he will confront his doctor with more questions. In order to deal successfully with the problem of having to answer the same basic questions over and over again, we have started to organize information and discussion sessions for groups of patients. In addition, they are also given information in writing. As a consequence, patient-doctor relationships have changed: instead of merely writing prescriptions we can now advise them specifically on their individual problems. In spite of the paucity of data, blood pressure self-recording seems to be not only an important and simple tool to facilitate the decision of whether or not to treat a patient, but has also improved the effectiveness and safety of treatment.

Conclusion

24-h blood pressure recordings and blood pressure self-monitoring are new, more sensitive tools for assessing hypertensives. They help us to make a correct decision whether or not to treat our patients more safely and with fewer side effects. It therefore appears appropriate to make the benefit of these techniques available to our patients.

References

1. Wetterer E, Kenner Th (1968) Grundlagen der Dynamik Arterienpulses. Springer, Berlin-Heidelberg-New York
2. Pickering GW (1972) Definitions, natural histories and consequencies. Am J Med 52: 570
3. Hypertension, Detection and Follow-up Program Cooperative Group: Five years findings of the Hypertension (1979) Detection and Follow-up Program. J Am Med Ass 242: 2562
4. Deubner, DC, Tyroler, HA, Cassel JC et al.: Attributable risk, population attributable fraction of death associated with hypertension in biracial population. Circulation 55: 901
5. Lew EA (1973) High blood pressure, other risk factors and longevity: Insurance viewpoint. Am J Med 55: 281
6. Centers for Disease Control (1982) Annual summary 1981: reported morbidity and mortality in the United States. Morbid. Mortal. Weekly Rep. 30: 54
7. Kannel WB, Sorlie P, Castelli WP, McGee DL (1980) Blood pressure and survival after myocardial infarction: The Framingham Study. Am J Cardiol 45: 326
8. Wolf PA, Kannel WB, Verter J (1984) Epidemiologic appraisal of hypertension and stroke risk. In: Guthrie G, (eds) Kotchen TA Hypertension and the Brain. Futura Publishing p 221
9. Kannel WB, Gordon T (1978) Evaluation of cardiovascular risk in the elderly: The Framingham Study. Bull N Y Acad. Med. 54: 573
10. Kannel WB, Dawber TR, McGee DL (1980) Perspectives on systolic hypertension: The Framingham Study. Circulation 61: 1179
11. Veterans Administration Cooperative Study Group on Antihypertensive Agents (1967) Effects of treatment on morbidity in hypertension. Results in patients with diastolic blood pressure averaging 115 through 129 mmHg. J. Am Med Ass 202: 166
12. Amery A, De Schaepdryver A (1973) European Working Party of High Blood Pressure in the Elderly (EWPHE); Organization of a double blind multicentre trial on antihypertensive therapy in elderly patients. Clin Sci Mol Med 45: 71

13. Robertson JIS (1980) Hypertension: primary and secondary prevention. In: Julian DG, O'Neal Humphries (eds), Preventive Cardiology Butterworths, London, pp 62—85
14. Robertson JIS (1980) The risk-benefit equation: when to initiate treatment. Br J Clin Pharmac 18: 181—185
15. Actuarial Society of America and the Association of Life Insurance Medical Directors (1925) Blood-pressure Study. New York
16. Australian National Blood Pressure Study Management Committee (1981) Treatment of mild hypertension in the elderly. Med J Austr 398
17. European Working Party on High Blood Pressure in the Elderly (1985) Mortality and Morbidity Results from the European Working Party on High Blood Pressure in the Elderly Trial. Lancet I, 1349
18. Helgeland, R (1980) The Oslo Study. Treatment of Mild Hypertension: A Five Year Controlled Drug Trial. Am Med 69: 725
19. IPPPSH Collaborative Group 1985 (1985) Cardiovascular risk and risk factors in a randomized trial of treatment based on betablocker Oxprenolol. J. Hypert 3: 379
20. Medical Research Council Working Party (1985) MRC trial of treatment of mild hypertension (1985) Principal results. Br Med J 291: 97
21. WHO/ISH Mild Hypertension Liaison Committee (1982) Trials of Treatment of Mild Hypertension: An Interim Analysis Lancet I, 149
22. Mancia G, Bertinieri G, Grassi G, et al (1983) Effects of blood pressure measurement by the doctor on patient's blood pressure and heart rate. Lancet 2: 695—697
23. Raftery EB (1987) Der sogenannte Praxisblutdruck — eine kritische Wertung. In: Magometschnigg D, Hrsg. Blutdruckselbstkontrolle Uhlen, Wien p 9
24. Mancia G (1987) Bewertung der Hypertonie mit Hilfe des Belalstungsblutdruckes, des 24-Stunden-Blutdruckprofils und der Blutdruckselbstmessung. In: Blutdruckselbstkontrolle, Magometschnigg (ed.), Uhlen, Wien, p 63.
25. Brunner H (1987) Selbstmessung und 24-Stunden-Blutdruckprofile als Grundlage für epidemiologische Schlußfolgerungen. In: Magometschnitt D, Hrsg. Uhlen, Wien 384
26. Arterial Hypertension Report of WHO Expert Committee: World Heath Organisation technical report series (1978) 628
27. Subcommittee on Definition and Prevalence of the 1984 Joint National Committee (1985): Hypertension Prevalence and the Statues of Awareness Treatment and Control in the United States. Hypertension 7: 457
28. Magometschnigg D, Hitzenberger G; (ed.) (1983) Blutdruckvariabilität, Uhlen, Wien
29. Pessina AC, Mormino P, Semplicini A, et al (1980) The blood pressure in labile and established hypertension. Computer analysis of the continuous blood pressure recording. ISAM 79, Academic Press, New York, p 253
30. Sokolow M, Werdegar D, Kain HK et al. (1966) Relationship between blood pressure measured casually and by portable recorders and severity of complications in essential Hypertension. Circulation 34: 279—298
31. Floras JS, Jones JV, Hassan MD, Osikowska B, Sever PS, Sleight P (1981) Cuff and ambulatory blood pressure in subjects with essential hypertension. Lancet 2: 107—109
32. Devereux R, Pickering TG, Harshfield GA et al. (1983) Left ventricular hypertrophy in patients with hypertension: importance of blood pressure response to regularly recurring stress. Circulation 68: 470—476
33. Parati G, Pomidossi G, Albini F, Malaspina D, Mancia G. Relationship of 24-h blood pressure mean and variability to severity of target organ damage in hypertension. J. Hypertens, in press
34. Mancia G, Parati G, Pomidossi G, Di Rienzo M (1985) Validity and usefulness of non-invasive ambulatory blood pressure monitoring. J. Hypertens 3, suppl 2: 5—11
35. Perloff D, Sokolow M, Cowan R (1983) The prognostic value of ambulatory blood pressures. I An Med Ass 249: 2792—2798
36. Mancia G, Parati G, Pomidossi G, Grassi G, Casadei R, Zanchetti A (1987) Alerting Reaction and Rise in Blood Pressure during Measurement by Physician and Nurse. J Hypertens 2: 209—215
37. McCall WC, McCall VR (1981) Diagnostic Use of Ambulatory Blood Pressure Monitoring in Medical Practice. J Fam Pract 13: 25
38. Perloff D, Sokolow M (1978) The representative blood pressure: usefulness of office, basal, home, and ambulatory readings. Cardiovasc Med 3/6: 655

39. Floras JS, Jones JV, Hassan MO, et al. (1981) Cuff and ambulatory blood pressure in subjects with essential hypertension. Lancet 2: 107
40. Kleinert HD, Harshfield GA, Pickering RB, et al. (1984) What is the value of home blood pressure measurement in patients with mild hypertension? Hypertension 6: 574
41. Edmonds D, Vetter W (1987) Verbessert die Selbstkontrolle die Zusammenarbeit des Patienten mit dem Arzt? In: Magometschnigg D (ed.) Blutdruckselbstkontrolle Uhlen, Wien: p 131

2. Ambulatory 24-h Blood Pressure Monitoring

History of telemetric automatic long-term blood pressure recording

B. Krönig

Innere Medizin, Ev. Elisabeth Krankenhaus, Trier, FRG

Introduction

As early as the turn of the century, Riva-Rocci (32), von Recklinghausen (30), and Korotkoff (16) introduced the indirect measurement of blood pressure with a cuff and mercury manometer, which has basically remained unchanged up to this day. With this method — and also in individual cases with precursor devices like the v. Basch apparatus (5) — it has been possible to gain fairly deep insights into the dynamic character of the variable "arterial pressure".

Changes in the sleep/wake rhythm, time of day, momentary emotional behavior, extent of physical activity and ultimately posture have been identified as causes for the daily variability in blood pressure. In addition, it has been demonstrated that the difference between diurnal and nocturnal blood pressure is directly proportional to the severity of hypertension (27) and that there is also a wider range in variability with increasing age (26).

With the introduction of automatic indirect long-term blood pressure measurement procedures (which are described in more detail by Anlauf in this book) it has been possible to systematize the studies on the diurnal and circadian blood pressure variability. A fairly concurrent result was a biphasic blood pressure curve with maximal values in the morning and evening hours, an indicated decrease in the midday hours, a pronounced minimal value in the early nocturnal hours and a slow renewed increase to the first peak in the morning (7, 31, 33).

However, these studies did not take into account blood pressure variances due to everyday or sport-related stress or to short-term vegetatively induced fluctuations (see 14). It seemed therefore useful to look for possibilities to take continuous long-term intra-arterial blood pressure measurements — if possible, of volunteers who move about freely. Based on the technically simpler ECG telemetry, Bachmann et al. introduced the "wireless transmission of continuous direct blood pressure recording" in 1967 (3).

Methods

Compared to the already wide-spread ECG telemetry, which hardly loses in importance because of a certain zero drift, the transmission of absolute values such as intraarterial blood pressure recording (besides a number of other cardiovascular parameters) necessitated the development of a temperature-stable integrated operational amplifier, accomplished by Zerzawy et al. (35, 37) of the Bachmann study group. In accordance with the cardiological orientation of the study group, other parameters such as aortic and pulmonary arterial pressure, ECG, and breathing were also registered.

The diagnostic possibilities and advantages of blood pressure telemetry as compared to discontinuous indirect long-term blood pressure recording as well as the continuous direct blood pressure recordings with patient-sided magnetic-tape registration (analogous to the long-term ECG) which was introduced at the same time in England, are given in Table 1. Telemetric transmission makes it possible to study everyday conditions and to avoid the "test stand situation" in the cardiovascular laboratory.
However, simultaneous registration of actual values in the stationary receiver unit (constant monitoring) permits direct intervention by the investigator whenever there are threatening blood pressure values or technical problems (e. g., occlusion/kinking of the measuring catheter).

Table 1. Diagnostic possibilities and advantages of blood pressure telemetry vs indirect and direct long-term measurement procedures without telemetry

Blood pressure telemetry
- everyday conditions
  (e. g., no "test stand"/cardiovascular laboratory)
  to register variad pressure changes due to
  - postural changes
  - psychic/physical stress
  - sport activities, during rehabilitation
  - diurnal/circadian rhythm (e. g., values during undisturbed sleep)
- detailed blood pressure analysis in regard to
  - "beat-to-beat"
  - variability
    - short-term ("blood pressure waves")
    - for a period of 24 h
- influence of antihypertensive treatment procedures
- registration of several variables (e. g., additionally HR, ECG, aortic/pulmonary arterial pressure)
- including constant observability of the values of volunteers

In detail, Bachmann et al. (3, 4) proceeded as follows: Using the Seldinger technique to puncture the femoral artery, a red Ödman-Ledin catheter is pushed as far as 20 cm into the common iliac artery. The catheter is then attached to a liquid-filled conduction system which establishes the connection with the pressure probe (Statham elements P23 Db and P37B were used) that is attached to the thorax in a ventral direction at the level of the heart. The catheter is intermittently flushed clear of any blood reflux at 20—30 min intervals via a three-way tap to prevent a loss of pressure amplitude.
In the pressure receiver the DC signal built up by the modulator is increased in proportion to the pressure and modulated to a subcarrier frequency. This frequency in turn modulates the carrier frequency of the transmitter (double frequency modulation). The energy for the patient unit is supplied by rechargeable nickel-cadmium cells. The total weight of the device kept in a carrying bag was approximately 3.5 kg. The stationary receiver unit consisted of a receiver, demodulator, band store, and registration unit and allowed the simultaneous recording and observation of measured values. The range of the transmitter is specified as 200—300 meters in a built-up area. The storage capacities were enough for a continuous measuring period of approximately 10 h. Although there were hardly any complications or restrictions in connection with the named method and the application of a large-caliber femoral catheter — e.g., at different sport activities —

we considered it necessary for the systematic examination of hypertensive patients and the resolution of basic problems (see below) to make a modification to the extent that, instead of a femorally applied Ödman-Ledin catheter, we used a percutaneously (without the Seldinger technique) applied brachial microcatheter. The 120 x 1.2 x 0.8 mm (length, inner and outer diameter) intraarterial indwelling cannula ("Intranüle" — Vyon, Aachen) consists of relatively rigid-walled polypropylene and an enclosed hollow steel needle which facilitates the percutaneous application after local anesthesia in the bend of the elbow. Pressure registration is done after inserting a liquid-filled plastic connective piece in a pressure receiver attached at the upper arm (Statham, P37B). The electric wiring leads from the pressure receiver to the patient-attached modulator including the electrical calibrating equipment and the actual high-frequency transmitter with the flexible antenna. The continuous pressure counter flow system (Fenwal unit) is placed parallel to the wiring system. An automatic reduction valve ("Intraflo", Sorenson, USA) guarantees a constant rinsing capacity of approximately 3 ml/h. The addition of 1000 E Heparin/100 ml rinsing fluid — analogous to Bachmann's procedure — serves as prophylaxis against the thrombosing occlusion of the microcatheter.

Apart from routine electrical calibrations, regular mechanical calibrations are necessary to check the accuracy of the ready-for-use equipment. The physical properties (e.g., inherent frequency and damping factor) should be performed on the ready-for-use equipment with the so-called pressure relief test. With the curves thus obtained we were able to calculate an inherent frequency of approximately 30 Hz and a damping grade of 0.50 for our apparatus, which approximatively reached up to the theoretically calculated values as well as the "ideals" (17). The other characteristics of our patient-sided equipment, like the stationary receiver unit with high-frequency receiver, demodulator, pulse integrator, peak indications for systolic and diastolic pressure (instead of an oscilloscope) and a four-channel thermodirect recorder, as well as a parallel-connected magnetic storage unit, approximately corresponded to those of the equipment used by Bachmann. Depending on the paper feed (or after a possible reproduction from the magnetic band registration) a very strongly compressed or stretched depiction of the curves can be obtained with the corresponding possibility for detail assessment. The evaluation of our measurement data from the compressed curves (at 0.5 mm/paper feed) is done by "geometrical" averaging for a period of one min at certain selected curve sections, and also during tolerance tests from summarized single pressure values.

Almost at the same time as the aforementioned technical developments of blood pressure telemetry according to the method by Bachmann and our modification, von Behr et al. (1969) introduced a microcatheter and pressure recording in the brachial artery which is comparable to our method, as well as an adapation of the Statham element on the upper arm. The results which were presented in the case reports of 10 patients with arterial hypertension or angina pectoris after myocardial infarction showed a considerable variability in blood pressure under everyday conditions (e.g., from 174/81 to approximately 250/150 mmHg during defecation).

Similar results in patients during rehabilitation after myocardial infarction were reported by Kobayashi et al. (15) in 1969. Further possibilities for the application of blood pressure telemetry with intraarterial recording of measurement data result from the anesthesiological monitoring of critically ill patients during surgery and in the perioperative phase (see 13). Irving et al. (12) have shown that blood pressure telemetry is also applicable for the differentiation of patients with borderline hypertension and established hypertension; the pressure is recorded in the radial artery in these examinations. In connection with the methods section special mention should also be made of the indirect, discontinuous long-term blood pressure monitoring with telemetric transmission of the measurement data, as presented by Pircher (29). With an automatic modification of the conventional cuff method, measurements taken at one-minute intervals in combat pilots revealed an enormous individual and intraindividual variability of the systolic and diastolic blood pressure response during different flight phases like start, flight, low-level flight, and landing.

Results

For reasons of clarity, only some of the results reported so far can be presented here as examples of the huge amount of data available in the literature. We will concentrate here on the telemetric blood pressure investigations performed by the Bachmann study group, who investigated the influence of sport activities on blood pressure, and we will present our own results obtained in hypertensives during standardized everyday activities (e.g., walking and climbing stairs) and the effect of antihypertensive drugs.

An interesting finding in this connection is the estimation of the blood pressure effect of various sport activities, which was revealed by Bachmann et al. (4) by interviewing gastroenterologists, general practitioners, and medical students (Fig. 1). All three groups greatly underestimated the blood pressure levels determined by intraarterial measurement and radio-telemetering in normotensives performing dynamic sports (e.g., jogging, swimming). On the basis of a mean resting value of 135/78 mmHg (in a sitting position), jogging led to an increase in blood pressure to 262/100 mmHg, as compared to an estimated blood pressure increase to about 160/90 mmHg. This example makes it clear that the blood pressure effect of everyday sport activities is severely underestimated, and that there is no clear notion of the effect on the cardiovascular system of actual everyday stress in normotensives.

A similar example illustrating the blood pressure effect of sport activities (Fig. 2) was presented by Zerzawy et al. (36), a member of the Bachmann study group. He showed that certain training components that used to be part of the so-called ''Bavarian fitness test'' led to considerable, short-term increases in blood pressure to peak levels of about 250/130 mmHg! The exercise-induced diastolic blood pressure increase thus corresponds to the level of the initial systolic resting value. The activities performed during the strain phases mainly consisted of isometric exercises, which, due to their blood pressure effect, lead to an excessive circulatory strain rather than an improvement of cardiovascular function, which is the aim of dynamic training. It is likely that the considerable increases in systolic and diastolic blood pressure during individual activity phases are, to a large extent, due to forced breathing. A similar phenomenon was observed by Zerzawy (34) in his study of bowlers (Fig. 3), who developed particularly high blood pressure levels when they were in a squatting position for releasing the ball and did not breathe with their mouths open.

Our more systematic studies performed in patients with different degrees of hypertension (17—23), in which we used continuous intraarterial measurements of up to 108 h, confirmed not only the well-known diurnal and circadian blood pressure rhythm but also the considerable blood pressure variability occurring during common everyday activities.

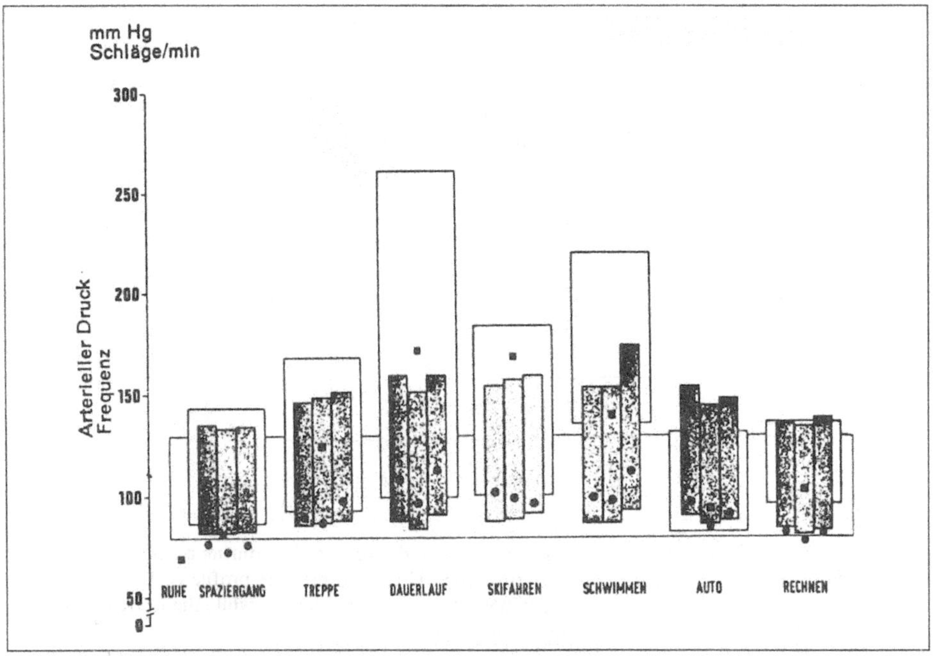

Fig. 1. Diagram of the estimated arterial blood pressure and heart rate in subjects with normal cardiovascular function under different forms of physiological stress, as compared to the values determined by telemetry. Values estimated by gastroenterologists (first dark column), general practitioners (second column), and medical students (third column) on the basis of a resting blood pressure of 130/80 mmHg and a heart rate of 70/min. Light columns represent actual values determined by telemetry; ● = estimated rate, ■ = actual rate (from (4)).

A good example to illustrate this phenomenon is that of a 43-year-old female with essential arterial hypertension (WHO stage II, Fig. 4). In this patient the resting blood pressure determined in a recumbent position was 175/95 mmHg. The simple task of climbing two flights of stairs led to a peak blood pressure level of 239/125 mmHg! Even walking on level ground resulted in a considerable blood pressure increase to 208/115 mmHg. These blood pressure levels correspond to those that occurred in the patient in her daily life (walking about the ward, eating). Overlapping with the pressure during defecation, however, may lead to a far greater, short-term increase in diastolic blood pressure (peak levels of 150 mmHg in this case). The day/night rhythm is preserved in over 90% of the patients with essential arterial hypertension; this was also true in this patient, as can be seen from her sleeping blood pressure of 114/62 mmHg.
A collective observation (Fig. 5) of the largest group of patients with WHO stage II hypertension investigated by our group showed that climbing two stairs increased blood pressure by 37.4 to 46.6/11.4 to 13.6 mmHg (systolic/diastolic). The strain-related hypertensive reaction was stronger at 1200 h and in the evening, at least systolically, than in the morning, a finding that might be explained by a potential role of the 24-h rhythm of the orthostatic posture (2).

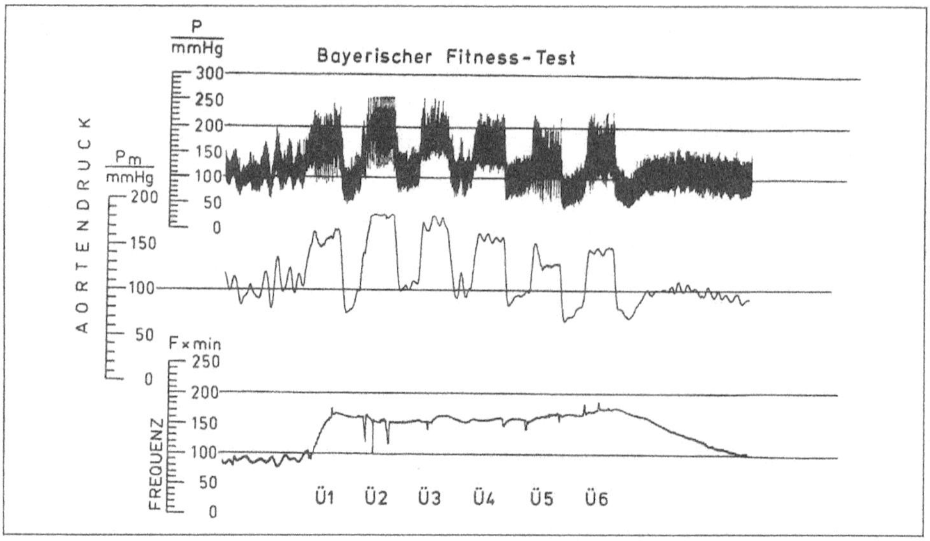

Fig. 2. Example of extreme circulatory strain in a 25-year-old sports student during a fitness test, which could only be demonstrated by blood pressure telemetry. The blood pressure profile is characterized by excessive values ranging between 200 and 250 mmHg during all six exercises, while the heart rate is at a fairly constant level of 155 to 175 beats/min (from (36)).

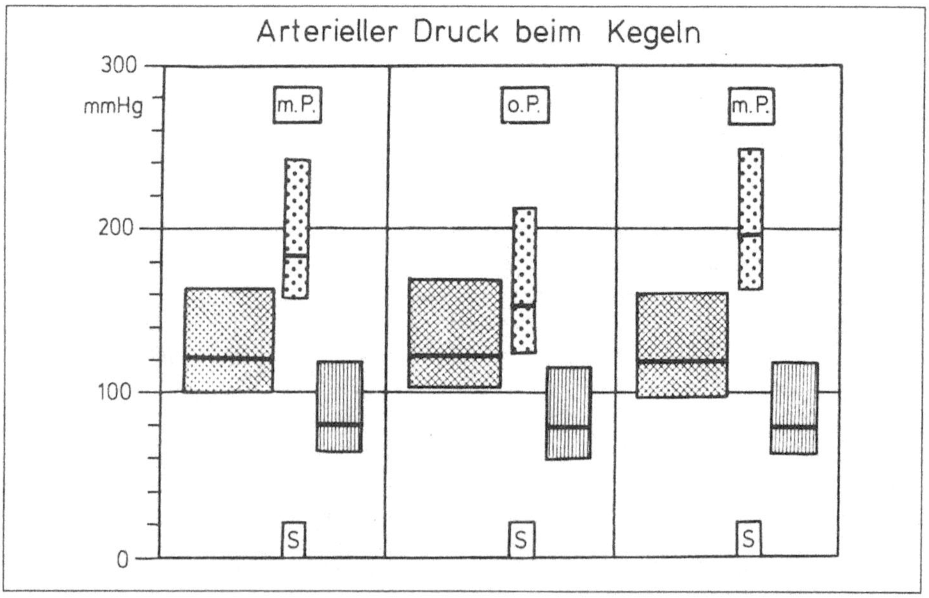

Fig. 3. Results of radiotelemetric measurements in nine normotensive members of a bowling club (ages 31—58 years), demonstrating the influence of forced breathing on blood pressure during bowling. Markedly higher blood pressure increases during phases of forced breathing (m. P.), e. g., when releasing the ball (S), than during a phase of conscious expiration (o. P.). L = run-up, A = straightening up after releasing ball.

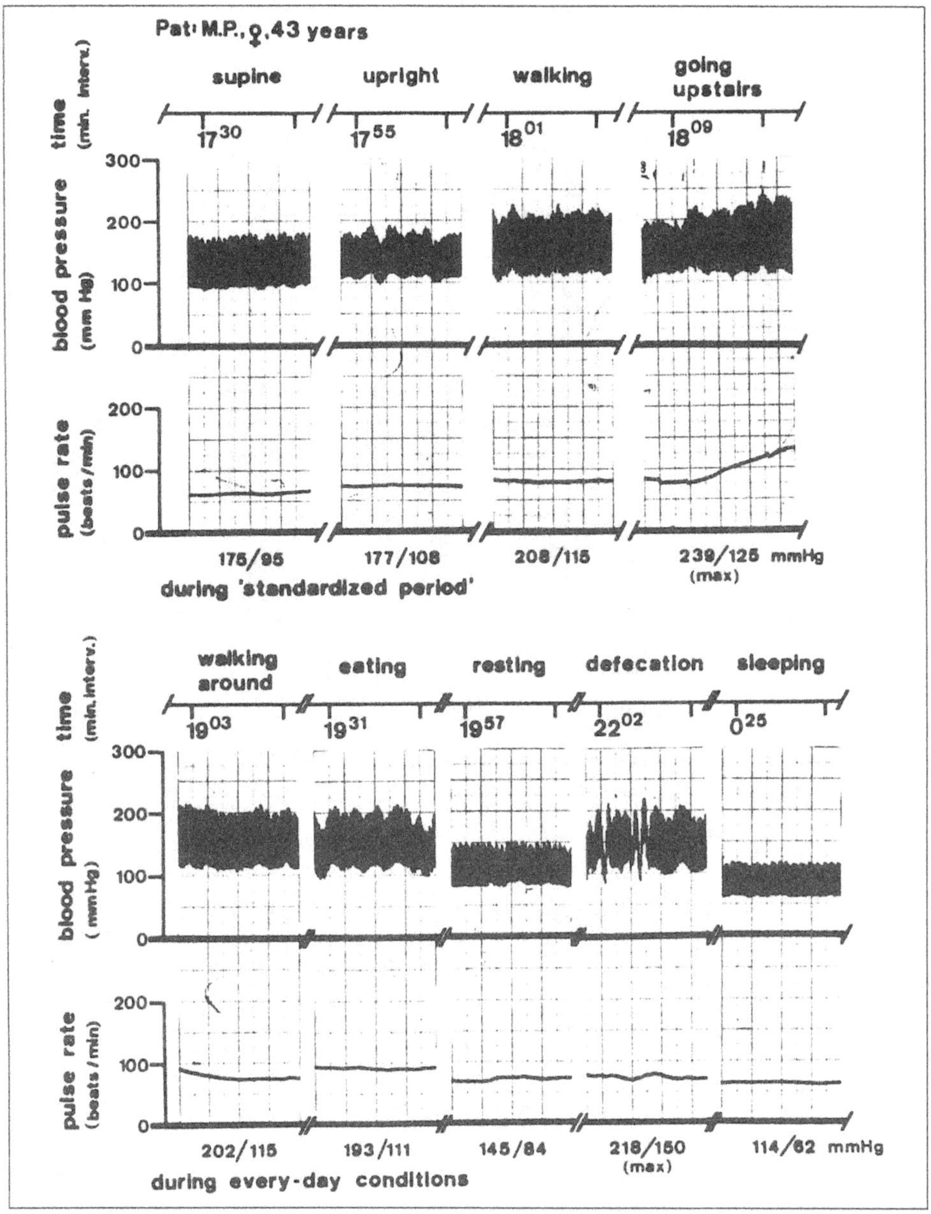

Fig. 4. Curve segments (80—100 s duration) from a long-term telemetric blood pressure reading in a 43-year-old female with essential hypertension, illustrating everyday blood pressure variation (from (17, 19)).

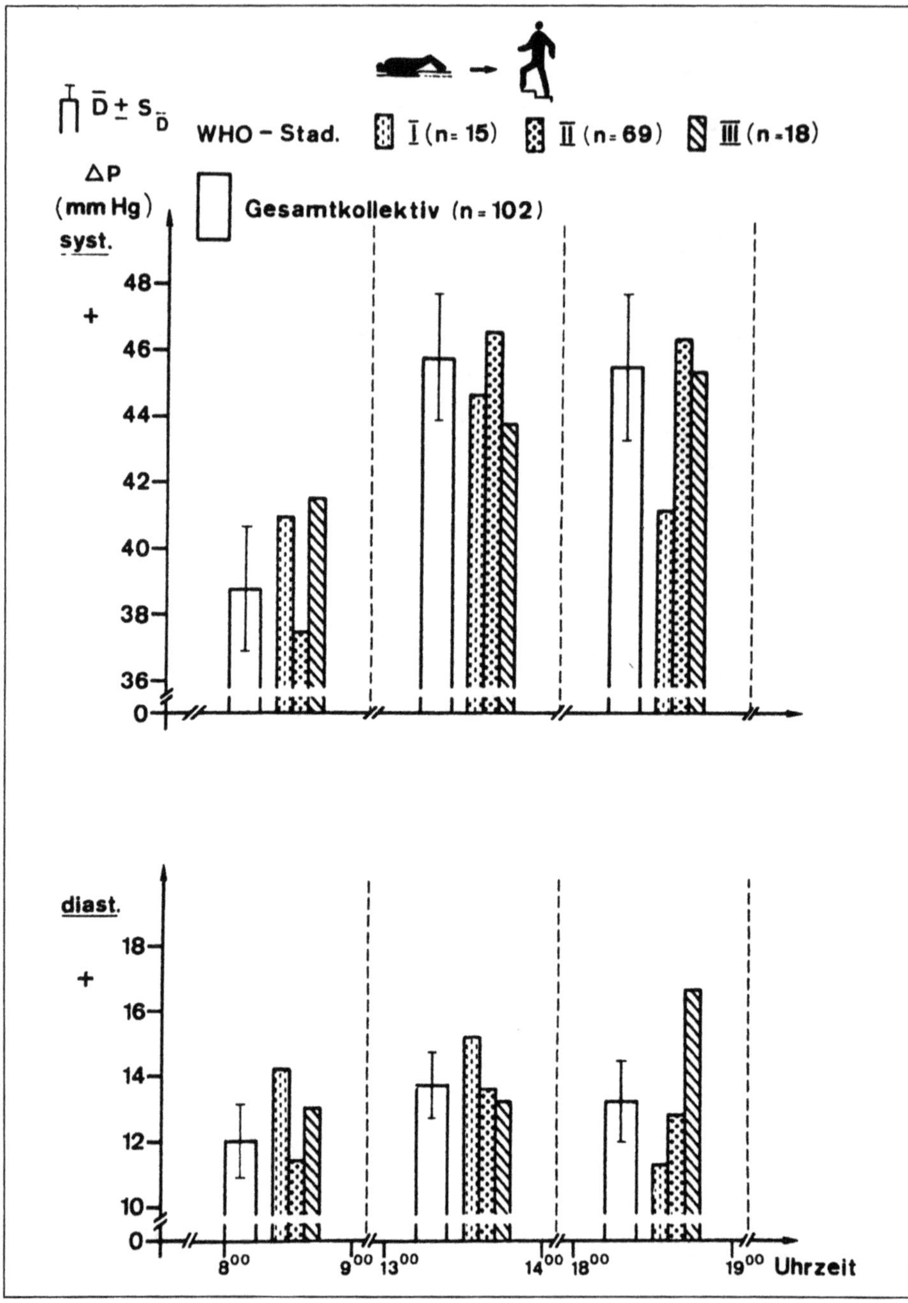

Fig. 5. Mean systolic (above) and diastolic (below) blood pressure differences (mmHg) between blood pressure during climbing several stairs and preceding resting pressure in a recumbent position; depicted separately for different times of measurement and WHO collectives, including the total collective (from (17)).

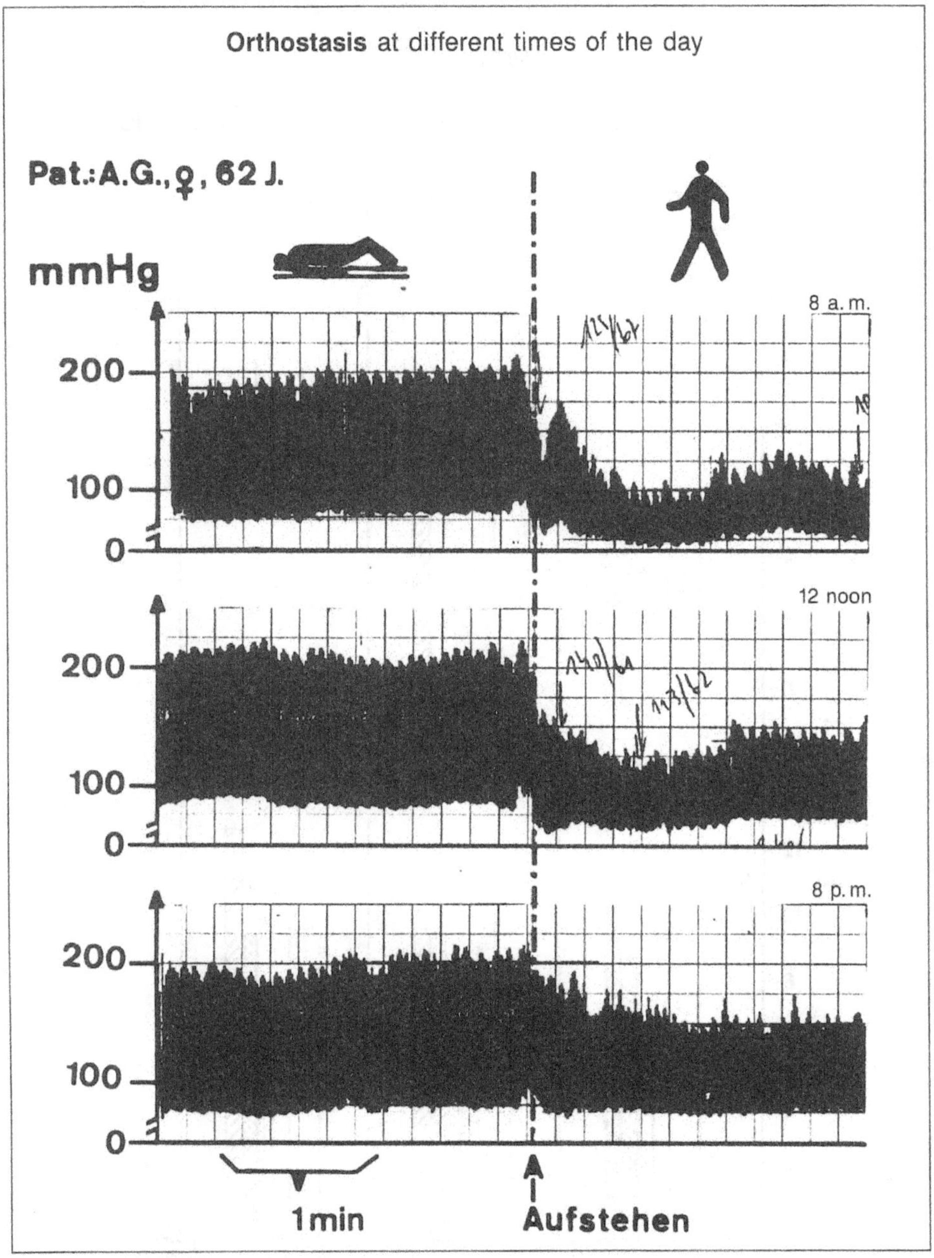

Fig. 6. Curve segment showing the transition from a recumbent position to active orthostasis at different times of day in a 62-year-old female with untreated essential arterial hypertension (WHO stage III). The orthostatic blood pressure decrease spontaneously becomes less pronounced towards evening (from (17)).

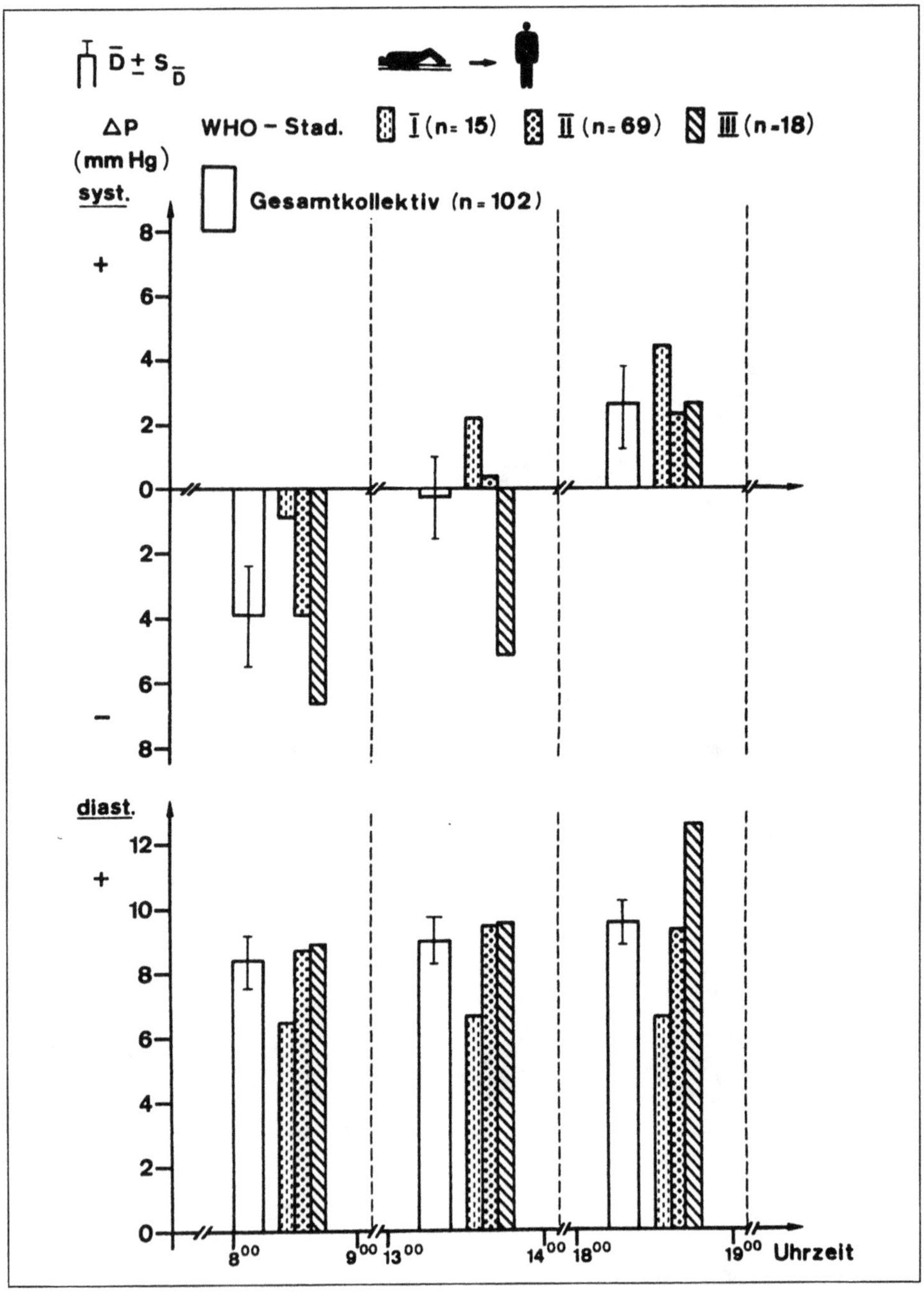

Fig. 7. Differences between resting blood pressure in a recumbent position and that during subsequent active orthostasis. Depicted separately for three different times of day and three WHO collectives. Additional depiction of the blood pressure variability observed in the total group of hypertensives (from (17)).

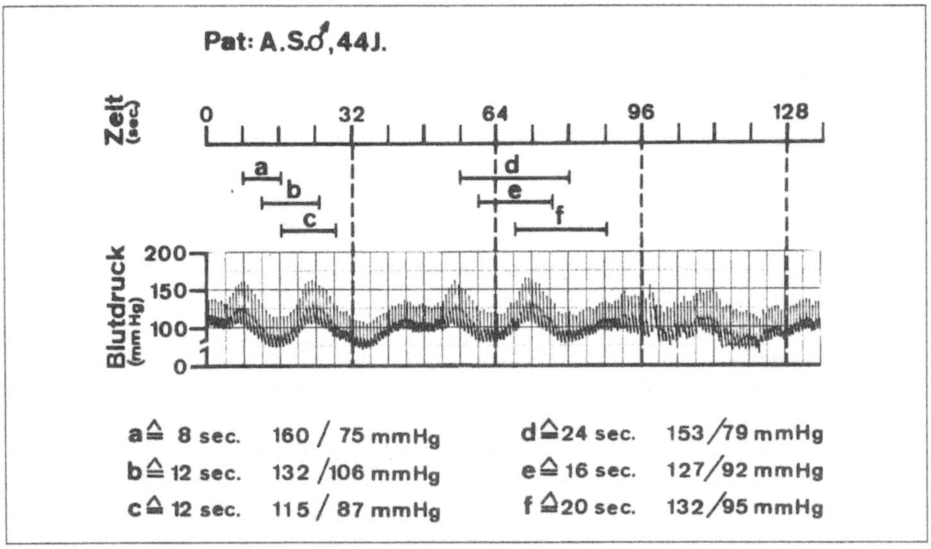

Fig. 8. Curve segment (stretched after magnetic tape reproduction) from a long-term telemetric blood pressure reading in a 44-year-old female with essential arterial hypertension during active orthostasis. Spontaneous short-term blood pressure variability may lead to fairly discrepant values in indirect measurements, depicted by lines a — f, due to the insufficient temporal resolution of the latter method (from (17)).

A good example to demonstrate the diurnal variability of orthostatic hypotension is that of a 62-year-old female (Fig. 6) with essential arterial hypertension: Compared to a fairly constant blood pressure in a recumbent position of approx. 200/80 mmHg, the blood pressure registered during active orthostasis in the morning, at 1200 h, and in the evening was 125/60, 145/65, and 160/75 mmHg, respectively. A similar trend can be observed when the values of all patients are taken together (Fig. 7): At all three WHO stages there was a certain morning decrease in systolic pressure (as compared to the preceding level measured in a recumbent position), which was completely reversed towards evening. The disturbance of orthostatic posture was most pronounced in patients with WHO stage III hypertension (17, 18, 22). Continuous intraarterial monitoring during orthostasis is well-suited for the demonstration of short-term, ''overlapping'' blood pressure variation, which is directly associated with the complex central and peripheral vegetative regulatory processes of the cardiovascular system. Figure 8 shows an example of such short-term, rhythmic blood pressure variation in a 44-year-old patient with essential hypertension (WHO stage I) measured in a standing position. This considerable, short-term blood pressure variation is very difficult to demonstrate by a single indirect measurement, since the latter may yield such diverse values as 115/87 and 160/75 mmHg, depending on the onset and duration of the measurement (cf. Fig. 8). In patients with suspected disturbances of vegetative regulation (e.g., during the labile phase of arterial hypertension), which have also been described by Koepchen (14), it is absolutely necessary to perform multiple standing blood pressure measurements in order to calculate the mean value and thus come close to the actual blood pressure.

Short-term blood pressure variation is also observed during undisturbed nocturnal sleep: Polygraphic monitoring with simultaneous EEG registration (cf. for example (9)) showed that blood pressure increases of approx. 30—40/20—30 mmHg (systolic/diastolic) of about 10—20 s duration occurred during the so-called dream phases of REM sleep.

Apart from systematic studies of the everyday blood pressure behavior in hypertensive patients during different rest and stress phases, microcatheter blood pressure telemetry was also used to investigate a number of additional problems. These investigations revealed that the informational value of the so-called basal blood pressure (1), which is relatively complicated to determine by indirect measurement, is only equivalent to that of the casual blood pressure determined in the morning or evening after 2—3 min in a recumbent position. The same holds true for the so-called relaxation blood pressure according to Meesmann et al. (25). Such special blood pressure values are therefore no longer required for the evaluation of individual blood pressure profiles and can thus be abandoned in favor of a large number of casual blood pressure readings or the results of indirect 24-h recordings. With respect to the age relation of blood pressure reactions to everyday stress (17), it could be shown that the age-related increase in systolic pressure during walking on level ground and climbing two flights of stairs was even more pronounced than originally assumed and that the stress peaks occurring in older subjects are therefore higher than expected on the basis of resting blood pressure measurements (Fig. 9).

In light of the assumption that frequent blood pressure peaks have a prognostically unfavorable influence on the cardiovascular system, the question as to whether these stress peaks can be influenced by adequate drug treatment gains particular importance. It was shown that, in the case of betasympathicolytics (such as metoprolol, Fig. 10) for example, the extent to which the hypertensive reaction was prevented was greater than expected from the resting blood pressure decrease: After a single morning dose of 100 or 200 mg metoprolol, the blood pressure recording phase at noon revealed a recumbent blood pressure decrease of 20.3/13.4 mmHg (syst./diastol.) in 10 hypertensives (WHO stage I and II), while strain pressure during stair climbing was decreased by 37.4/16.8 mmHg. It was thus shown that the blood pressure profile of hypertensives is "smoothed" by betasympathicolytics. One may speculate that betasympathicolytic therapy could also, at least partially, reduce the pronounced early morning blood pressure increase prior to waking up (as compared to the absolute 24-h minimum registered during deep sleep), which has frequently been demonstrated by 24-h recordings. Some results of the MILIS-study (28) seem to support this assumption: It was shown that the early morning peak in the incidence of acute myocardial infarction did not occur in patients treated with betablockers.

Future perspectives

Blood pressure telemetry with intraarterial recording and wireless transmission of the values to a stationary receiver unit makes it possible to analyze blood pressure behavior under everyday conditions by means of short-term measurements (beat-to-beat analysis) or long-term recordings over several days. It is thus possible to obtain basic data on the short-term variability (so-called "blood pressure waves") away from the circulatory laboratory. This method also yielded information on the effect of various forms of psychic

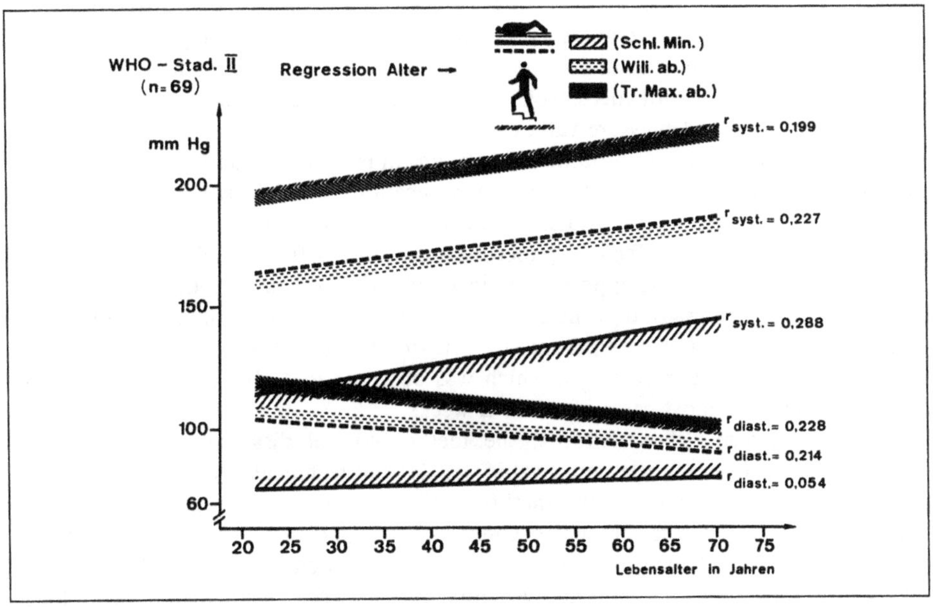

Fig. 9. Correlation between age and different resting blood pressure levels (Schl.Min. and Wili.ab) as well as a stress level occurring when climbing two storeys (Tr.Max.ab) in 69 patients with WHO stage II hypertension (from (17)).

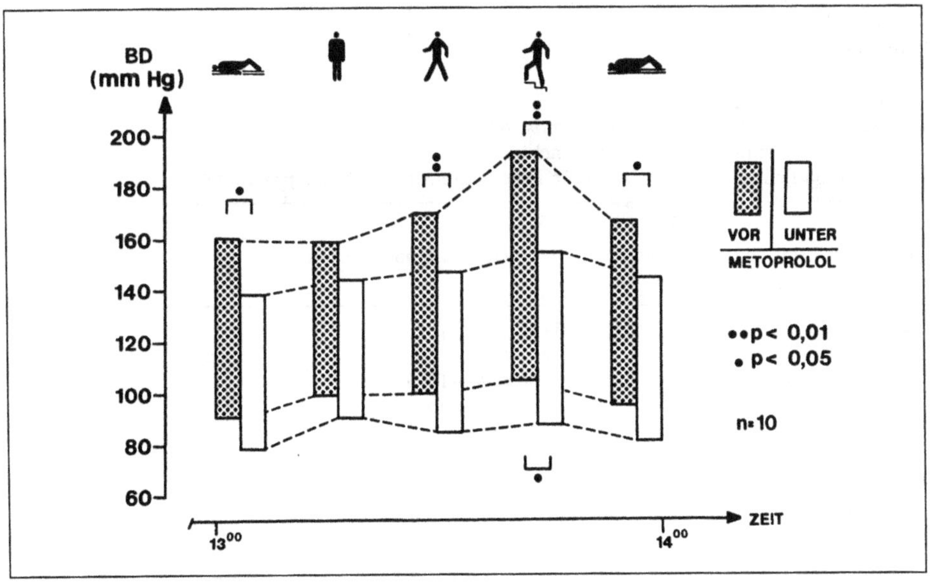

Fig. 10. Varying blood pressure-lowering effects of chronic metoprolol therapy (approx. four h after a single morning dose of 100 or 200 mg). The blood pressure increase induced by everyday actitivies, such as climbing stairs, is inhibited more strongly than expected from the resting blood pressure decrease (from (17, 19)).

and physical stress, as well as changes in body posture, the influence of different sport activities, and especially information on the diurnal and circadian blood pressure rhythm including the behavior during undisturbed sleep. This method also made it possible to study the influence of antihypertensive therapeutic measures in more detail than by analysis of resting blood pressure values alone.

Criticism that the invasive procedure with an indwelling intraarterial cannula is associated with too high a rate of serious complications is not justified: Serious complications were not seen in the studies performed by Bachmann et al., nor in our own investigations. As shown in Table 3, puncture was unsuccessful in 4.1% of our patients and had to be repeated at the opposite arm in 17.2% of the cases. The 4.8% rate of subcutaneous after-bleeding given in the table was primarily due to an initially insufficient manual compression after termination of long-term registration. Neuritic irritation (especially of the nervus medianus), which was observed in 4.1% of the cases, disappeared completely in most cases after 1—2 weeks.

Despite these undisputed advantages, the methodological disadvantages cannot be ignored (Table 2). It is however conceivable that further technical development will improve the practical application of this method in that, for instance, the use of miniaturized catheter tip pressure receivers makes counter-flow superfluous, that miniaturization of the patient-attached modulator/transmitter unit considerably reduces the size and weight of the apparatus, and that improvements in the area of high-frequency technology enlarge the range of the signal. The advances made in the analysis of data recorded on magnetic tapes have been recognized for years, as will be shown in the following chapter which presents the studies performed by Raftery.

Table 2. Methodological disadvantages of (micro-)catheter blood pressure telemetry.

Blood pressure telemetry
— invasive procedure
— extensive procedure
— spatial limitation (action radius of approx. 600 m)
— expensive and requires a lot of personnel
— application limited to specific scientific investigations (no „routine procedure“)

Table 3. Problems and complications in 414 telemetric blood pressure measurements using the microcatheter method (according to (17)).

Blood pressure telemetry using a microcatheter		
Study period:	1971—1975	
Duration of measurement:	approx. 4—108 h	
Total number:	414 examinations	
	n	%
— puncture unsuccessful	17	4.1
— puncture of contralateral arm	71	17.2
— discontinuation		
— apparatus-related	19	3.6
— subject-related	6	1.5
— complications		
— subcutaneous after-bleeding	20	4.8
— thrombophlebitis	2	0.5
— neuritic irritation	17	4.1

Conclusion

1. Previous findings on blood pressure variation, which were obtained by careful indirect measurements and showed that this variation was more pronounced in hypertensives, led to the introduction of blood pressure telemetry in the late 1960s and early 1970s. Apart from individual studies in which the cuff method was used for indirect measurement, pressure was recorded by an intraarterial catheter (a. femoralis, a. brachialis, a. radialis). The patient-sided technical equipment of the system comprised the pressure-recorder, which had to be placed approximately at heart level, and a still fairly unwieldy modulator and transmitter unit, which transmitted the pressure values to a stationary receiver unit by so-called double frequency modulation.
2. Blood pressure telemetry permits continuous intraarterial long-term blood pressure monitoring in subjects moving about freely with simultaneous observability of the values. Blood pressure reactions to everyday psychic and physical stress and the effects of sport activities, as well as questions concerning circadian and diurnal blood pressure rhythm can thus be studied in detail.
3. Serious complications or permanent damage did not occur in any of the over 1000 examinations reported in the literature.
4. Disadvantages are the technically complex system, the invasive procedure, and the low range of the high-frequency signal, which limits the subject's movement radius (this can possibly be improved by further technical developments).
5. Direct long-term recording with patient-sided tape recording (Oxford-Medilog system) has proved to be an effective alternative to blood pressure telemetry. The results of blood pressure telemetry promoted the application of indirect 24-h blood pressure recording, which has meanwhile become an almost routine procedure.

References

1. Alam GM, Smirk FH (1943) Casual and Basal Blood Pressures. II. In Essential Hypertension. Brit Heart J 5: 156
2. Aschoff J, Aschoff J (1969) Tagesperiodik der orthostatischen Kreislaufreaktion. Pflügers Arch 306: 146
3. Bachmann K, Thebis J, Heynen HP, Graf N (1967) Die drahtlose Blutdruckregistrierung unter physiologischen Belastungen. Verh dtsch Ges Kreisl-Forsch 33: 185
4. Bachmann K, Zerzawy R, Riess PJ, Zölch KA (1970) Blutdrucktelemetrie — kontinuierliche, direkte Blutdruckmessungen im Alltag und beim Sport. Dtsch med Wschr 95: 741
5. von Basch S (1881) Über die Messung des Blutdruckes beim Menschen. Z klin Med 2: 1
6. Behr K, Duner H, Malmström G (1969) Intraarteriellt blodtryck. Kontinuerlig registrering med telemetrisk Dataöverföring. Nordisk Medicin 82: 1014
7. Bock KD, Kreuzenbeck W (1965) Über die Tagesschwankungen des arteriellen Blutdrucks. In: Heilmeyer L, Holtmeier HJ (Hrsg) Hochdruckforschung. Thieme, Stuttgart, S 72
8. Brash HM, Irving JB, Kirby, BJ, and Donald KW (1976) Transmitter for radiotelemetry of intra-arterial pressure in man. Med Biol. Engineer 14: 61
9. Coccagna G, Mantovani M, Brignani F, Manzini A, Lugares E (1971) Arterial Pressure Changes during Spontaneous Sleep in Man. Electroenceph clin Neurophysiol 31: 277
10. Dufey K, Krönig B, Fries G, Gunkel R, Walter U, Wolff HP (1975) Beeinflussung des Blutdruckprofils Hochdruckkranker durch Prindolol unter besonderer Berücksichtigung der Belastungsreaktion und der Plasmareninaktivität. Dtsch med Wschr 100: 1726

11. Dufey K, Krönig B, Wolff HP (1975) Effekt von Minoxidil auf Ruhe- und Belastungsdrucke bei schweren arteriellen Hypertonien. Ergebnisse telemetrischer intraarterieller Langzeitmessungen. Verh dtsch Ges inn Med 81: 1047
12. Irving JB, Brash HM, Kerr, Kriby BJ (1976) The Value of ambulatory monitoring in borderline and established hypertension. Postgrad Med J 52: (Suppl 7), 137
13. Klein FF, Davis DA (1976) A 4-Channel Telemetry System for Hospital Patient Monitoring. Biotelemetry 3: 98
14. Koepchen HP (1962) Die Blutdruckrhythmik. Steinkopff, Darmstadt
15. Kobayashi T, Takenchi M, Koro T, Tawara T (1969) Radio-telemetering of electrocardiogram and blood pressure. Mal cardiovasc 10: 129
16. Korotkow NS (1905) K voprosu o metodakh issledonaiya krovianogo davleniya. Izv Voen-med Akad 11: 365
17. Krönig B (1976) Blutdruckvariabilität bei Hochdruckkranken — Ergebnisse telemetrischer Langzeitmessungen. Hüthig, Heidelberg
18. Krönig B (1981) Telemetrische Untersuchungen zum Ausmaß des Belastungsblutdrucks unbehandelter und behandelter Hochdruckkranker: In Franz IW (eds): Belastungsblutdruck bei Hochdruckkranken. Ausmaß, Bedeutung und Konsequenz für die Praxis, p 125—138. Springer, Berlin-Heidelberg-New York
19. Krönig B (1984) Blutdruckvariabilität bei Hochdruckkranken. I. Ausmaß unter Ruhebedingungen. II. Praktische Konsequenzen, prognostische Bedeutung und therapeutische Aspekte. Therapiewoche 34: 5947—72
20. Krönig B, Dufey K, Moergel K, Michaelis J, Jahnecke J (1974) Telemetrische Untersuchungen zur Wertigkeit eines Basalblutdruckes bei Hochdruckkranken. Klin Wschr 52: 3054
21. Krönig B, Dufey K, Reinhardt P, Jahnecke J, Wolff HP (1974) Long term telemetry of direct arterial blood pressure in unrestricted hypertensives. Biotelemetry 1: 117
22. Krönig B, Knappen F (1977) Spezielle Aspekte der Blutdruckvariabilität Hochdruckkranker. Herz/Kreisl 9: 499
23. Krönig B, Knappen F, Dufey K, Wolff HP (1976) Blood pressure response to physical activity in hypertensive subjects at different times of the day. Clin Sci Molec Med 51: 6775
24. Krönig B, Parade D, Schwarz W, Witzel U, Klemeit R, Jahnecke J, Wolff HP (1972) Blutdrucktelemetrie beim Menschen mit der Mikrokathetermethode. Klin Wschr 50: 898
25. Meesmann W, Stöveken HJ, Billing CP (1970) Die Bestimmung des Basisblutdruckes in der Praxis durch die Ermittlung des sogenannten Entspannungswertes. Dtsch med Wschr 95: 734
26. Menzel W (1941) I. der 24-Stunden-Rhythmus des menschlichen Blutkreislaufes. Ergebn inn Med Kinderheilk 61: 1
27. Müller C (1921) Die Messung des Blutdrucks am Schlafenden als klinische Methode speziell bei der gutartigen (primären) Hypertonie und der Glomerulonephritis. I. und II. Acta med scand 55: 381
28. Muller JE et al./Milis Study Group (1985) Circadian Variation in the frequency of onset of acute myocardial infarction. N Engl J Med 313: 1315
29. Pircher L (1972) Belastung des Kreislaufs beim Fliegen von Kampfflugzeugen. Schweiz med Wschr 102: 444
30. Recklinghausen H von (1901) Über Blutdruckmessung beim Menschen. Arch exp Path Pharm 46: 78
31. Richardson DW, Honour AJ, Fenton GW, Stott FH, Pickering GW (1964) Variation in Arterial Pressure throughout the Day and Night. Clin Sci 26: 445
32. Riva-Rocci S (1896) Un nuova sfigmomanometro. Gazz med Torino 47: 981
33. Shaw DB, Knapp MS, Davies DH (1963) Variations of Blood Pressure in Hypertensives during Sleep. Lancet 1963/I: 797
34. Zerzawy R (1984) Wertigkeit unterschiedlicher Belastungsformen für den Hochdruckpatienten. In: Holzgreve H und Rost R (eds): Aktuelles und Kontroverses aus der Hochdruckforschung. MMV München, S. 141
35. Zerzawy R, Bachmann K (1970) Anwendung neuer Halbleiterbauelemente für die Signalübertragung in der Blutdrucktelemetrie. In: Demling L und Bachmann K (eds.) Biotelemetry. Thieme, Stuttgart, S. 202
36. Zerzawy R, Bachmann K (1979) Telemetrie von arteriellem Druck und Herzfrequenz unter alltäglichen und sportlichen Belastungen im Vergleich zur Fahrradergometrie. Z Kardiol 9: 617
37. Zerzawy R, Bachmann K, Hennig A (1971) Technik und Anwendung einer neuen Vierkanal-Telemetrieanlage. Z Kreisl-Forsch 60: 162

The direct intra-arterial method for ambulatory blood pressure recording: present status and future applications

E.B. Raftery

Northwick Park Hospital and Clinical Research Centre Watford Road
Harrow, Middlesex, UK

Introduction

The indirect method for blood pressure recording devised by Riva-Rocci has not changed substantially since the first description. The technique is known to be inaccurate and slow-moving, and there are no satisfactory explanations for most of the observed and measured inaccuracies (6, 14). In contrast, the direct methods for measuring blood pressure have steadily increased in accuracy and sophistication, and it is recognised that these techniques are precise and rapid-moving. The direct techniques are the only available methods for accurate recording of blood pressure, and the Oxford technique developed by Scott and his colleagues (1) in the laboratories of Sir Georg Pickering is of particular importance because it remains the only way of obtaining accurate information on blood pressure variability in the ambulant individual subject. The technique has been shown to be safe (10), but it is invasive and this factor limits its application to a few centers engaged in research with the resources to ensure continued safety.
However, there can be no doubt that the Oxford technique has made an important and highly significant contribution to our understanding of blood pressure and its variation both in normal and hypertensive subjects. Many descriptive studies have demonstrated the way in which blood pressure responds to the activities of daily life (7, 20), but the most significant observations have stemmed from the application of statistical methods to the plethora of data yielded by the technique.

Circadian variation of blood pressure

Application of the technique of coherent averaging to long-term recordings of intra-arterial blood pressure have confirmed the presence of a long-suspected circadian rhythm (12) with the highest readings in the morning and the lowest at night (Fig. 1). This rhythm has been shown to be highly reproducible in groups of subjects both in the short- and long-term (5, 15) and that it is not affected by the administration of placebo (Figs. 2 and 3) (9). Crucial to this description is the rise in pressure between the nadir at 0300 hours. and the hour of awakening; regrouping the data around the hour of awakening has confirmed that this rise is a true event and is distinct from the behavior of heart rate, which continues to fall until the hour of awakening (Fig. 4). Further observations have confirmed that the circadian rhythm is not due to a simple alternation of activity and inactivity (8) and recordings in patients with fixed-rate pacemakers have confirmed the divergence of behaviour between blood pressure and heart rate (4). These observations

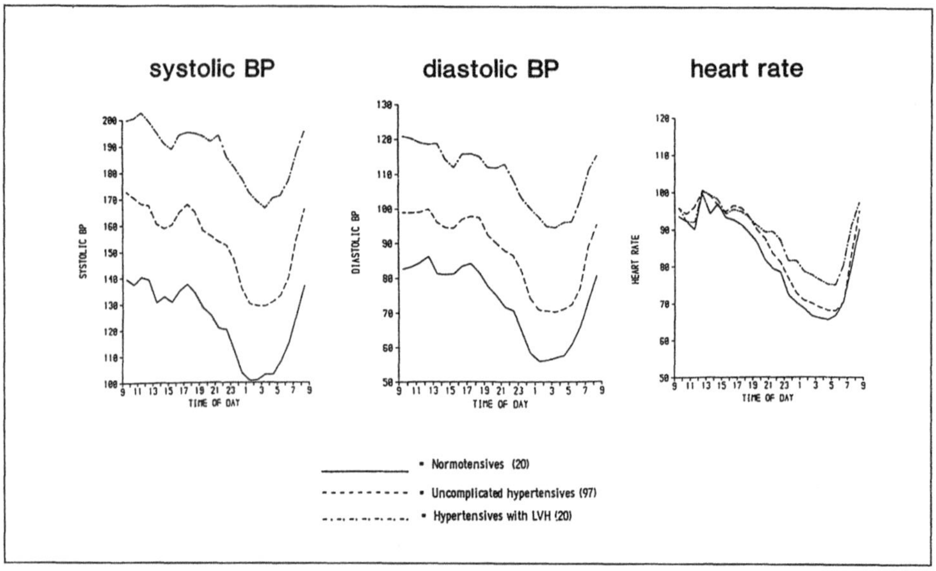

Fig. 1. Circadian variation of blood pressure and heart rate in normotensive and hypertensive subjects, displayed by the technique of coherent averaging of hourly means. Note the two peaks of blood pressure and the rise of blood pressure and the rise before the hour of awakening. By way of contrast, heart rate peaks once, at a different time, and does not change until the time of awakening.

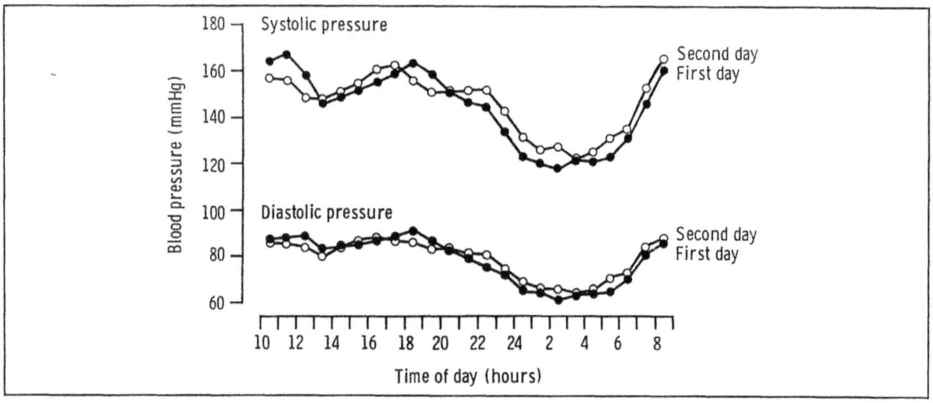

Fig. 2. Comparison of the circadian blood pressure curves in a group of patients in whom a full 48-h of recording was available. Note the marked similarity of the curves for the first and secound 24-h periods.

fit well with other evidence of increased sympathetic activity during the morning (19) and have focussed attention upon the possibility that blood pressure may be reflecting a series of physiological events which might be responsible for the increased incidence of stroke (2) and myocardial infarction (13) at this time of day.

Further support is added by the finding that central (9) and peripheral sympathetic denervation produces a reversal of this rhythm, with highest pressures during the night and lowest during the day (Fig. 5). This suggests that the circadian rhythm is imposed by the

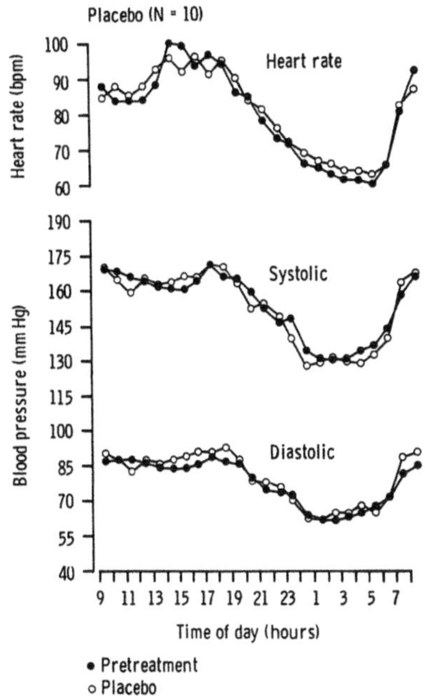

Fig. 3. Comparison of circadian blood pressure curves before and after 6 weeks of placebo administration. This demonstrated the long-term repeatability of the curves and the lack of placebo effect.

sympathetic nervous system, and the finding of a similar reversal in patients after heart transplant raises the interesting possibility that the stimulus for this sympathetic activity may originate in the heart itself.

More sophisticated analyses (17) of 24-h ambulatory intra-arterial recordings have shown that four basic rhythms can be defined (Fig. 6):

1. The 24-h circadian rhythm
2. Slow base-line fluctuations
3. Rapid transients
4. Cyclic variations due to respiration and baro-receptor activity.

The physiological significance of these rhythms and the role they play in the pathogenesis of cardiovascular disease remains to be defined.

Which blood pressure?

For the practising clinician, the question of prognosis still remains the most important issue in deciding the correct management for an individual patient. Blood pressure is a powerful and independent predictor for cardiovascular disease, but there are indications that the number and the timing of recordings may increase predictive accuracy. A recent study (11) of the predictive accuracy of casual and 24-h intra-arterial blood pressure recordings for target organ damage and cardiovascular events over a one-year period has confirmed the power of casual blood pressure readings, but has also shown that the 24-h

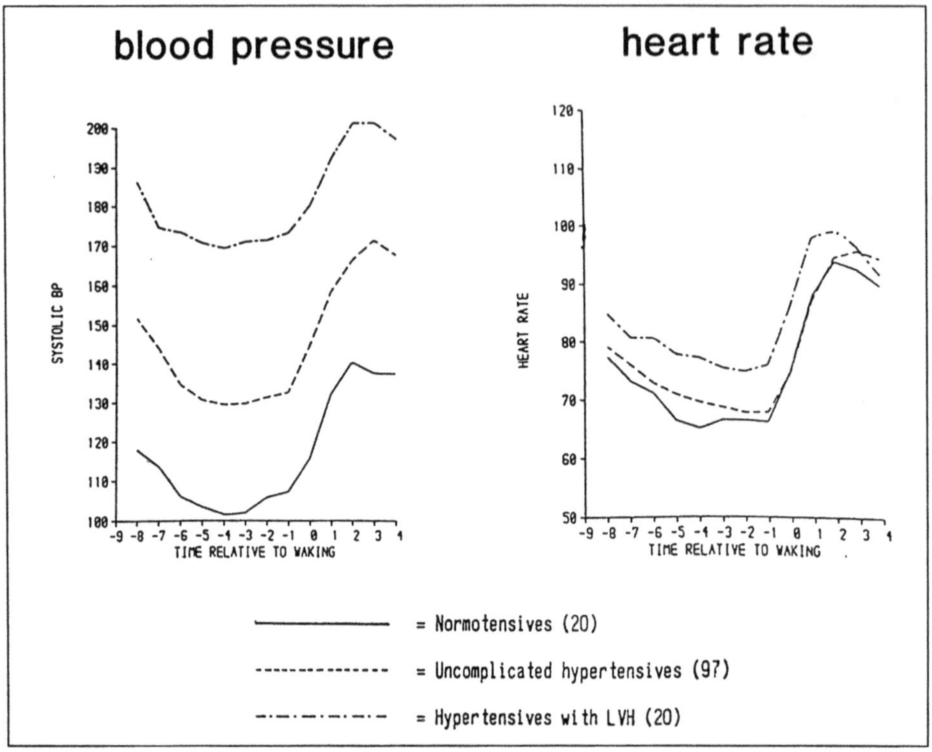

Fig. 4. The same data as in Fig. 1 orientated around the hour of awakening (0). Note that the rise of pressure is still present, but heart rate does not begin to change until the hour of awakening.

mean blood pressure increases this power dramatically (Fig. 7). The most interesting part of this study is the suggestion that the 24-h mean is a better predictor of developing morbid events than the casual pressure. Breakdown of the 24-h cycle into four 6-h periods has shown that most of this predictive power resides in the mean pressures between 0000 and 0600 hours and 0600 and 1200 hours. This data supports the work of Smirk (18) in stressing the importance of nocturnal blood pressure and must provide a powerful stimulus to the efforts to produce a method of accurately recording blood pressure at this time of day. This study is too small to be considered as anything but a "pilot" but the findings are powerful enough to provoke a bigger and more intensive investigation, which has now been mounted.

Ischemic heart disease

The technique of direct recording of ambulatory blood pressure has also been applied to studying the mechanisms of angina and silent myocardial ischemia (3). A system for accurate simultaneous recording of the ST-segment of the electrocardiogram and systemic blood pressure on the same recorder has been devised and used to record the hemodynamic changes during exercise-induced and "spontaneous" ischemic episodes in

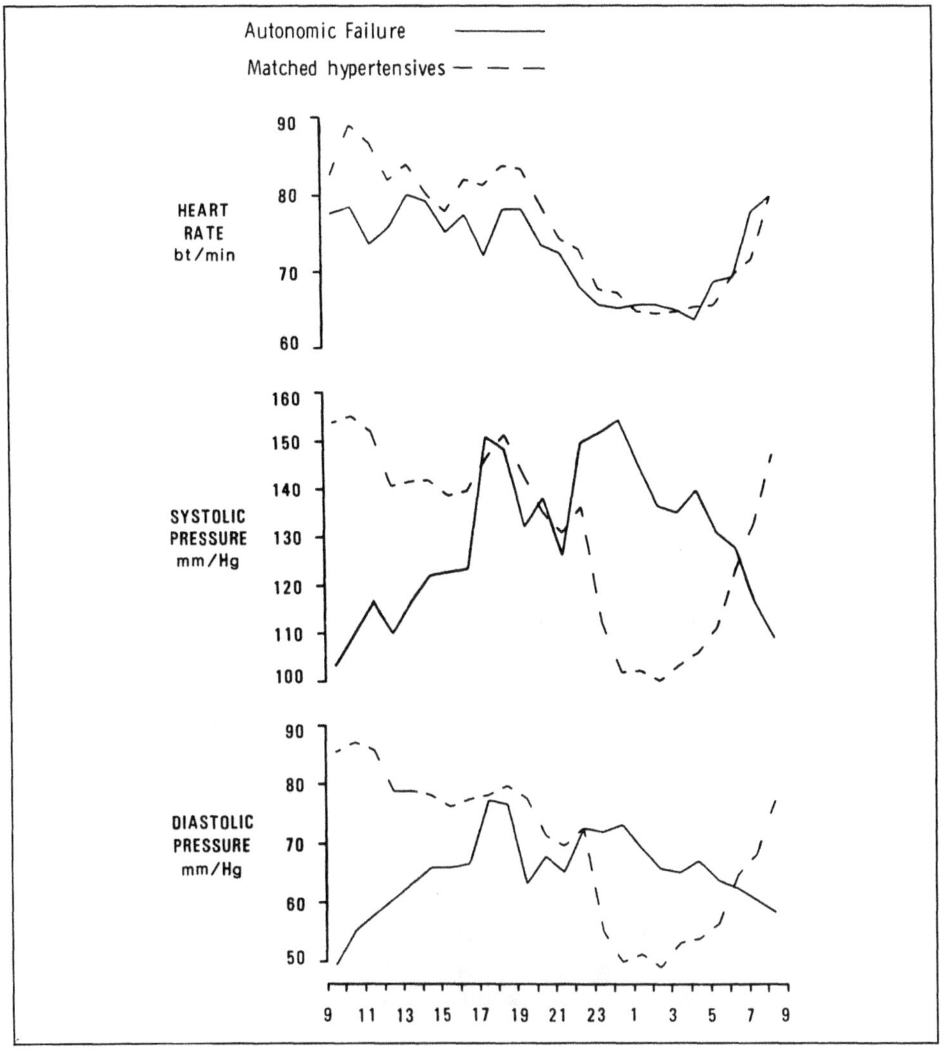

Fig. 5. The circadian rhythm in a group of patients with Shy-Drager Syndrome (central automatic denervation), compared with an age-and sex-matched group of hypertensive subjects. Note the complete inversion of the rhythm.

patients with obstructive coronary artery disease. This study has clearly shown that the development of ischemia in the two situations is very different (Figs. 8 and 9). During exercise-induced angina, ST-segment depression does not occur until significant changes in heart rate, blood pressure, and the "double product" are well established. During "spontaneous" angina, none of these changes occur until after the ST-segment has become depressed. Furthermore, the peak double-product during "spontaneous" angina is lower than during exercise-induced angina, and there are no significant differences between silent and painful episodes of ST-segment depression.

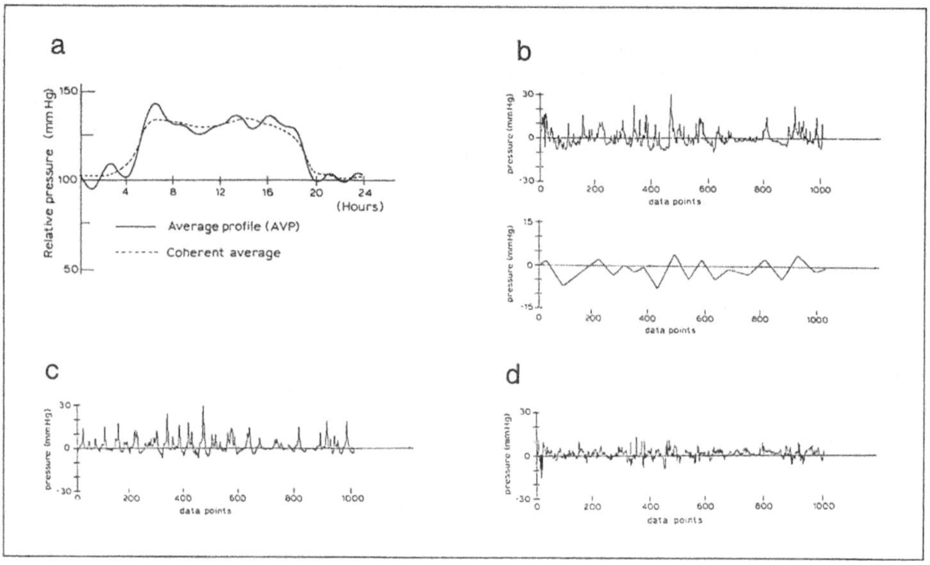

Fig. 6. The four basic rhythms of blood pressure which have been described: (a) Circadian; (b) slow baseline drift; (c) rapid transients; (d) vasomotor components.

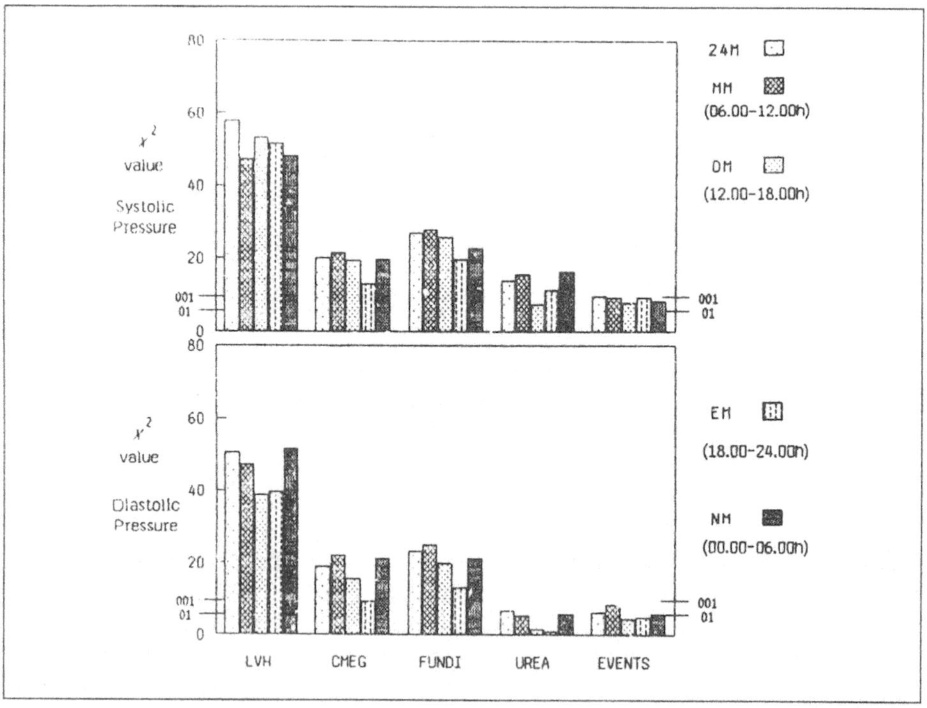

Fig. 7. The predictive value of the casual and 24-h intra-arterial blood pressure for target organ damage and morbid events. Note the power of the casual blood pressure, but the much greater power of the intra-arterial 24-h mean pressure.

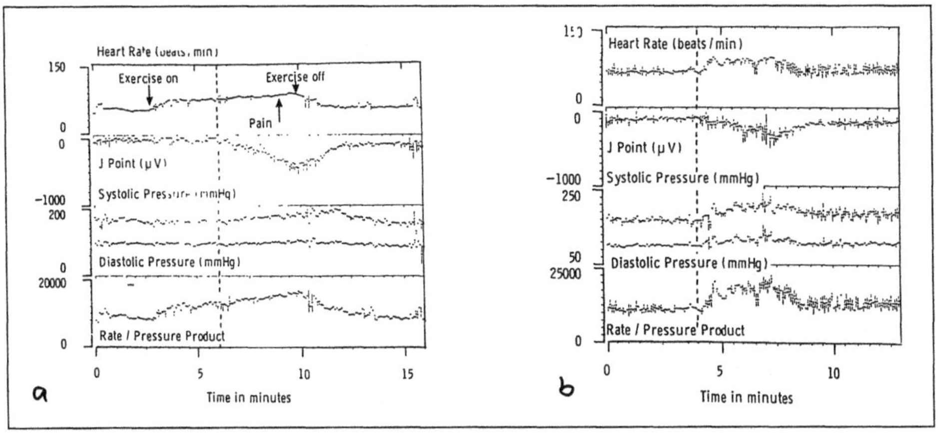

Fig. 8. Trends of blood pressure, heart rate, ST-segment and double product during exercise-induced and "spontaneous" angina. Note that all the hemodynamic changes start after the onset of ST depression in "spontaneous" angina.

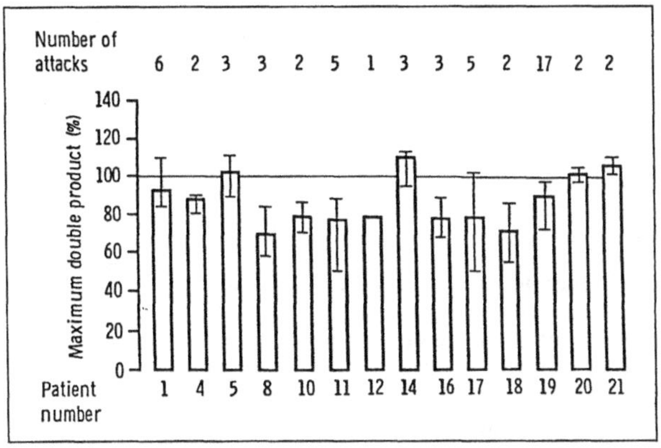

Fig. 9. Maximal double product during "spontaneous" angina expressed as a proportion of the double product during exercise-induced angina. The "spontaneous" double product is usually less than the exercise induced value.

All of which indicates that the classical "supply-and-demand" theory of obstructive coronary heart disease does not tell the whole story. Other mechanisms such as coronary spasm must also be at work, and these are bound to have important therapeutic implications for the management of ischemic heart disease.

Heart failure

Similar studies of ambulatory blood pressure in patients with documented chronic heart failure due to ischemic heart disease have clearly shown that the nocturnal fall in blood pressure is abolished. Coherent averaging reveals a remarkably flat 24-h cycle with little variation in blood pressure or heart rate. Furthermore, there is a significant relationship between the degree of myocardial damage, as measured by the resting ejection fraction and pulmonary capillary wedge pressure, and all the indices of blood pressure variability which have been devised todate (unpublished data). These findings lend strong support to the concept of the heart as a powerful central organ with a significant part to play in the regulation of the circulation. Recent attention to the endocrine function of the heart (20) points in the same direction.

Conclusions

The Oxford technique for ambulatory intra-arterial blood pressure recording has been successfully applied to normal and hypertensive subjects to describe the circadian rhythm of blood pressure and the changes produced by disease states. Long-term studies are emphasising the importance of nocturnal and morning blood pressure in the pathogenesis of cardiovascular disease states. The technique has also been applied to studies of angina and silent myocardial ischemia which have highlighted the differences between ischemia induced by exercise and that which occurs "spontaneously" in a natural environment. Studies in heart failure have provided evidence which points to the heart as a central regulating organ in the circulation and not just a pump which responds to outside controlling influences. Despite the considerable contribution which the direct technique has made, it remains a research tool for application in only a few centers and strictly controlled conditions. The search for an equally accurate indirect method has not been very fruitful, but must go on since the need for such a technique is self-evident.

References

1. Bevan AT, Honour AJ, Scott FH (1969) Direct arterial pressure recording in unrestricted man. Clin Sci 36: 329—344
2. Bock KD, Kreuzenbeck W (1966) Spontaneous blood pressure variations in hypertension: the effect of anti-hypertensive therapy and correlations with the incidence of complications. In: Gross F (ed) Antihypertensive therapy. Principles and Practice. Springer, Berlin Heidelberg, pp 224—228
3. Davies AB, Bala Subramanian V, Cashman PMM, Raftery EB (1983) Simultaneous recording of continuous arterial pressure, heart rate, and ST segment in ambulant patients with stable angina pectoris. Br Heart J 50: 85—91
4. Davies AB, Gould BA, Cashman PMM, Raftery EB (1984) Circadian rhythm of blood pressure in patients dependent on ventricular demand pacemakers. Br Heart J 52: 93—98
5. Gould BA, Mann S, Davies AB, Altman DG, Raftery EB (1981) Does Placebo Lower blood Pressure? Lancet II: 1377—1381
6. Gould BA (1982) An evaluation of indirect methods of ambulatory blood pressure recording. MD Thesis, University of London, pp 54—55
7. Littler WA, Honour AJ, Sleight P (1974) Direct arterial pressure, pulse rate, and electrocardiogram during micturation and defaecation in unrestricted man. Am Heart J 88: 205—210
8. Mann S, Millar Craig MW, Melville D, Bala Subramanian V, Raftery EB (1979) Physical activity and the circadian rhythm of blood pressure. Clin Sci 57 (Suppl 5): 375a—377s
9. Mann S, Altman D, Raftery EB, Bannister R (1983) Circadian variation of blood pressure in autonomic failure. Circulation 68: 477—483
10. Mann S, Jones RI, Millar Craig MW, Wood C, Gould BA, Raftery EB (1984) The Safety of Ambulatory intra-arterial Pressure Monitoring: A Clinical Audit of 1000 Studies. Int J Cardiol 5: 585—597
11. Mann S, Millar Craig MW, Raftery EB (1985) Superiority of 24-hour-measurement of blood pressure over clinic values in determining prognosis in hypertension. Clin Exp Hypertens 7: 279—281
12. Millar Craig MW, Bishop CN, Raftery EB (1978) Circadian variation of blood pressure. Lancet I: 795—797

13. Myers A, Dewar HA (1975) Circumstances attending 100 sudden deaths from coronary artery disease with Coroners Necropsies. Br Heart J 37: 1133—1143
14 Raftery EB, Ward AP (1968) The Indirect Method of Recording Blood Pressure. Cardiovasc Res 2: 210—281
15. Raftery EB, Millar Craig MW (1979) Blood Pressure Variation: Information derived from direct 24-hour Recordings. Proceedings International Conference on Blood Pressure Variation. University of Ghent. MTP Press, Lancaster, UK, pp 53—65
16. Rudolf EL, Unger T, Ganten D (1987) Atrial Natriuretic Peptide: a New Factor in Blood Pressure control. Hypertension 5: 255—272
17. Sayers B McA, Cicchiello LR, Raftery EB, Mann S, Green H (1982) The assessment of continuous ambulatory blood pressure records. Med Inform 7: 93—108
18. Smirk FH (1964) Observations on the mortality of 270 treated and 199 untreated grade 1 and 2 hypertensive patients followed in all instances for 5 years. N Z Med J 63: 413—443
19 Turton MB, Deegan T (1974) Circadian variations of plasma catecholamines, cortisol and imunoreactive insulin concentrations in supine subjects. Clin Chim Acta 55: 389—397
20. Wertheimer L, Bandul I, Amarsinghe S (1977) Blood Pressure in normal subjects. Proceedings Second International Symposium on Ambulatory Monitoring. Academic Press, London, pp 143—148

Non-invasive ambulatory blood pressure recording

U. Scherrer, B. Waeber, J. Nussberger, H.R. Brunner

Division d'Hypertension, Centre Hospitalier Universitaire Vaudois, Lausanne, Switzerland

Introduction

Arterial hypertension is still a major public health problem. The disorder affects about 10% to 15% of the population in industrialized countries and represents one of the main risk factors for the development of cardiovascular complications. The diagnosis of arterial hypertension is usually established on the basis of repeated blood pressure measurements at the doctor's office (1). Unfortunately, the blood pressure levels thus registered do not always reflect the levels prevailing during the patient's daily routine outside the medical environment. In addition, the level above which blood pressure values have to be considered elevated is arbitrary, and, from an epidemiological point of view, there is no clearcut differentiation between normotension and hypertension. These problems involved in the registration of actual blood pressure values and in the clear definition of hypertension explain the difficulties encountered in making a therapeutic decision in individual patients (2).

Today, non-invasive ambulatory blood pressure recording permits us to recognize those patients who will very probably profit from antihypertensive treatment. The aim of the present study is to assess the clinical value of this method in the diagnosis and treatment of hypertension.

Ambulatory blood pressure recorders

Various portable blood pressure recorders have been introduced in recent years (3, 4). Three of these devices have been tested on a larger scale. They allow multiple, non-invasive registration of blood pressure during the patient's daily routine. The first of these devices is now marketed under the brand name of Remler M2000. This is a so-called semi-automated device, which means that the patient has to self-inflate the cuff using a hand pump. This method registers Korotkoff's sounds; decodation is laborious and requires a special reading device, the Remler M3000. The great advantage of this method is the fact that the quality of the registered values can be checked by a direct acoustic method during decodation, thus allowing elimination of false blood pressure values resulting from artifacts produced by other sounds. The accuracy of the Remler recorder was assessed in comparative studies with simultaneously recorded non-invasive (5, 6) and intraarterial (7) blood pressure levels.

In addition, there are fully automated blood pressure recorders which are automatically switched on at predetermined intervals. These recorders are equipped with a pump, which holds true for both the Del Mar Avionics recorder (8) and the Spacelabs system (9). In both cases, the registered values are analyzed by a computer. Though this procedure accelerates assessment, it is not possible to subsequently eliminate artifact-induced errors of measurement. Nevertheless, the Del Mar Avionics blood pressure recorder yields blood pressure profiles which show good agreement with those obtained by non-invasive and invasive procedures (8, 10—12). Concerning the reliability of the Spacelabs recorders, comparison with conventionally obtained auscultatory blood pressure values (9, 11) yielded satisfactory results.

Are there reasons to prefer one device to another? The Remler M2000 is much lighter and less bulky than other fully automated recorders. The latter, however, make it possible to register blood pressure not only during the waking phase but also during the sleeping phase, but the information derived from analysis of nocturnal blood pressure profiles is relatively limited. For physiological reasons, blood pressure is higher during the waking period than during sleep. This night-day profile remains intact in hypertensives (13). There are only few pathological conditions in which nocturnal blood pressure levels deviate from this physiological pattern and this holds true for patients who have undergone cardiac transplantation (14) as well as for orthostatic hypotension secondary to diseases of the autonomous nervous system (15) and preeclampsia (16). Furthermore, blood pressure values registered during sleep appear to be less precise than those obtained during the waking phase (10).

It might be expected that the inflation of the cuff, either automatic or manual, leads to an alarm reaction and thus increases the patient's blood pressure. It was, however, shown that this is not the case (17). Irrespective of the system used it is necessary that the blood pressure recorder be carefully fixed by specially trained staff members who are also able to give the patient a minimum of necessary instructions. High-quality blood pressure readings can be obtained only by strict adherence to these guidelines.

Ambulatory, non-invasive blood pressure recording yields a large number of blood pressure values. How are they to be evaluated to gain valuable information? Analysis of the blood pressure profile as a whole may already yield useful information. Some patients, for instance, have elevated blood pressure during a few hours of the day only, while others show hypotension during a certain period of the day. If such situations occur in patients under antihypertensive therapy, they can frequently be avoided by changing the dose and/or time of drug intake. In many cases, it may also be helpful to analyze individual blood pressure values and correlate them with the patient's activity at the time of measurement. For this kind of analysis, the patient has to record his psychic condition (calm or agitated), his physical or intellectual activities and his body position for each individual measurement over the entire period of ambulatory blood pressure recording. The mean of all registered blood pressure values can be calculated to obtain general information about the predominant blood pressure of one day. It is obvious, in this connection, that the values registered during sleep have to be considered separately. Although the mean value thus calculated is based on a relatively low number of individual values, it is very close to that which would result from including all values occurring during that measurement period. This holds true as long as the intervals between individual measurements remain below 30 min (18).

Difference between blood pressure values measured in the presence and absence of the physician

The majority of normotensive and hypertensive subjects show an increase in blood pressure in the physician's office (19—22) which is usually more pronounced at the beginning of the consultation than at the end (20). This increase tends to recur irrespective of whether the measurement is repeated after a few days or a few months (21, 22). Measurement of the blood pressure by a nurse likewise leads to an elevation, which is, however, less pronounced than that provoked by the physician. As a rule, ambulatory blood pressure values in hypertensive patients under antihypertensive therapy are markedly lower than those measured by the physician (23, 24).
Difficulties arise from the fact that ambulatory blood pressure values measured during the patient's normal activities by no means show a systematic deviation from the levels determined by the physician. Although, in a non-selected patient collective, ambulatory arterial (systolic and diastolic) blood pressure values were, on the average, about 10 mmHg below those measured at the physician's office (21), it cannot be concluded that an individual patient's blood pressure outside the physician's office can simply be obtained by subtracting 10 mmHg from the value measured by the physician. The differences between both methods can indeed be highly variable. Deviations of over 40 mmHg are occasionally seen in normotensives. Even wider deviations between both methods frequently occur in hypertensives (23). It is also important to note that a not insignificant minority of normotensives and hypertensives have higher blood pressure levels in the physician's absence than in his presence (21, 23). It should be emphasized that it is impossible to predict an individual patient's blood pressure during normal daily activity on the basis of blood pressure levels determined by the physician (19, 21, 23).

Ambulatory blood pressure readings and assessment of cardiovascular risk

Does the ambulatory blood pressure profile yield reliable information about the individual cardiovascular risk? This is a key question since the criteria presently used for the definition of normotension are based upon the blood pressure levels determined at the physician's office (1), where it was possible to demonstrate a favorable effect of antihypertensive measures on the prevention of cardiovascular disease. But it cannot be denied that the therapeutic decisions based on these tradional diagnostic methods are often difficult to make and that they yield disappointing results (2, 25, 26). There are probably many patients who take antihypertensive drugs for years without any benefit. Any drug treatment, whether it is justified or not, may involve considerable side-effects. A physician treating hypertensive patients should therefore always bear in mind that the borderline between normal and high blood pressure is purely arbitrary. The relationship between arterial blood pressure and the likelihood of cardiovascular complications is a continuous one. There is justified hope now that the blood pressure values determined outside the physician's office are better suited for identifying those patients who are more likely to benefit from antihypertensive treatment (27—31).
Various retrospective studies support the assumption that ambulatory blood pressure readings allow a more accurate prediction of the risk of future cardiovascular complications than blood pressure values determined at the physician's office. Some of these

studies are based on intraarterial determinations (19, 32, 33), while others used non-invasive procedures (34—36). In these investigations, different diagnostic procedures were used to look for damage to various organs (fundus oculi, electrocardiography, chest x-ray, echocardiography, and/or determination of kidney function). The most convincing results are those obtained in a long-term study including over 1000 patients who were followed up for a period of up to 10 years (37). This study, in which the Remler system was used, has shown that the probability of developing of cardiovascular complications or dying because of them is all the greater the smaller the difference between the ambulatory blood pressure level and that determined at the physician's office. The observations made in this study therefore seem to suggest that patients with low blood pressure values outside the physician's office are at a low risk for cardiovascular complications.

It is presently not possible to give a borderline for ambulatory blood pressure levels above which a patient has to be considered hypertensive. Establishment of normal values for this type of blood pressure recording would require the registration and subsequent follow-up of thousands of patients who would have to do without antihypertensive treatment during the study period. Ethical reasons, of course, forbid the performance of such a study. But is there still a possibility of using ambulatory blood pressure readings as a practical aid in making a therapeutic decision? What appears to be important is to bear in mind that there is a difference between ambulatory blood pressure and the levels determined at the physician's office. In cases where ambulatory blood pressure is markedly below office blood pressure readings, it appears to be justified for the pyhsician to assume a wait-and-see attitude and not to initiate therapy too soon (37).

Ambulatory blood pressure recording for the evaluation of antihypertensive treatment

The use of ambulatory blood pressure recording in evaluating the effectiveness of antihypertensive drugs is desirable for several reasons (28, 38). For instance, it is important to know whether a specific treatment lowers the blood pressure constantly or whether it only prevents the blood pressure increase otherwise occurring in the presence of the physician. Analysis of the blood pressure profile can be useful for adjusting therapy in patients who develop symptomatic side-effects (e.g., orthostatic hypotension). "Overtreatment" of hypertensives can often be prevented by ambulatory blood pressure recording (23), an aspect that has recently been confirmed in a prospective study (39). This is likely to reduce the frequency of side-effects and to improve compliance. Another important point is that too strong a blood pressure reduction may disturb the circulation of individual organs, especially the heart (40).

Portable blood pressure recorders have also proved useful in the study of antihypertensive drugs (38): the blood pressure values are no longer influenced by the investigating physician and — what is even more important — ambulatory blood pressure values appear to not be subject to any placebo effect (41, 42). It is indeed highly advantageous to be able to investigate the effectiveness of antihypertensive drugs without a preceding placebo phase. Another possible advantage offered by ambulatory blood pressure recording might be the fact that it allows us to demonstrate considerable blood pressure reductions even in very small patient collectives (43).

References

1. Gross F, Pisa Z, Strasser T, Zanchetti A (eds) Guide pratique à l'usage des médecins et du personnel paramédical. Organisation Mondiale de la Santé, pp 1—73
2. Sleight P (1985) High blood pressure: what level to treat?. J Cardiovasc Pharmacol 7 (Suppl 1): 109—111
3. Tcherdakoff P (1987) Enregistrement ambulatoire de la pression artérielle. Editions R. Dacosta, Paris, pp 5—102
4. Pagny JY, Corvol P (1986) Les mesures ambulatoires de la pression artérielle. Laboratoires Squibb, Paris, pp 1—45
5. Hinman AT, Engel BT, Bickford AF (1962) Portable blood pressure recorder: accuracy and preliminary use in evaluating intradaily variations in pressure. Am Heart J 63: 663—668
6. Kain HK, Hinman AT, Sokolow M (1964) Arterial blood pressure measurements with a portable recorder in hypertensive patients. I. Variability and correlation with "casual" pressures. Circulation 30: 882—892
7. Gould BA, Hornung RS, Kieso HA, Altman DG, Cashman PMM, Raftery EB (1984) Evaluation of the Remler M2000 blood pressure recorder. Comparison with intraarterial blood pressure recordings both at hospital and at home. Hypertension 6: 209—215
8. Harshfield GA, Pickering TG, Laragh JH (1979) A validation study of the Del Mar Avionics ambulatory blood pressure system. Ambulatory Electrocardiography 1: 7—12
9. Dembrowski T, MacDougall TM (1984) Validation of the Vita-Stat automated non-invasive blood pressure recording device. In: Herd JA, Gotto AM, Kaufman PC, Weiss SM (eds) Cardiovascular instrumentation: applicability of new technology to biobehavioral research. National Institutes of Health, Bethesda MD, pp 55—78
10. Palatini P, Sperti G, Cordone L, Mormino P, Di Marco A, Bastanzetti M, Pessina AC (1985) Reliability of indirect blood pressure monitoring for the evaluation of hypertension. Clin Exp Hypertension A7: 437—443
11. Harshfield GA, Pickering TG, Blank S, Lindahl C, Stroud L, Laragh JH (1984) Ambulatory blood pressure monitoring: recorders, applications, and analysis. In: Weber MA, Drayer JI (eds) Ambulatory blood pressure monitoring. Springer, New York, pp 1—7
12. Mallion JM, De Gaudemans R, Debru JL, Doyon B, Perdrix A, Morin B, Cau G (1979) Mesure de la pression ambulatoire par méthode automatique. Arch Mal Coeur Band suppl: 95—101
13. Reeves RA, Johnson AM, Shapiro AP, Traub YM, Jacob R (1984) Ambulatory blood pressure monitoring methods to assess severity of hypertension, variability and sleep changes. In: Weber MA, Drayer JI (eds) Ambulatory blood pressure monitoring. Springer, New York, pp 27—34
14. Reeves RA, Shapiro AP, Thompson ME, Johnson AM (1986) Loss of nocturnal decline in blood pressure after cardiac transplantation. Circulation; 73: 401—408
15. Mann S, Millar-Craig MW, Altman DG, Raftery EB, Hunyor SN (1985) Blood pressure variability in health, hypertension and autonomic failure. Clin Exp Hypertension, A7: 187—194
16. Sawyer MM, Lipshitz J, Anderson GD, Dilts PV, Halperin L (1981) Diurnal and short-term variation of blood pressure: comparison of preeclamptic, chronic hypertensive and normotensive patients. Obstet Gynecol; 58: 291—296
17. Pomidossi G, Parati G, Casadei R, Mancia G (1985) Absence of alarm reactions with use of non-invasive blood pressure monitoring devices. Clin Exp Hypertension; A7: d 429—436
18. Di Rienzo M, Grassi G, Pedotti A, Mancia G (1983) Continuous versus intermittent blood pressure measurements in estimating 24 hour average blood pressure. Hypertension; 5: 264—269
19. Floras JS, Jones JV, Hassan MO, Osikowska B, Sever PS, Sleight P (1981) Cuff and ambulatory blood pressure in subjects with essential hypertension. Lancet; 2: 107—109
20. Mancia G, Bertinieri G, Grassi G, Mancia G, Pomidossi G, Bertinieri G, Grassi G, Di Rienzo M (1983) Effects of blood pressure measurement by the doctor on patient's blood pressure and heart rate. Lancet; 2: 695—698
21. Jacot des Combes B, Porchet M, Waeber B, Brunner HR (1984) Ambulatory blood pressure recordings: Reproducibility and unpredictability. Hypertension; 3: C110—C115
22. Mancia G, Parati G, Pomidossi G, Grassi G, Casadei R, Zanchetti A (1987) Alerting reaction and rise in blood pressure during measurement by physician and nurse. Hypertension: 9: 209—215

23. Porchet M, Bussien JP, Waeber B, Nussberger J, Brunner HR (1986) Unpredictability of blood pressure recorded outside the clinic in the treated hypertensive patient. J Cardiovasc Pharmacol; 8: 332—335
24. Rion F, Waeber B, Graf HJ, Jaussi A, Porchet M, Brunner HR (1985) Blood pressure to antihypertensive therapy: ambulatory versus office blood pressure readings. J Hypertension; 3: 139—143 and 3: 521
25. Kaplan NM (1981) Whom to treat: the dilemma of mild hypertension. Am Heart J; 101: 867—870
26. Alderman MH, Madhavan S (1981) Management of the hypertensive patient: a continuing dilemma. Hypertension; 3: 192—197
27. Brunner HR, Waeber B, Nussberger J (1985) Blood pressure recording in the ambulatory patient and evaluation of cardiovascular risk. Clin Sci; 68: 485—488
28. Pickering TG, Harshfield GA, Devereux RB, Laragh JH (1985) What is the role of ambulatory blood pressure monitoring in the management of hypertensive patients? Hypertension; 7: 171—177
29. O'Brien E, Fitzgerald D, O'Malley K. Blood pressure measurement: current practice and future trends. Br Med J 1985; 290: 729—734
30. Mallion JM, Debru JL, De Gaudemaris R, Dimitriou R, Perdrix A, Cau G (1985) Mesure ambulatoire de la pression artérielle: intérêt diagnostique, prognostique et thérapeutique. Presse Med; 14: 151—155
31. Health and public policy committee of the American College of Physicians. Automated ambulatory blood pressure monitoring. (1986) Ann Intern Med; 104: 275—278
32. Rowlands DB, Ireland MA, Glover DR, McLeay RAB, Stallard TJ, Littler WA. The relationship between ambulatory blood pressure and echocardiographically assessed left ventricular hypertrophy. Clin Sci 1981; 61: 101 s—103 s
33. Mann S, Millar-Craig MW, Raftery EB (1985) Superiority of 24-hour measurement of blood pressure over clinic values in determining prognosis in hypertension. Clin Exp Hypertension; A7: 279—281
34. Sokolow M, Werdegar D, Kain JK, Hinman AT (1966) Relationship between level of blood pressure measured casually and by portable recorders and severity of complications in essential hypertension. Circulation; 34: 279—298
35. Devereux RB, Pickering TG, Harshfield GA, Kleinert HD, Denby L, Clark L, Pregibon D, Jason M, Kleiner B, Borer JS, Laragh JH (1983) Left ventricular hypertrophy in patients with hypertension: importance of blood pressure response to regularly recurring stress. Circulation; 68: 470—476
36. Pessina AC, Palatini P, Sperti G, Cardone L, Libardoni M, Mos L, Mormini P, Di Marco A, Dal Palu C (1978) Evaluation of hypertension and related target organ damage by average day-time blood pressure. Clin Exp Hypertension: A7: 267—278
37. Perloff D, Sokolow M, Cowan R (1983) The prognostic value of ambulatory blood pressure. JAMA; 249: 2792—2798
38. Waeber B, Nussberger J, Brunner HR (1984) Are surgery blood pressure measurements adequate to evaluate the efficacy of antihypertensive drugs? J Hypertension 2: 449—451
39. Waeber B, Scherrer U, Petrillo A, Bidiville J, Nussberger J, Waeber G, Hofstetter JR, Brunner HR (1987) Are some hypertensive patients overtreated? Results of a prospective study of ambulatory blood pressure recordings. Lancet ii: 732—734, 1987
40. Stewart ID (1979) Relation of reduction in pressure to first myocardial infarction in patients receiving treatment for severe hypertension. Lancet i: 861—865
41. Gould BA, Mann S, Davies AB, Altman DG, Raftery EB (1981) Does placebo lower blood pressure? Lancet; ii: 1377—1381
42. Drayer JIM, Weber MA, De Young JL, Brewer DD (1983) Long-term blood pressure monitoring in the evaluation of antihypertensive therapy. Arch Intern Med; 143: 898—901
43. Schaller MD, Nussberger J, Waeber B, Porchet M, Brunner HR (1985) Transdermal clonidine therapy in hyptertensive patients: effects on office and ambulatory recorded blood pressure values. JAMA; 253: 233—235.

Methodological developments and problems of recorders for automatic, indirect, ambulatory 24-hour monitoring of blood pressure

W. Meyer-Sabellek, K.-L. Schulte, A. Distler, R. Gotzen

Medizinische Klinik und Poliklinik, Klinikum Steglitz, Freie Universität Berlin, Berlin

Introduction

Blood pressure is a dynamic parameter subject to short-term (e. g., beat-to-beat) and long-term (e. g., circadian rhythm) variation. As early as 1898, Hill (1) was able to register daily blood pressure variations and a permanent blood pressure decrease during sleep by means of **indirect palpitation** with the aid of a sphygmograph. The **auscultation** of Korotkoff sounds above the brachial artery (2) — first described in 1905 — and its combination with an occlusion cuff according to Riva-Rocci (3) has become the most widely used procedure for the quantitative assessment of arterial blood pressure in daily routine. Stationary devices use auscultatory procedures by means of a microphone, Doppler sonography or oscillometry introduced by von Recklinghausen (5) in 1940 and different tonometric methods (piezofoils) (Table. 1).

Table 1. Methods of 24-h blood pressure monitoring

Direct continuous	Intra-arterial brachial catheter
Indirect intermittent	Auscultation by microphone(s) in an occlusive arm cuff
	Oscillometry by amplitude detection in an adjusted arm cuff
	In a finger cuff by plethysmography
Indirect continuous	Plethysmography and photoelectrically, finger volume clamp by Peñáz
	Palpation method, piezo foils on the radial artery (?)

Direct intraarterial blood pressure measurement was first used for continuous ambulatory measurement in 1966 by Bevan et al. (6) and has since been described by numerous study groups (7—10). This method not only permits beat-to-beat analyses but also statistical assessment of the circadian blood pressure profile on the basis of more than 100,000 measurement point within 24-h. The application of this method is limited to research purposes: the risk of bleeding, infection and nerve lesion does not allow the use of this procedure in daily routine.

Today, for clinical research, semi-automatic and fully automatic devices are available as portable, indirect, non-invasive long-term blood pressure recorders (8—10, 13—23). Fully automatic blood pressure recorders investigated by our study group are listed in Table 2. While semi-automatic procedures (e. g., Remler 2000) require the patient to press a button to trigger the measuring process, fully automatic devices record the blood pressure at predetermined intervals of 2—60 min (e. g., Physioport, P IV) with individual adjustment for day and night over a 24-to 48-h period for blood pressure and pulse rate measurement. The well-known method according to Riva-Rocci with an upper arm cuff is auscultatorily (Korotkoff phase V) combined with an integrated directional microphone.

Table 2. Weight, methods and ECG-monitoring in indirect ambulatory automatic 24-h blood pressure devices

monitors	weight (g)	methods		ECG	
		auscult.	oscillom.	gating	monitoring
* SL 90202 (90207) (SpaceLabs, USA)	480 (380)	—	+	—	+
* Physio-Port (Natic, BRD)	990	+	—	(+)	(+)
* Accutracker (II) (Suntechn. USA)	1100 (480)	+	—	(+)	+
ABPM-630 (Colin, Japan)	780	+	+	—	—
Medilog (Oxford, GB)	600	+	—	+	+
TM-2420 (A & O), Japan	490	+	—	—	—
* Pressurometer IV (Del Mar Avioncs, USA)	780	+	—	(+)	+

* accepted by AAMI & PTB

Since background noises may occur (e.g., muscle contraction) some devices are equipped with ECG leads to register Korotkoff sounds in a R-wave gating manner, which requires application of three electrodes to the chest. This instrumentation restricts the patient and is therefore generally less well tolerated than devices without ECG electrodes (Fig. 1). In addition, these electrodes do not prevent auscultatory inaccuracy in patients with dysrhythmias (e.g., absolute or especially respiratory arrhythmias). Some devices allow one to choose the ECG leads (P IV, Accutracker). One of the recorders using the auscultation procedure additionally permits oscillometric determination, which is used when the auscultatory results cannot be evaluated (s. Table 2).

New development: oscillometry

The successful application of recorders which allows one to choose between auscultatory and oscillometric blood pressure measurement and the demand for even smaller, portable devices for ambulatory use has led to a further development. A purely oscillometric monitor (SpaceLabs 90207) is the smallest and lightest device available and it has a high data throughput (Fig. 2). Internal algorithms are used to register oscillations. Systolic and diastolic blood pressure are calculated via premaximal and postmaximal oscillations of an inflated, occluding upper arm cuff, respectively. This method has been described (24—26) previously and has been severely criticised in the past because pulse pressure

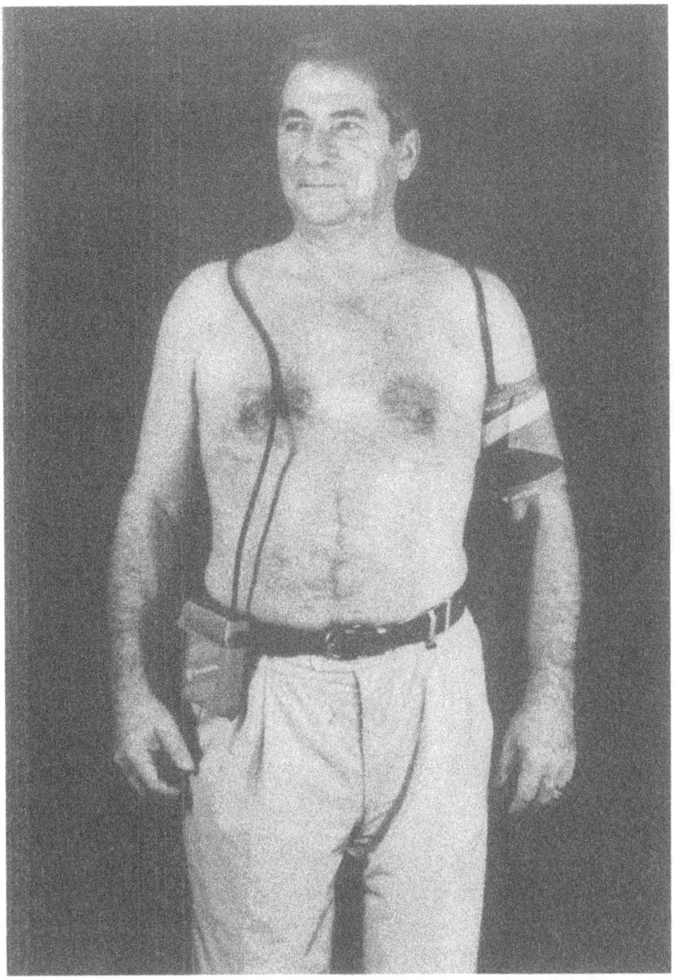

Fig. 1. Ambulatory patient with an oscillometric monitor (Spacelaps 90202)

is influenced by cardiac output (e.g., cardiac insufficiency), peripheral resistance (e.g., vasadilating drugs), and anatomy of the artery (e.g., arteriosclerosis, especially stationary waves due to stenoses). Nevertheless, this procedure is now routinely used in some stationary devices (e.g., Dinamap). Basically, the criticism holds true for all indirect procedures; the ambulatory usefulness of oscillometry remains to be evaluated (47, 48). In addition, this light device may be combined with the 24-h electrocardiogram (ECG). Simultaneous registration and evaluation of 24-h profiles of blood pressure and ECG will be available in 1989 and so far the problem is one of hardware.

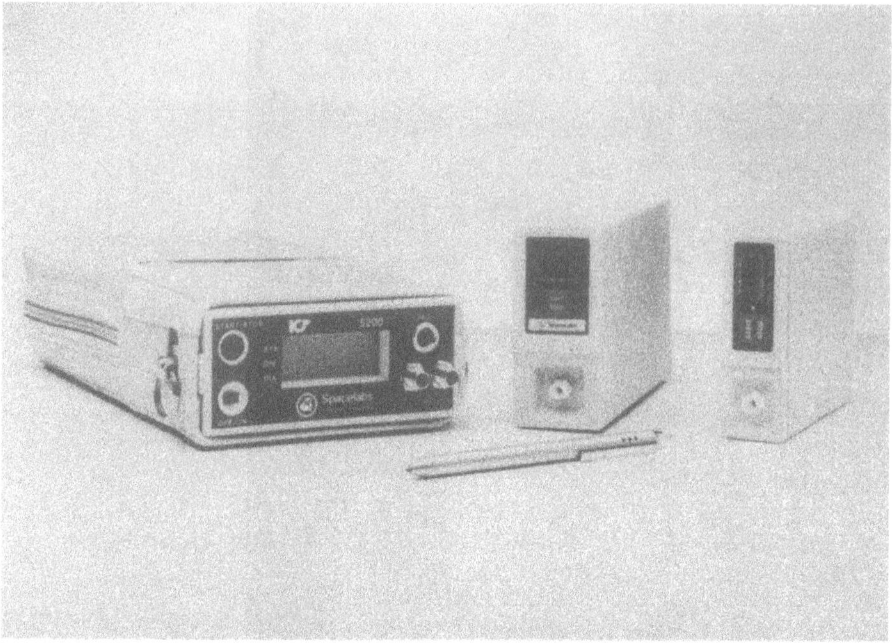

Fig. 2. Development of ambulatory monitors (SL 5200 in 1984, SL 90202 in 1986, SL 90207 in 1989)

Data storage unit

Systolic and diastolic blood pressure and pulse rate are registered and stored by a portable recorder of different weight (s. Table 2). While the device used in the past recorded the data on tape, all newer ones have a solid memory. This so-called permanent memory (operated by an 8-bit CMOS microprocessor or a similar device) stores the data (e. g., 32K RAM) until the batteries are empty or changed. The data have to be transferred to a computer via an interface. The batteries have a life of a few days. The storage capacity of the devices varies between 100 and 300 measurement points per 24—48 h. If it is assumed that 15-min measurement intervals are sufficient for diagnostic purposes, 96 measurement points can be evaluated, which allows one to register the three parameters, systolic and diastolic blood pressure and heart rate. Devices with a high storage capacity or with exchangeable energy sources and data storage units are required for the registration of two continuous 24-h cycles. The availability of accustic copplers, which have to be licensened in some countries (e. g., FRG), allow to transmit data via telephone. Data from portable monitors may be transfered, stored, pooled and statistically analyzied from different peripheral centres into a central unit.

Data display

All devices are equipped with segment liquid crystal displays that can be programmed to announce each measurement process by an alarm signal, and show the data after each measurement cycle. A renewed display of the data on the monitor is not possible. Errors are also indicated in an encoded form (e. g., defective microphone) and can be corrected by the patient to a limited extent (e. g., position of the cuff) after getting in touch with the laboratory.

Energy source

Company-owned or commercially available rechargeable accumulators (nickel cadmium batteries) still present a problem, although considerable improvements have been achieved. First, they comprise up to 50% of the total weight of the portable recorder, and secondly, they do not allow reliable registration of more than 50 24-h profiles, although the manufacturer indicates that they last for 1000 measurements. After that, they cannot be recharged at all, or only insufficiently, or fail during the ambulatory registration, which may result in the loss of all data. It is not possible to determine precisely the point of time at which the accumulators have to be exchanged. Commercially available accumulators should basically be exchanged after a maximum of twenty 24-h profiles, which causes considerable costs and environmental pollution. By utilizing a CO_2, cartridge for cuff pressurization one system (TM 2410) decreased noise level (< 40 dB) and weight, but only 60 measurements per 24 h are available (52).

Pump noise

Besides the batteries, long-stroke or centrifugal pumps comprise the largest space and highest weight, which substantially limits the development of lighter devices. It takes approximately 10 s to inflate the cuff until occlusion pressure is reached (generally 20 mmHg above the last systolic value). It does not, as frequently assumed, lead to alarm reactions with an increase in blood pressure (27). Some devices announce the measurement process by a programmable alarm sound several seconds prior to inflation. Nevertheless, some patients refuse to use the device at their workplace or in public (e. g., on a bus). More severe problems are caused by the fact that the pump noise and cuff pressure of all devices lead to sleep disorders (46) (Fig. 3). In few cases, the measurement process was interrupted at night, which makes it impossible to assess the circadian blood pressure variability or that during the wake-up period.

Side effects

As expected, there are few objectifiable side effects associated with this method. We performed 1100 examinations and observed allergic exanthema in the area of the cuff in three cases, one of which involved formation of urticaria caused either by the material (rubber) or detergent in the fabric cuff. In one further case, petechia formation in the

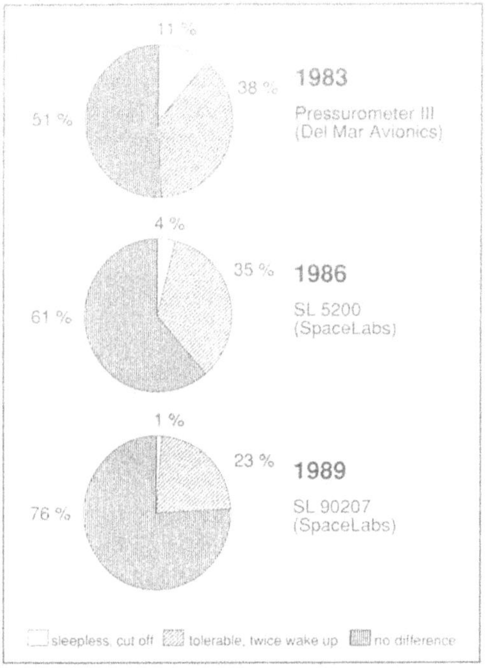

Fig. 3. Improved subjective assessment of sleep during initial 24-h monitoring with different devices.

sense of a positive Rumpel-Leede phenomenon occurred, which led to the further clarification of an idiopathic thrombocytopenia. Additional fixation of the microphone, electrodes or tubes caused plaster allergies in three cases. Phlebitis of the arm vein, which was described in a case report in the literature (28), was not observed.

Data transfer

With the aid of an interface, the recorded data can be transferred to a computer for analysis and assessment. The manufactures offer different assessment programs which exclude illogical data (e.g., systolic equal to diastolic pressure) from the data bank, but partly include artefacts (see below), such as pulse rates of 30 min. Determination of mean hourly values on the basis of two (30-min recording) to six (10-min recording) measurement points is prone to errors that falsify the results. More and more manufacturers offer compatible interfaces so that it is no longer necessary to purchase a new computer system and monitor. Almost all computer systems, especially IBM-compatible, can therefore be used to store and display (graphics, statistics) the data.

Accuracy of measurement: sensitivity and sensibility

Doubt has frequently been expressed about the accuracy of these devices and has induced comparative studies with intraarterial measurements, which have confirmed their accuracy (12, 29). It has to be taken into consideration, however, that auscultation yields a lateral pulse pressure curve of an arterial wall rather than a laminar pressure gradient like intraarterial measurement, which requires a different method. In view of the fact that the measuring procedures used here are not based on so-called beat-to-beat analyses, but variations of more than 20 mmHg may occur in systolic and up to 10 mmHg in diastolic pressure, the same limits are obvious for sphygmomanometric techniques. For these reasons, the simple correlation calculations reported in the literature have frequently been questioned (12) and the necessity for variance analyses expressed. Comparative investigations using standardized mercury manometers yielded significant correlations (30—33). The limits and possible errors (e.g., caused by displacement of the microphone) are discussed elsewhere (34).

Preliminary studies showed a good correlation between oscillometric systems and simultaneous intraarterial measurements, as well as conventional auscultatory techniques. A standard deviation of ± 7 mmHg and ± 4 mmHg was seen for systolic and diastolic pressure, respectively, with the largest deviation occuring in subjects with high blood pressure or blood pressure values with a high amplitude. It should be noted, however, that the deviation was not greater than the difference between the values measured by two different examiners (so-called interobserver error) and that it was only slightly different from individual sensibility (so-called intraobserver error).

Measurement values and calibration

The duration of the measurement process depends on individual blood pressure and ranges between 20 and 60 s. Systolic pressure is registered up to approx. 270 mmHg and the cuff is inflated to a pressure 20 mmHg above the systolic blood pressure last recorded. Diastolic pressure is recorded up to 150 mmHg with only minor differences between presently available devices. Deflation rate is controlled by the microprocessor and should not exceed 2—3 mmHg/s. In oscillometric measurement, the cuff is inflated until the maximal pulse pressure amplitude is reached and deflated at intervals.

The correct cuff size — different sizes are available — is mandatory (49). In addition, the individual anatomy and the course of the brachial artery must be considered when applying the cuff. Upper-arm circumferences exceeding 39 cm lead to considerable artifacts, registration possibly being rendered more difficult by dislocation of the cuff or the integrated microphone in obese persons and of the fixed microphone in muscular ones. If the side differences of blood pressure, left vs. right, are not significant, the measuring cuff should be applied to the non-dominant, usually left arm. On applying the long-term measuring apparatus, care should be taken that the registered systolic and diastolic blood-pressure values do not deviate from a standarized sphygmomanometer by more than 5 mmHg. The application can be optimized by establishing the point of maximum impulse of auscultation using a Doppler stethoscope and checking the blood pressure values with a Y-tube after application. Oscillometric systems installed with an auto-zero system require integrated computerized calibration.

License for use in clinical practice

Although long-term blood pressure measuring devices are used as an aid in establishing the diagnosis and assessing the therapy of arterial hypertension in different countries and the costs are settled with the health insurances, they have not yet all been licensed for use in clinical practice. In addition, daily blood pressure profiles, not only exemplary invasive but also indirectly determined data sets, are required for the licensing of new antihypertensive drugs by the American control agency, the Food and Drug Administration (FDA), but not yet by the German Federal Health Agency (Bundesgesundheitsamt, Berlin).

Patient instruction and protocol

Detailed instruction of the patient leads to fewer artifacts (see below) in the registration. Movement of the arm during the measuring procedure should be avoided as far as possible. Some devices interrupt and repeat the measuring procedure after 2 min in order to maintain the preprogrammed measuring times. The patient is asked to keep a 24-h protocol in order to provide additional information on physical activity, stress situation (stay in hospital), working time and sleeping phase. In this connection, the times of drug intake are also necessary for the evaluation of antihypertensive therapy. As opposed to oscillometric devices, precise positioning of the directional microphone is requisite for the auscultatory procedure and thus a removal of the cuff (e.g., taking a shower) can lead to incorrect measurements. The reinstallation of the cuff without instruction is easier with oscillometric monitors.

Reproducibility

Reproducibility of the circadian blood pressure profile is a necessary prerequisite for observations of the course and for long-term investigations. This has been confirmed by different groups of investigators (21, 35), although a certain adaptation cannot be excluded here (36). Comparative remeasurements should, however, be performed under comparable daily routine conditions; attention should be given in this connection, for example, to the duration and commencement of working hours. Profiles registered at the weekend should not be compared with circadian profiles of days during the week. Ultradian (i.e., less than 24 h) and infradian (i.e., more than 24 h, e.g., seasonal fluctuations) rhythmus (37) of the blood pressure can be taken into account in this connection.

Artifacts

A reliable technical system is the first prerequisite for the reduction of artifacts. Energy sources (see above) were partially responsible for artifacts; in addition, cable failures through material fatigue must be considered. As already mentioned, data obtained during active physical exercise (e.g., running; Fig. 4) can only be assessed in a limited sense, if at all. Secondary sounds engendered by muscular contractions or external sounds at the place of work (e.g., engine noise or vibrations transmitted into the arm via the steering wheel (Fig. 5)) can lead to unverifiable blood pressure values which, in case of doubt, should not be used in the evaluation. In addition to the programmed error sorting, this necessitates renewed examination of the raw data (e.g., on the screen). The different body positions (lying, sitting, standing) are not taken into account.

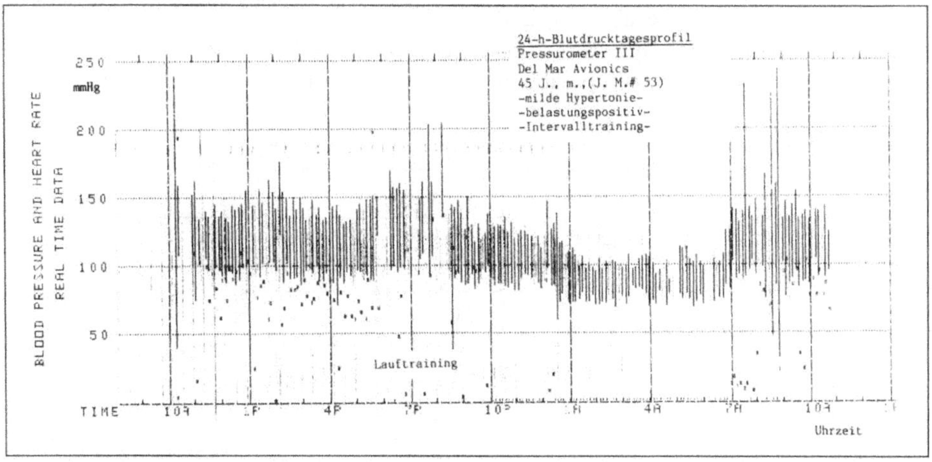

Fig. 4. Auscultatory 24-h-ABPM during excercise (Lauftraining = jogging)

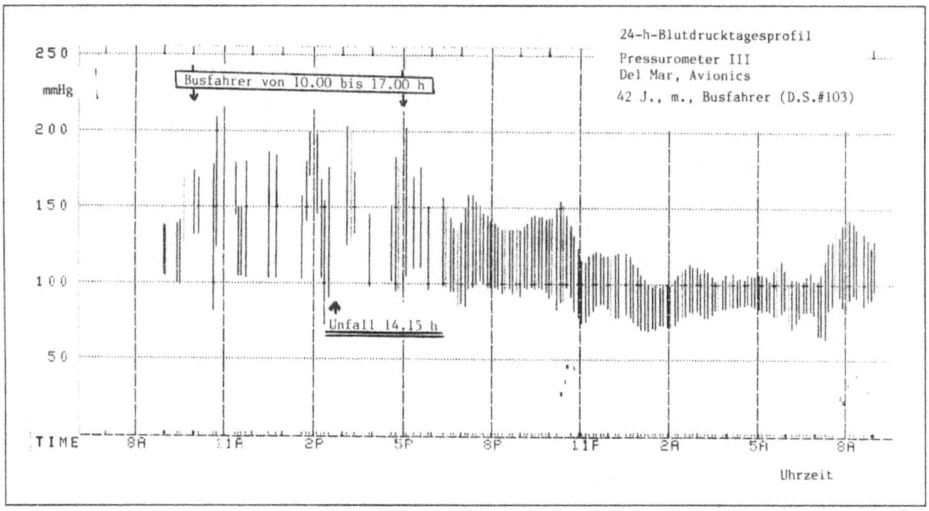

Fig. 5. Auscultatory 24-h-ABPM during work (Busfahrer = busdriver)

The normal diurnal blood pressure profile

The inadequate informational value of a single blood pressure measurement in practice has been widely known ever since the classical study of AymanH and Goldshine (38) in

1940. A whole series of published investigations are devoted to the establishment of "normal casual blood pressure".

A "normal" circadian blood pressure profile can certainly not be given in standardized form, since a role is played in this dynamic parameter by individual factors and endogenous rhythms (37) that cannot be dealt with statistically (39). Nevertheless, every study group has to provide its own normal collective. Compared to the standardized casual blood pressure, the absolute and mean hourly values in the circadian blood pressure profile are markedly lower in this connection (40, 41). Despite different measuring systems, the values are comparable according to data in the literature (s. Table 3).

Table 3. Normal values of 24-h blood pressure profiles

sex	age	24-h	day	night	2 h-wake up
♂	< 60 y.	116 ± 9 73 ± 7	122 ± 11 77 ± 8	101 ± 9 67 ± 8	123 ± 10 78 ± 7
	> 60 y.	118 ± 12 75 ± 11	124 ± 13 79 ± 10	106 ± 11 73 ± 10	121 ± 14 76 ± 12
♀	< 60 y.	108 ± 9 71 ± 10	113 ± 10 76 ± 10	98 ± 11 67 ± 9	113 ± 11 75 ± 10
	> 60 y.	112 ± 9 74 ± 9	116 ± 10 78 ± 9	104 ± 9 65 ± 8	114 ± 12 75 ± 9

It must be considered that blood pressure is subject to a biphasic circadian rhythm (i.e., comprising a nearly 24-h period) (37) that can be detected invasively and, as a rule, noninvasively as well. This rhythm can be detected in normotensives and essential hypertensives but may be abolished during the measuring procedure by outward circumstances (e.g., intake of sedatives (42), shift work (43, 44)) and by various diseases (e.g., coarctation (20), autonomic insufficiency (45) or post heart and renal transplantation (46, 47) and in secondary hypertension (48)) as well as by sleep disturbances (49). Sleep disturbances caused by the measuring procedure occur in more than a third of the patients (see Fig. 3) and have to be taken into account in the statistical assessment of the total collective.

Assessment and statistical parameters

The following statistical parameters can be derived from the noninvasive 24-h measurement of the systolic and diastolic blood pressure and the heart rate:

1. Casual values
2. Maximum and minimum values
3. Mean hourly values and standard deviation (or median and quantiles)
4. Total 24-h blood pressure
5. 2-h matutinal (wake-up) blood pressure
6. Diurnal (or waking-phase) blood pressure (mean value and standard deviation or histogram)

7. Nocturnal (or sleeping-phase) blood pressure
The discussion in the literature is controversial with regard to additional data such as the percentage specification of increased blood pressure values above an arbitrary line, spectroscopic analyses or cosinor analyses for evaluation of infra- and circadian rhythms; new statistical analyses make it possible to gain an insight into blood pressure and heart rate modulation (50, 51).

Conclusion

Investigations in extensive normal collectives and comparisons with conventional standardized blood pressure measuring techniques (e. g., ergometry) show the value of noninvasive ambulatory 24-h blood pressure measurement in daily blood pressure assessment. Follow-ups of many years' duration have to be done to analyze in greater detail the early prognostic informational value of a circadian blood pressure profile with regard to secondary organ damage in patients with boderline and mild hypertension and also to determine the value of such a profile in comparison to standardized casual measurements and/or repeated self-measurement of blood pressure. On the basis of the many blood pressure values obtained outside the practice, long-term blood pressure measuring procedures are able to provide a more reliable assessment of blood pressure and thus possibly also of cardiovascular risk.
Technically, the portable monitors still need some improvements: the weight must be further reduced and the pump noise cut down. The reliability of the energy sources and the recording efficiency must be improved. It will not be possible, however, to apply these measuring systems unrestrictedly. In more than 24% third of those examined, sleep disturbances occur due to the cuff pressure or pump noise and complicate assessment of the circadian profile. It is under discussion whether only the waking-phase should be used for the antihypertensive assessment. However, the blood pressure values in the early morning hours and in the wake-up phase are also of particular interest in assessing the cardiovascular risk. This is substantiated by more recent investigations that demonstrate a matutinal (8.00—10.00 h a. m.) peak in the incidence of myocardial infarction (53, 54). The significance of these observations for cardiovascular or cerebrovascular diseases and the increased incidence of angina pectoris or cerebral ischemias during the relatively hypotensive nocturnal phases make it necessary to carry out reliable long-term blood pressure measurements during the night as well (55).
Hypertensives with confirmed left ventricular hypertrophy show an increased incidence of complex ventricular arrhythmias (56) and sudden heart death: this makes it necessary to have ambulatory measuring assessment which permits simultaneous long-term electrocardiography and blood pressure measurement, which will be available for clinical research in the near future.

References

1. Hill L (1898) On rest, sleep, and work and the concomitant changes in the circulation of blood. Lancet I: 282—285

2. Korotkoff NC (1905) To the question of methods of determining the blood pressure (from the Clinic of CP Federoff). Reports of the Imperial Military Medical Acedemy II: 365—367
3. Riva Rocci S (1896) Un nuovo sfingmomanometro. Gaz med Torino 47: 981
4. Addis T (1922) Blood pressure and pulse rate levels. Arch Intern Med 29: 539—542
5. Recklinghausen H v (1940) Blutdruckmessung und Kreislauf in den Arterien des Menschen. Steinkopff, Dresden, Leipzig
6. Bevan AT, Honour AJ, Stott FH (1969) Direct arterial pressure recording in unrestricted man. Clin Sci 36: 329—344
7. Krönig B, Dufey K, Reinhardt P, Jahnecke J, Wolff HP (1974) Long-term telemetry of direct arterial pressure in unrestricted hypertensives. Biotelemetry 1: 117—131
8. Millar-Craig MS, Hawes B, Whittington J (1978) A new system for continous arterial pressure measurement in man. Med Biol Emg Comp 16: 727—731
9. Raftery EB (1984) Understanding hypertension. The contribution of direct ambulatory blood pressure monitoring. In: Weber MA, Drayer JIM (eds) Ambulatory Blood Pressure Monitoring. Steinkopff Darmstadt 105—116
10. Hinman AT, Engel BT, Bickford AF (1962) Portable blood pressure recorder: accuracy and preliminary use in evaluating intradaily variations in pressure. Am Heart J 63: 663—667
11. Jacot des Combes B, Porchet M, Waeber B, Brunner HR (1984) Ambulatory blood pressure recordings. Hypertension 6: 110—114
12. Gould BA, Hornung RS, Kieso HA, Altman DG, Cashman PM, Raftery EB (1984) Evaluation of Remler M2000 blood pressure recorder: comparison with intraarterial blood pressure recordings. Hypertension 6: 209—215
13. Kain HK, Hinman AT, Sokolow M (1964) Arterial blood pressure measurements with portable recorder in hypertension patients. Variability and correlations with casual pressures. Circulation 30: 882
14. Richardson DW, Honour AY, Fenton GW, Stott FD, Pickering GW (1964) Variations in arterial pressure throughout the day and night. Clin Sci 26: 445—460
15. Schneider RA (1968) A fully automated portable blood pressure recorder. J Appl Physiol 24: 115—119
16. Thornton W, Wallace J (1984) Aerospace applications of ambulatory blood pressure monitoring. In: Weber MA, Drayer JIM (eds) Ambulatory blood pressure monitoring. Steinkopff, Darmstadt, pp 129—136
17. Harshfield GA, Pickering TG, Kleinert HD, Blank S, Laragh JH (1982) Situational variations of blood pressure in ambulatory hypertensive patients. Psychosomatic Medicine 44: 237—244
18. Horan MJ, Kennedy HL, Padgett NE (1981) Do borderline hypertensive patients have labile blood pressure. Ann Int Med 94: 466—468
19. Drayer JIM, Weber MA, DeYoung JL, Wyle FA (1982) Circadian blood pressure pattern in ambulatory hypertensive patients. Am J Med 73: 493—499
20. Meyer-Sabellek W, Sehested J, Schulte KL, Gotzen R (1984) Clinical significance of cardiovascular rhythms and applicability of invasive, and non-invasive methods for 24-h blood pressure monitoring. In: Kimmich HP, Klewe H-J (eds) Biotelemetry VIII. Drönig, Braunschweig, pp 183—186
21. Weber MA, Drayer JIM (1984) The circadian blood pressure pattern in ambulatory normal subjects. Am J Cardiol 54: 115—119
22. Sheps SG, Schirger A, Spiekerman RE, Harman TR, O'Brian PC, Kleven K, Kremer-Simpson K (1985) Evaluation of pindolol dosage in hypertension by automatic indirect BP monitoring. Arch Int Med 145: 54—57
23. Frielingsdorf J, Stricker M, Hany S, Förster CC, Vetter W (1985) 24-h-Blutdruckmessung bei Hypertonikern verschiedener Schweregrade. Schweiz Rundsch Med Prax 74: 1260—1265
24. Hildebrandt A, Hildebrandt G (1958) Oszillographische Praxis. Bosch und Speidel, Jungingen
25. Forster FK, Turley D (1987) Oscillometric determination of diastolic, mean and systolic blood pressure — a numerical model J Biomech Eng 108: 359—364
26. Friesen RH, Lichtor JL (1981) Indirect measurement of blood pressure in neonates and infants utilizing an automatic noninvasive oscillometric monitor. Anesth Analg 60: 742—745
27. Parati G, Pomidossi G, Casadei R, Mancia G: Lack of alerting reactions to intermittent cuff inflations during non-invasive blood pressure monitoring. Hypertension 7: 597—601
28. Creevy PC, Burris JF, Mroczek WJ: Phlebitis associated with noninvasive 24-hour ambulatory blood pressure monitor. JAMA 254, 2411

29. Palatini P, Pessina AC, Sperti G (1982) Comparison between an indirect and direct method of ambulatory blood pressure monitoring. In: Scott FD (ed) Intern. Symp. on Ambulatory Monitoring. Academic Press, London, pp 491—503
30. Harshfield GA, Pickering TG, Blank S, Lindahl C, Stroud L, Laragh JH (1984) Ambulatory blood pressure monitoring: recorders, applications and analyses. In: Weber MA, Drayer JIM (eds) Ambulatory blood pressure monitoring. Steinkopff, Darmstadt, S 1—8
31. Dembrowski T, MacDougall TM (1984) Validation of the Vita-Stat automated noninvasive blood pressure recording device. In: Herd YA, Gotto AM, Kauman PC, Weiss SM (eds) Cardiovascular instrumentation: applicability of new technology to behavioral research. Bethesda NIH, pp 55—78
32. Harshfield GA, Pickering TG, Blank S, Lindahl C, Stroud L, Laragh JH (1979) A validation study of the Del Mar Avionics automatic ambulatory blood pressure system. Ambulatory Electrocardiol 1: 7—12
33. Sheps SG, Elveback LR, Close EL, Kleven MK, Bissen C (1981) Evaluation of the Del Mar Avionics automatic ambulatory blood pressure-recording device. Mayo Clin Proc 56: 740—743
34. Anlauf M, Weber F (1987) Automatische Registrierung der Korotkow-Geräusche: Klinische Erfahrung mit automatischen Blutdruckmeßgeräten im Vergleich zu auskultatorischen Methode. In: Meyer-Sabellek W, Gotzen R (Hrsg) Indirekte 24-Stunden-Blutdruckmessung. Steinkopff, Darmstadt, S 29—35
35. Fitzgerald DJ, O'Malley K, O'Brien ET (1984) Reproducibility of ambulatory blood pressure recordings. In: Weber MA, Drayer JIM (eds) Ambulatory blood pressure monitoring. Steinkopff, Darmstadt, pp 71—74
36. Pessina AC, Palatini P, Sperti G, Cordone L, Ventura F, Dal Palu PC (1984) Adaptation to non-invasive continous blood pressure monitoring. In: Weber MA, Drayer JIM (eds) Ambulatory blood pressure monitoring. Steinkopff, Darmstadt, pp 57—64
37. Halberg F, Halberg E, Halberg J, Halberg F (1984) Chronobiologic assessment of human blood pressure variation in health and disease. In: Weber MA, Drayer JIM (eds) Ambulatory blood pressure monitoring. Steinkopff, Darmstadt: pp 137—156
38. Ayman D, Goldshine AD (1940) Blood pressure determinations by patients with essential hypertension. I. The difference between clinic and home readings before treatment. Am J Med Sci 200: 465—474
39. Mancia G, Zanchetti A (1986) Blood pressure variability. In: Zanchetti A, Tarazi RC (eds) Handbook of Hypertension, Vol. 7. Elsevier, Amsterdam: pp 125—152
40. Kennedy HL, Horan MJ, Sprague MK, Padgett NE, Shriver KK (1983) Ambulatory blood pressure in healthy normotensive males. Am Heart J, 106: 717—722
41. Drayer JIM, Weber MA (1985) Definition of normalcy in whole-day ambulatory blood pressure monitoring. Clin Exper Hypertension A7: 195—204
42. Seidel WF, Roth T, Roehrs T, Zorick F, Dement WC (1984) Treatment of a 12-hour shift of sleep schedule with benzodiazepines. Science 244: 1262—1264
43. Sundberg S, Kohvakka A, Gordin A (1988) Rapid reversal of circadian blood pressure rhythm in shift workers. J. Hypertens 6: 393—396
44. Baumgart P (1989) Diurnal blood pressure rhythm: dependence on internal and external time triggers. In: Meyer-Sabellek W, Anlauf H, Gotzen R, Steinfeld L (eds) Blood pressure Measurement. New techniques in automatic indirect monitoring. Steinkopff, Darmstadt, Springer, New York, pp 253—259
45. Brevetti G, Bonaduce G, Breglio R, Canonico V, Izzo A, Chiariello M (1985) Blood pressure ambulatory monitoring and autonomic dysfunction. In: Germano C (ed) Blood pressure recording in the clinical management of hypertension. L. Pozzi, Rom, pp 77—82
46. Reeves RA, Shapiro AP, Thompson ME, Johnsen AM (1986) Loss of nocturnal decline in blood pressure after cardiac transplantation. Circulation 73: 401—408
47. Meyer-Sabellek W, Schulte K-L, Gotzen R (1989). Bedeutung der Langzeitblutdruckregistrierung für die Diagnostik und Therapiebeurteilung der arteriellen Hypertonie. Mitt klin Nephrologie XXIII: 42—50.
48. Meyer-Sabellek W, Schulte K-L, Streitberg B, Gotzen R (1988) Two-year follow-up of 24-hour indirect blood pressure monitoring: an open study. Evaluation of once-daily and twice-daily regimens of carvedilol. Drugs 36 (Suppl 6) 106—112
49. Meyer-Sabellek W, Schulte K-L, Gotzen R (1989) Technical possibilities and Limits of indirect twenty-four-hour blood pressure devices. J Hypertension 7 (Suppl 3): 21—24

50. Streitberg B (1987) Analyse der zirkadianen Bludruckprofile. Bemerkungen eines Statistikers. In: Meyer-Sabellek W, Gotzen R (Hrsg) Indirekte 24-Stunden-Blutdruckmessung. Steinkopff, Darmstadt, S 117—124
51. Streitberg B, Meyer-Sabellek W, Baumgart P (1989) Analysis of 24-hour blood pressure profiles. J. Hypertension 7 (suppl 3): 11—18
52. Tochikubo O, Kaneko Y, Yokoi H, Yukinori (1985) A new portable device for recording 24-h indirect blood pressure in hypertensive outpatients. J. Hypertens 3: 355—357
53. Muller JE, Stone PH, Turi ZG, Rutherford JD, Czeisler CA, Parker D, Poole K, Passamani E, Roberts R, Robertson T, Sobel BE, Willerson JT, Braunwald E (1985) Circadian variation in the frequency of onset of acute myocardial infarction. N Engl J Med 313: 1315—1322
54. Willich SN, Levy D, Rocco MB, Tofler GH, Stone PH, Muller JH (1987) Circadian variation in the incidence of sudden cardiac death in the Framingham Heart Study population. Am J Cardial 60: 801—806
55. Pickering T (1987) Strategies for evaluation and treatment of hypertension and some inplications of blood pressure variability. Circulation 76: I-77—I-82
56. McLenachen JM, Henderson E, Morris KI, Dargie HJ (1987) Ventricular arrhythmias in patients with hypertensive left ventricular hypertrophy. N Engl J Med 317: 787—792

Analysis of circadian blood pressure profiles: some remarks from a statistician

B. Streitberg[1], W. Meyer-Sabellek[2]

[1]Institut für Statistik, Hamburg, Hamburg, FRG
[2]Medizinische Klinik und Poliklinik, Klinikum Steglitz, Freie Universität Berlin, Berlin, FRG

Introduction

Voltaire once defined a boring man as one who tells you everything he knows. I will therefore confine myself to a few remarks on three topics only: the spectral analysis of blood pressure profiles, the specification of descriptive models for them and methods for their comparison. The paper can be regarded ar a light-hearted introduction to some of the statistical problems of these data, which have recently been discussed in detail (5).
In the last section, a new statistical test is proposed which allows a computationally inexpensive determination of exact p-values for the comparison of a patient's profile with a given data base of profiles.

Spectral analysis of profiles

Blood pressure is an essentially continuous phenomenon. For indirect blood pressure monitoring, however, pressures can be recorded at discrete time intervals only. The determination of the length of these sampling intervals or, equivalently, the sampling frequency

$$f_s = \text{No. of samples/time unit}$$

is largely a matter of compliance considerations and clinical relevance. A certain mathematical rationale is provided by Shannon's sampling theorem: a continuous function h(t) of time can be reconstructed completely from samples spaced $1/f_s$ time units if the Fourier transform of h:

$$H(f) = \int_{-\infty}^{+\infty} h(t) \exp(i2\pi ft)\, dt$$

is band limited by $f_s/2$, i.e.

$$H(f) = 0 \text{ for } |f| \geqq f_s/2.$$

Expressed less formally: if we consider the signal to be composed of sinusoidal frequency components and assume that f is the highest frequency which appears in the signal, a sampling frequency of 2f is sufficient to capture the signal completely.
Blood pressure is certainly not band limited in the relevant frequency range, as witnessed by several investigations of high frequency variation of invasively recorded blood pressure data (1). For low frequency variation, however, an indication of possible reduc-

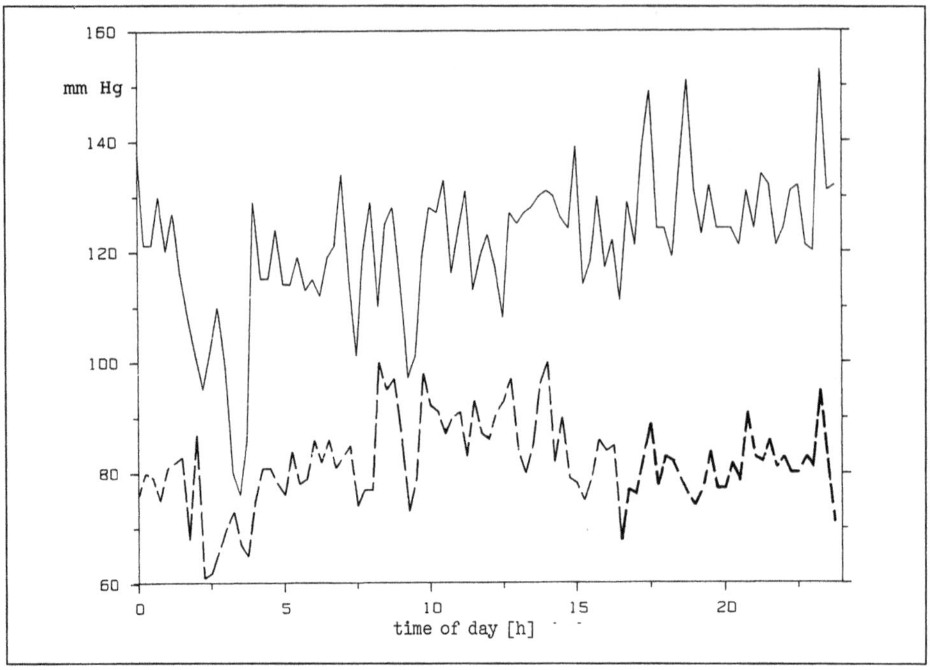

Fig. 1. Typical profile (systolic and diastolic 8 p)

tions in sampling frequency can be obtained by spectral analysis of relatively coarsely sampled data. A typical profile from a hypertensive patient is shown in Fig. 1.

The profile reveals the characteristic spectral shape of circadian blood pressure series. There is a clear circadian frequency peak (period approx. 24 h) and a somewhat less pronounced ultradian frequency peak (period 80 to 120 min). The other peaks in this spectrum seem to be spurious and could not be verified consistently across subjects (see Fig. 2).

The spectrum was estimated by smoothing the FFT with a Gaussian kernel of bandwidth 3 cycles/day. For these and other methods of spectrum estimation, see ref. (2).

Since areas under the curve represent proportions of signal variance, the tail cumulated spectrum gives the proportion of variance which is aliased if a sampling frequency lower than twice the Nyquist frequency were chosen.

Even if a proportion of 0.1 were tolerable, the sampling frequency could only be lowered to about 30 = 2 x 35 cycles/day, corresponding to a sampling interval of about 20 min.

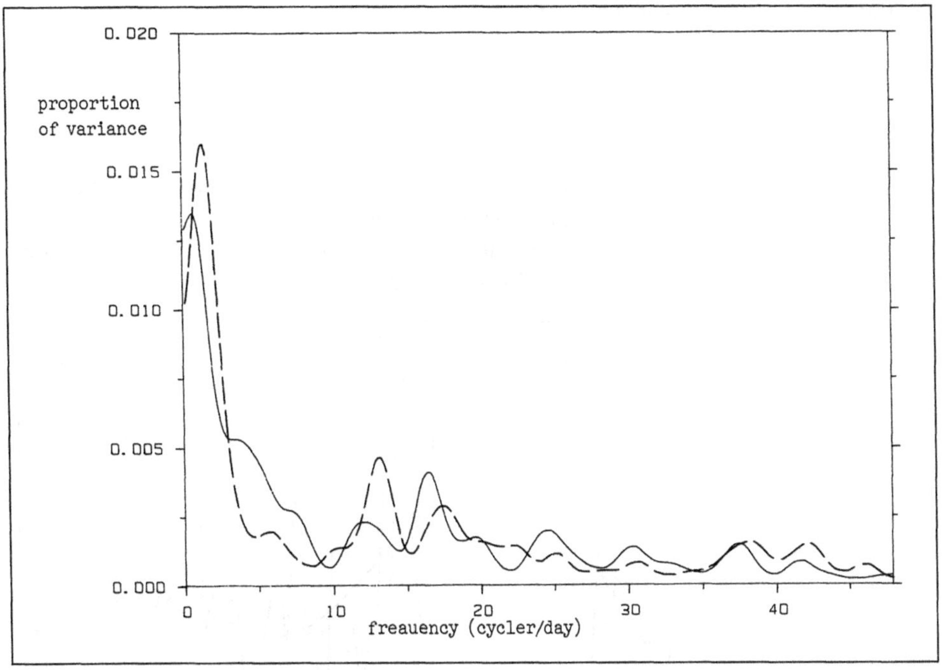

Fig. 2. Spectral density of profile

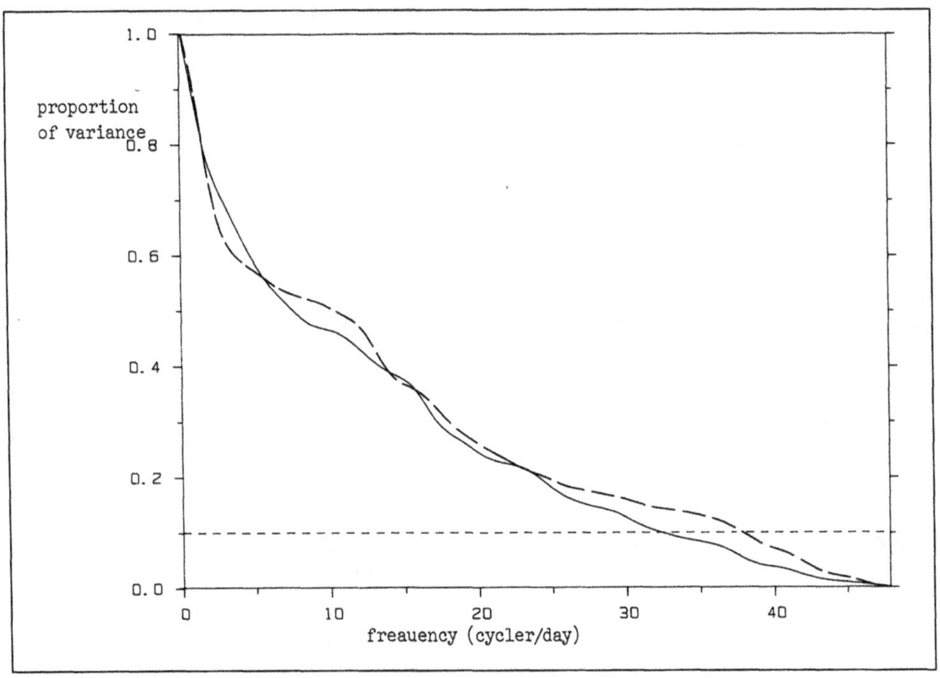

Fig. 3. Tail comulated spectral density

Descriptive models for circadian profiles

For profile smoothing, descriptive models like degree-k polynomials

$$f(t) = a_o + a_1 t + a_2 t^2 + \dots + a_k t^k$$

are often used. The direct estimation of these models by least squares, as in Fig. 4 where k = 7 was used, has a small but undesirable consequence, however.
This can be seen if one repeats the signal and its estimate over a period of 48 h, where a visible discontinuity appears at T = 24 h (see Fig. 5).

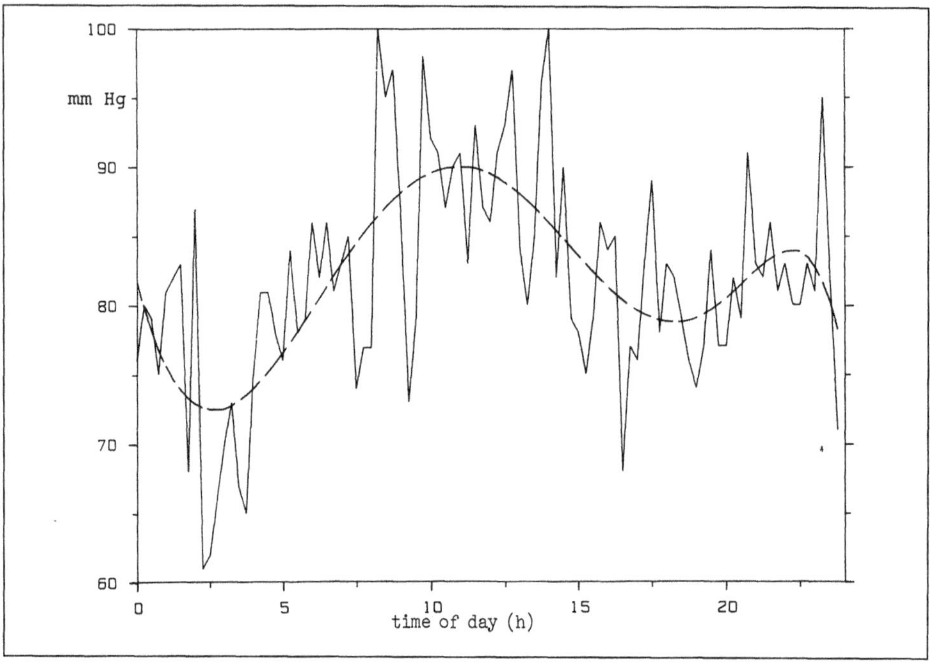

Fig. 4. Smoothed diastolic 8b profile

Circadian profiles are defined not on the real axis R, but on the circle $R/T \cdot Z$ (with circumference T). It is therefore advisable to impose certain circularity conditions, namely
(1) Continuous signal : $f(T) = f(o)$
(2) Continuous derivative : $f'(T) = f'(o)$
(3) Continuous curvature : $f''(T) = f''(o)$.

Models of this type can be estimated by least squares with linear restrictions:
If the unrestricted model is given by $f = Xa$ and the restrictions are represented by $Ra = 0$, the problem to minimize the squared norm $| y - X a |^2$ of the signal's y deviations from the model Xa subject to $Ra = 0$, is solved by

$$\hat{a} = (X'X)^{-1}X'y - (X'X)^{-1} R' (R (X'X)^{-1} R')^{-1} R (X'X)^{-1} X'y.$$

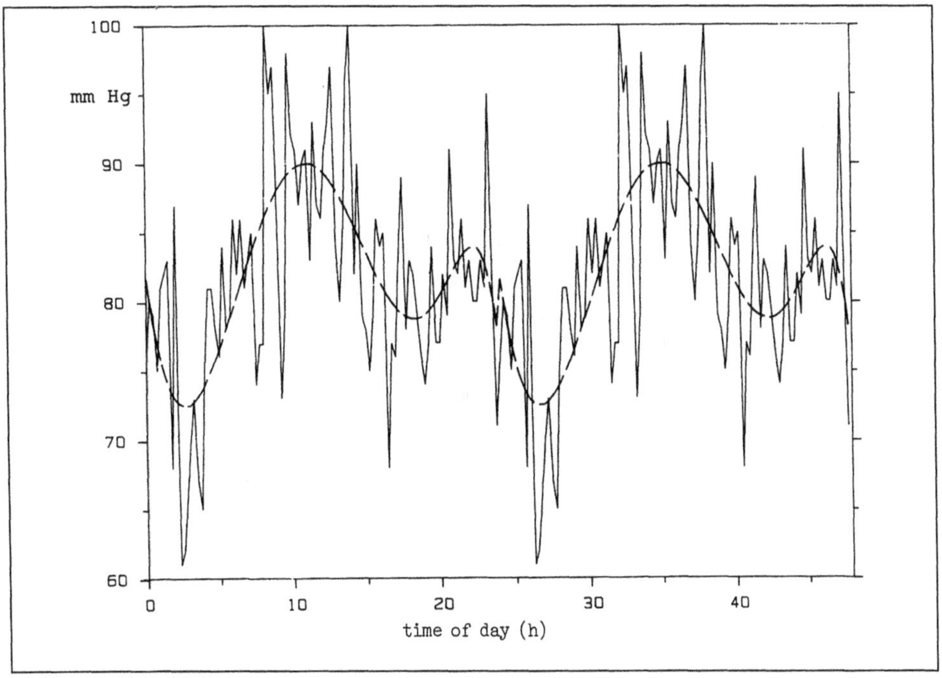

Fig. 5. Smoothed profile with periodicity

The estimated signal, with k = 7, is shown in Fig. 6.
The degree k of the polynomial can be estimated consistently by minimizing one of the recently developed model selection criteria, e.g., the Bayesian information criterion (BIC). Here

$$\text{BIC}(k) = \ln(\sigma^2(k)) + (k-2)\frac{\ln(n)}{n}$$

is computed for k = 3, 4, 5, ... and k with a minimum value of BIC (k) is chosen. The error variance is

$$\sigma^2(k) = \frac{1}{n}|y - X\hat{a}|^2$$

and n is the length of the profile (96 in our example). In our example, BIC is minimized by k = 7.

Note that this example is not meat as a recommendation of polynominal smoothing. A better approach is detailed elsewhere (5).

Comparison of profiles

There are two basic approaches to statistical testing — the parametric one, usually based on the normal distribution, and the nonparametric approach. Mathematicians believe in the normal distribution, because they think it is a fact of natural science, and natural scientists believe in the normal distribution, because they think mathematicians have

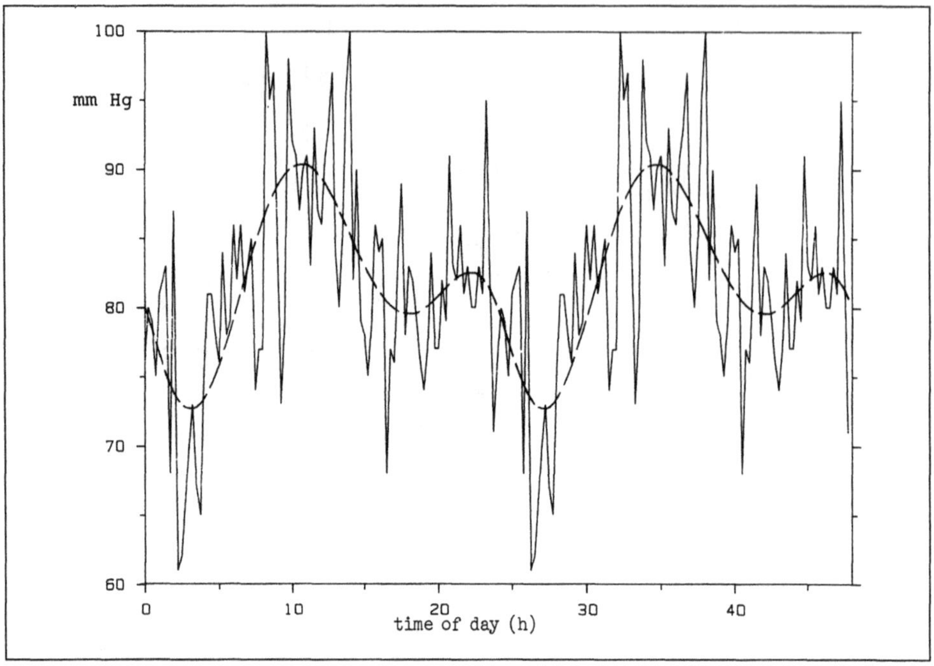

Fig. 6 Smoothed profile without periodicity

proved it. In biological practice, however, normally distributed data practically never appear. Blood pressure data are one of the very few biological parameters, which are at least approximately normal. In Fig. 7 a nonparametric density estimator with Gaussian kernel (s = 3) was applied to the data of Fig. 1. Note that the smoothing seems adequate for the diastolic pressures and too weak for the systolic ones.

Nevertheless, many statisticians would, even for these data, prefer a nonparametric approach to the problem of comparing blood pressure profiles between, say, normo- and hypertensive subjects or treated and untreated patients. The reason for this preference is the much greater flexibility of nonparametrics in choosing parameters dictated not by statistical considerations, but by clinical judgement.

An example is provided by a new class of tests, presented here for the first time. These tests are applicable to the following problem:

A data base of standard profiles has been built up, consisting, for instance, of typical normotensive profiles. In routine application of this data base, profiles of new patients are compared with the data base in order to determine profiles which deviate from the typical normotensive profile.

Let the data base consist of profiles X_1, X_2 ..., X_n and the patients profile be denoted by X. In nonparametrics, the null hypothesis that the patients profile does not deviate from the profiles in the data base, would be expressed as

H_0: X, X_1, ..., X_n are exchangeable.

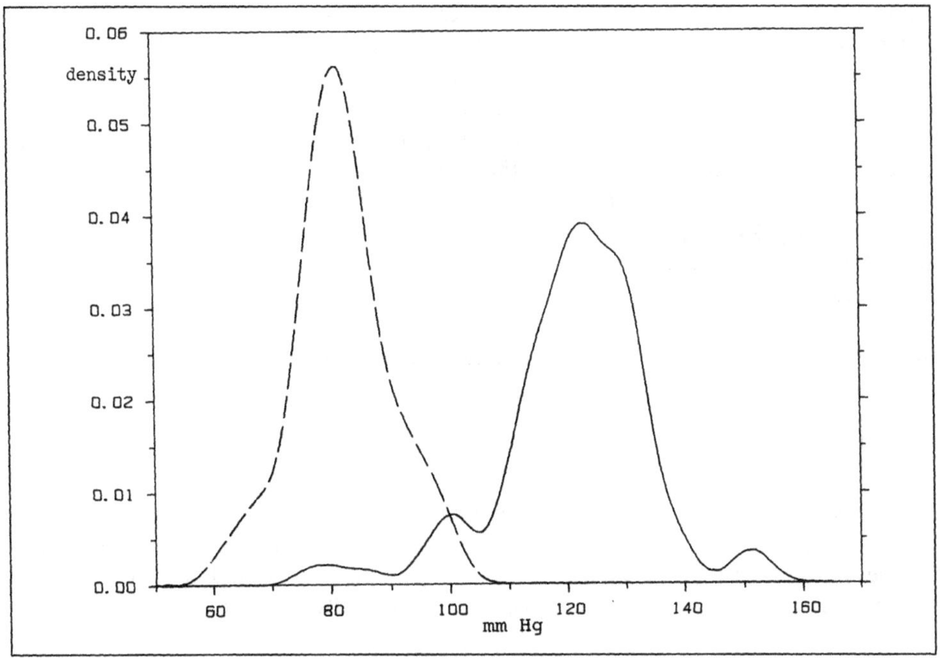

Fig. 7. Density extimates for BP data

Mathematically, this means that the joint distribution of $X, X_1, \ldots, X_n$ is invariant under all permutations of the $n + 1$ profiles.
Now the physician is free to choose a test statistic, i.e., a measure of how far X deviates from $X_1, \ldots, X_n$. Some possible choices are

$$\Delta_o = \frac{1}{n} \sigma_{i=1}^{n} d\,(X, X_iY)$$

or

$$\Delta_o = \max_i \,(d\,(X, X_i))$$

where $d\,(X, X_i)$ is any distance measure for comparing two individual profiles. But, in general, any function $\Delta_o = \Delta\,(X \mid X_1, \ldots, X_n)$ could be used.
A general principle of nonparametrics (the permutation principle, see (4) for an explanation of recent developments) shows that an exact nonparametric p-value for assessing the significance of Δ_o can be obtained as follows:
Permute $X, X_1, \ldots, X_n$ in all possible ways and compute for each of these $(n + 1)!$ permutations the value of Δ.
Then the p-value p is the proportion of these values, which are at least as big as the actually observed value Δ_o. Since the number of permutations grows very rapidly with n, this principle can only be applied to very small data bases in general.

If however, we impose the following natural restriction on Δ, such that Δ is symmetric in the profiles of the data base, i.e. the test statistic does not express any preferences for particular profiles in the data base, the exact p-value can be obtained very easily. Note that the above examples do fulfil this restriction.
For symmetric Δ, all permutations which only permute the data base itself, leave the value of Δ unchanged. Therefore, only the $n + 1$ values

$$\Delta_o = \Delta(X \mid X_1, X_2, \ldots, X_n)$$
$$\Delta_1 = \Delta(X_1 \mid X, X_2, \ldots, X_n) \ldots$$
$$\Delta_n = \Delta(X_n \mid X_1, X_2, \ldots, X)$$

are obtained if we apply all permutations. Since these values occur with equal frequency, the p-value is determined by computing

$$\Delta_0, \Delta_1, \ldots, \Delta_n$$

in one pass through the data base and counting the proportion of values at least as big as Δ_o among these $n + 1$ values. If, for example, in a data base of 199 profiles, only 5 values not smaller than Δ_o were observed, the p-value of Δ_o would be $6/200 = 0.03$. This method is computationally unexpensive and generally applicable.

References

1. Akselrod S, Gordon D et al (1985) Hemodynamic regulation: investigation by spectral analysis. Am J Physiol
2. Schlittgen R, Streitberg B (1987) Zeitreihenanalyse. 2nd ed. Oldenbourg, München
3. Streitberg B, Roehmel J (1986) Exact Nonparametrics. Statistical Software Newsletter
4. Winfree A (1980) The geometry of biological time. Springer, Berlin
5. Streitberg B, Meyer-Sabellek, W, Baumgart P (1989) Statistical analysis of circadian blood pressure profiles in controlled clinical trials. Journal of Hypertension 7 (3) 11—18

Ambulatory blood pressure — direct and indirect

B.A. Gould, R.S. Hornung, P.M.M. Cashman and E.B. Raftery

Department of Cardiology and Divisions of Bioengineering and Clinical Sciences, Northwick Park Hospital and Clinical Research Centre, Harrow, Middlesex, UK

Introduction

Blood pressure is a continually varying parameter which cannot be characterized by the occasional outpatient (office) indirect recording. Serial measurements throughout the day and night are required. Such measurements may be obtained by ambulatory blood pressure monitoring; however, these methods have not been assessed for accuracy in operation away from the hospital environment. We have used the Oxford system for intra-arterial ambulatory blood pressure monitoring as the standard against which the indirect techniques could be compared. We evaluated self-recorded blood pressures, the Remler M2000, and the Avionics 1978 pressurometer. In addition we have assessed how well self-recorded blood pressures (as measured by epidemologists) on awakening and on going to bed reflected the daytime blood pressures. We have also compared the recorded reductions during trials with anti-hypertensive agents.

Methods

Each method of non-invasive measurement was assessed separately.

Home blood pressures

Fifty-seven patients with essential hypertension were recruited but two were unable to learn the technique of self-recorded blood pressure measurement; 35 were on no medication. The group consisted of 17 females, and 38 males with a mean age of 51.8 (range 23—70) years.

The patients attended a special session of the Hypertension Clinic where an indirect measurement was recorded using the Hawkesley random zero sphygmomanometer (Gelman Ltd.). They were taught the technique of self-recording using a calibrated anaeroid gauge, standard techniques of measurement (1) and phase V for diastolic pressure. The patient's recordings were checked using a double-listening stethoscope but none were excluded from the study on the grounds of inaccurate recordings. Home blood pressures were recorded after a 5-min rest in the sitting position, four times daily at 8—9 am, 1—2 pm, 5—7 pm, and at bedtime for 10 days.

During this period, intra-arterial ambulatory blood pressure monitoring was undertaken. Patients were freely ambulant in their normal environment and over 2 days (2) only attended hospital at 12-h intervals for calibration and equipment checks. During these visits indirect recordings of the blood pressure were made by the physician using a random zero sphygmomanometer, followed by a check on the patient's technique using a double listening stethoscope.

The intra-arterial tape recording was marked with an event signal whenever an indirect reading was taken, both at home and in the hospital. Indirect measurements were made on the dominant arm and intra-arterial recordings on the contralateral arm. The pressure difference between the arms was assessed by two observers recording the pressure in each arm simultaneously. One random zero sphygmomanometer was connected to two blood pressure cuffs. A series of paired readings on each arm were recorded and repeated after switching the cuffs, providing a total of eight paired readings.

Remler, M2000

Twenty-eight patients volunteered to wear the Remler M2000 for 1 day in addition to the Oxford system for ambulatory intra-arterial recording. There were seven females and 21 males with a mean age of 50 years (range 23—67 years). Ten patients were receiving anti-hypertensive therapy.

Simultaneous readings of intra-arterial, clinic and Remler M2000 pressure were recorded on three occasions in the hospital. The Remler M2000 was linked via a Y connector to a random zero sphygmomanometer and the clinic pressure auscultated using a standard stethoscope in the usual position. Thus simultaneous clinic and Remler pressures were recorded from the same arm whilst intra-arterial pressures were recorded from the contralateral arm. Pressures were recorded hourly at home in the sitting position and the intra-arterial tape was marked with an event signal.

Avionics, 1978 Pressurometer

Twenty patients were recruited from those undergoing intra-arterial recording. The only difference in the protocol from that for the Remler was that a standard mercury sphygmomanometer was used in place of the random zero sphygmomanometer, which could not be used with the Avionics Pressurometer as this instrument "searched" for the systolic pressure.

Morning and evening self-recorded blood pressures

Fourteen patients additionally measured their blood pressures in the supine position on awakening (defined as morning pressures) and in the supine position on going to bed (defined as evening pressures).

Self-recorded blood pressures during a clinical trial with verapamil and prazosin

Ten patients who were undergoing a clinical trial with the calcium ion antagonist verapamil were asked to record their blood pressures as described, before and after treatment with verapamil. A further 12 patients who were undergoing a clinical trial with prazosin also recorded their pressures.

Data Analysis

A hybrid computer was used to compute hourly mean intra-arterial blood pressure (3) and also a 1-min average systolic and diastolic pressure (3) and also a 1-min average systolic and diastolic pressure at each selected time marked by the event signal. Analysis was divided into assessment of pressures recorded away from hospital and clinic pressures recorded whilst attending hospital. A system to mark events on the intra-arterial tape was added mid-way through the home blood pressure study, enabling 27 patients to have clearly identifiable event marks corresponding to the exact time they recorded their blood pressure at home. In the laboratory, event marks were initially produced by disconnecting the intra-arterial transducer from the tape-recorder for a short period immediately prior to the indirect measurement.

The analyses of the Remler and Avionics recorders followed similar lines. Three pressures were selected at random from the home recordings and the corresponding 1-min mean intra-arterial pressure was digitized using the computer. The scope of this paper limits us to presenting data from the first of these three recordings. For each comparison the following information was calculated: mean and standard deviation of measurements by each method; mean, standard deviation and frequency distributions of between-method differences (the mean difference is referred to as the mean discrepancy). Only the lines of identity are shown on the scatter plots; regression lines and correlation coefficients are not presented. These are a measure of assocation only, and by definition the different methods of recording the blood pressure must be associated. Correlation gives no measure of the agreement of the different methods of blood pressure measurement nor information on precision or accuracy, and if misused may give misleading results (4). Differences between two methods were also assessed by Student's paired t-test.

Similarly, morning and evening self-recorded blood pressures were compared to mean daytime self-recorded and to intra-arterial blood pressures. The reductions in blood pressure as recorded by patients, the physician and intra-arterial measurement were similarly assessed.

Results

Analysis of the inter-arm differences showed that no patient had a mean difference greater than 10 mmHg and most had differences of less than 5 mmHg. In order to assess our methods of validation (i. e., the use of a 1-min mean intra-arterial pressure) we took records from 28 patients and for each patient a single reading was randomly selected. The systolic and diastolic points which were marked on the intra-arterial trace corresponded with the first Korotkoff sound and the point of dissappearance of Korotkoff sounds. These intra-arterial pressures were then compared with the average intra-arterial pressure over 1-min from which they were selected. The mean discrepancy was —2/2 mmHg (Table 1).

Table 1. Comparison of home, clinic and intra-arterial blood pressures

	Mean	SD	Mean Diff. A—B	SD of Diff.	P	N	Fig. No.
Systolic							
A. IABP (1-min mean)	162	28.7	—2	2.9	< 0.001	28	—
B. IABP (Beat-to-beat)	164	28.8					
A. Clinic BP	156	25.6	—13	16.2	< 0.001	55	1
B. IABP	169	26.6					
A. Home BP	164	37.8	0	23.0	> 0.9	27	2
B. IABP	164	32.6					
A. Patient BP	171	34.3	—2	5.9	> 0.5	31	3
B. Clinic BP	173	35.2					
Diastolic							
A. IABP (1-min mean)	88	15.4	—2	2.1	< 0.001	28	—
B. IABP (beat-to-beat)	90	15.2					
A. Clinic BP	95	17.7	1	13.0	> 0.5	55	1
B. IABP	94	13.0					
A. Home BP	97	14.4	3	16.7	> 0.2	27	2
B. IABP	94	16.5					
A. Patient BP	103	21.6	2	7.0	> 0.1	31	3
B. Clinic BP	101	19.4					

NB. Mean values have been rounded to whole numbers, thus the difference between mean values in column one may not correspond exactly with the mean difference in column 3. BP = blood pressure; IABP = intra-arterial blood pressure

Clinic blood pressure — intra-arterial blood pressure

The mean discrepancy for this comparison was —13/1 mmHg (Table 1). The scatter plot (Fig. 1) showed that the majority of systolic points lay above the line of identity whilst the diastolic points were more evenly distributed.

Home blood pressures

Blood pressures recorded by patients at home ("Home BP-Intra-arterial BP") compared to simultaneous intra-arterial blood pressure gave a mean discrepancy value of 0/3 mmHg (Table 1). The plot of "Home BP — Intra-arterial" (Fig. 2) showed a wide scatter of points. The number of patients included in this analysis was limited to 27, due to the late addition of the event marking systems.

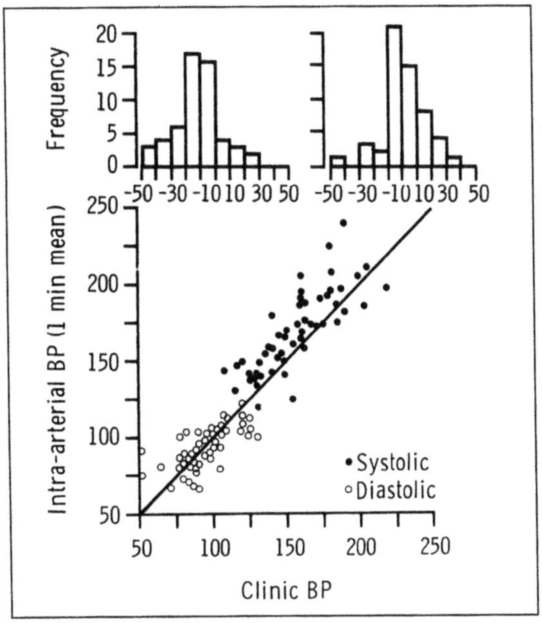

Fig. 1. Frequency histogram and scatter plot of Clinic BP — Intra-arterial BP (1 min mean). Frequency histogram: Systolic BP: 36% within ± 10 mmHg of the intra-arterial BP. Diastolic BP: 65% within ± 10 mmHg

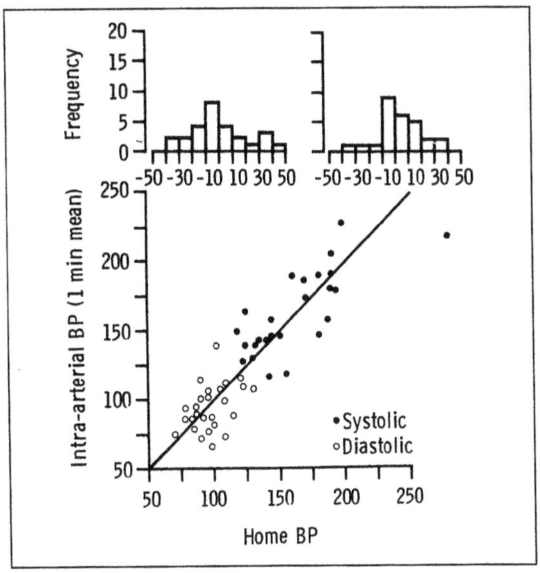

Fig. 2. Frequency histogram and scatter plot of Home BP — Intra-arterial BP (1 min mean). Systolic BP: 47% within ± 10 mmHg. Diastolic BP: 55% within ± 10 mmHg.

Comparison of the physician and patient recorded pressure (using a double listening stethoscope and anaeroid gauge) showed very good agreement with a mean discrepancy value "Patient BP — Clinic BP" of —22/2 mmHg (Table 1) confirmed by the scatter plot (Fig. 3).

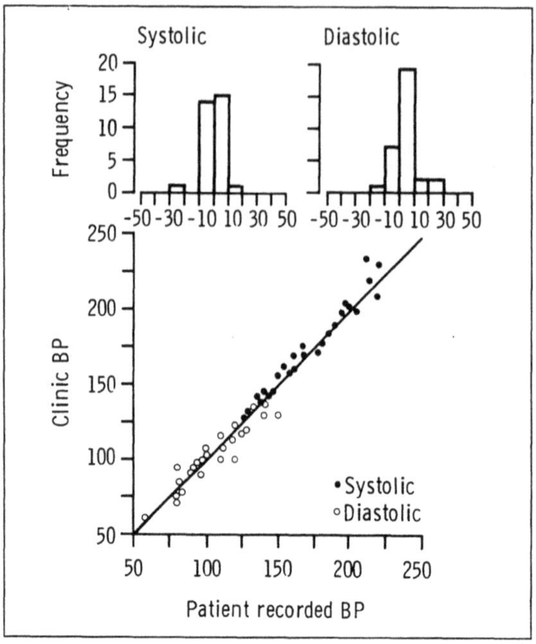

Fig. 3. Frequency histogram and scatter plot of patient-recorded BP — Clinic BP. Systolic BP: 93% within ± 10 mmHg. Diastolic BP: 83% within ± 10 mmHg.

Remler M2000

Away from the hospital environment the mean discrepancy "Intra-arterial BP — Remler was 1/2. mmHg (Table 2). The scatter plot (Fig. 4) showed wide deviation of the points from the line of identity but diastolic points were distributed more evenly. The mean discrepancy "Clinic BP — Remler" was —2/4 mmHg (Table 2). The plot was similar to Figure 4 and showed modest scatter around the line of identity with the majority of diastolic points lying below the line.

Avionics, 1978 Pressurometer

The pressurometer overestimated intra-arterial diastolic pressures at home with mean discrepancy values of —2/—11 mmHg (Table 2). The scatter plot, which was similar to that in to Fig. 4, showed even distribution of the systolic points around the line of identity but diastolic points lay above the line of identity, indicating higher Avionic recorded diastolic pressures.

The pressurometer overestimated indirect pressures. Table 2 shows that the mean discrepancy of the "Avionics pressurometer BP — Clinic BP" was 3/8 mmHg. The scatter plot was similar to Fig. 3 and showed fairly close grouping, but there were two systolic and three diastolic points which deviated widely.

Table 2. Comparison of Remler M2000, Avionics 1978 Pressurometer and intra-arterial blood pressure

	Mean	SD	Mean Diff. A—B	SD of Diff.	P	N	Fig. No.
Systolic							
A. IABP	159	31.2	−1	15.5	> 0.5	28	4
B. Remler	158	32.6					
A. Clinic BP	163	27.8	−2	9.9	> 0.05	28	—
B. Remler	163	30.3					
A. IABP	148	25.7	−2	15.9	> 0.05	18	—
B. Avionics	150	28.0					
A. Clinic BP	165	28.2	3	12.6	> 0.1	18	—
B. Avionics	162	32.3					
Diastolic							
A. IABP	93	22.4	2	11.6	> 0.2	28	4
B. Remler	92	17.8					
A. Clinic BP	99	15.6	4	5.9	< 0.001	28	—
B. Remler	95	14.1					
A. IABP	88	17.6	−11	12.3	< 0.01	18	—
B. Avionics	99	18.1					
A. Clinic BP	102	13.2	8	18.3	> 0.05	18	—
B. Avionics	94	16.9					

Abbreviations as in Table 1.

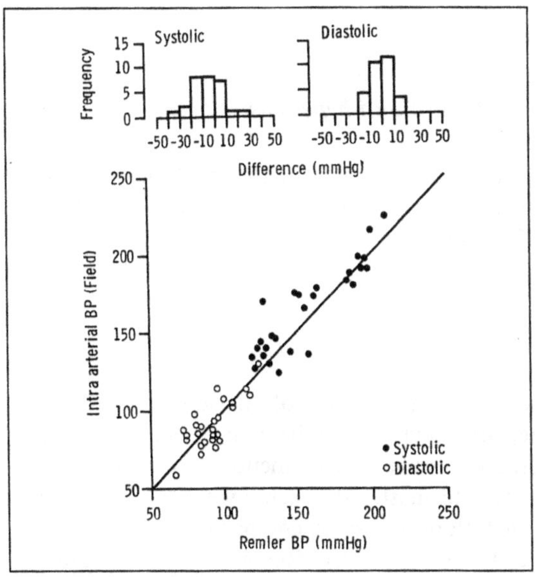

Fig. 4. Frequency histogram and scatter plot of Remler M2000 — Intra-arterial BP. Systolic BP: 54% within ± 10 mmHg. Diastolic BP: 78% within ± 10 mmHg.

Morning and evening pressures

The scatter plot (Fig. 5) and data (Table 3) demonstrated that the mean differences for morning supine Home BP and evening supine Home BP, compared with mean daytime home blood pressure, were not accurately reflected as far as the individual was concerned.

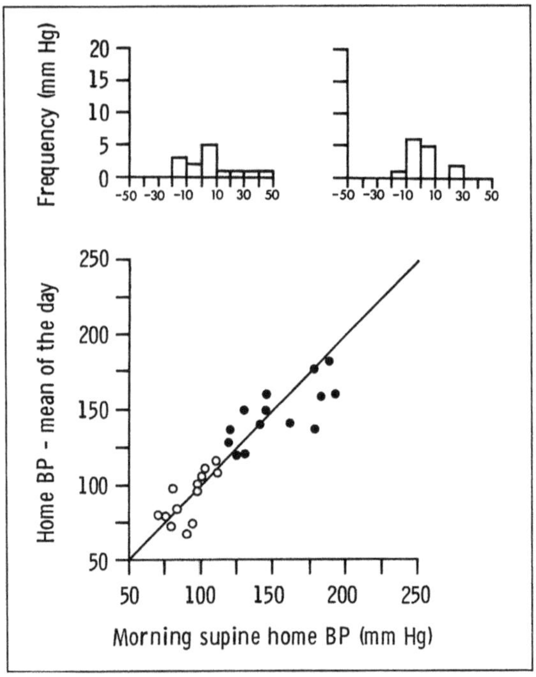

Fig. 5. Frequency histogram and scatter plot of morning supine blood pressure — Home blood pressure mean of that day. Systolic BP: 50% within ± 10 mmHg. Diastolic BP within ± 10 mmHg.

Self-recorded pressures, during a clinical trial of anti-hypertensive agents

Generally, there was poor agreement between different methods of blood pressure measurement in individual patients but as far as the group was concerned generally good agreement was observed (Fig. 6 and Table 4).

Discussion

Despite the limited information concerning the accuracy of the indirect methods of ambulatory blood pressure monitoring, these methods are being increasingly advocated (5, 6). In the study of self-recorded blood pressure measurements, no patients were excluded and only two patients were unable to master the technique. There was a wide variation in the accuracy of self-recorded blood pressures compared with intra-arterial recordings with occasional individual differences of nearly 50 mmHg. There was no dif-

Table 3. Means and mean differences of morning and evening supine home blood pressures

	N	Mean	SD	Mean Difference	SD of Differences	P
a. Morning Supine						
Systolic						
Morning	14	153	27.2	5	19.0	> 0.2
HBP (mean of day)		147	19.5			
Morning	14	153	27.2	—9	21.6	> 0.2
IABP (mean daytime)		162	27.4			
Diastolic						
Morning	14	92	12.7	0	10.9	> 0.9
HBP (mean of day)		92	15.9			
Morning	14	92	12.7	7	11.1	< 0.05
IABP (mean daytime)		85	11.4			
b. Evening Supine						
Systolic						
Evening	10	149	20.0	0	13.3	> 0.9
HBP (mean of day)		149	24.8			
Evening	10	149	20.0	—12	17.8	> 0.05
IABP (mean daytime)		161	29.6			
Diastolic						
Evening	10	88	16.7	—3	7.9	> 0.2
(mean of day)		91	18.2			
Evening	10	88	16.7	6	12.1	> 0.1
IABP (mean daytime)		82	12.3			

Abbreviations as in Table 1.

Table 4. Changes, in blood pressure recorded by different methods: after treatment with verapamil (n = 10) and with prazosin (n = 12)

	Verapamil		Prazosin	
	Mean change	SD	Mean change	SD
Intra-arterial	23/19	112.3/10.1	18/5	19.2/9.6
Clinic BP	38*/20	13.6/10.1	28/18*	21.5/8.5
Home BP	24/16	17.9/7.3	21/6	20.5/13.7

* $p < 0.05$; ** $p < 0.01$

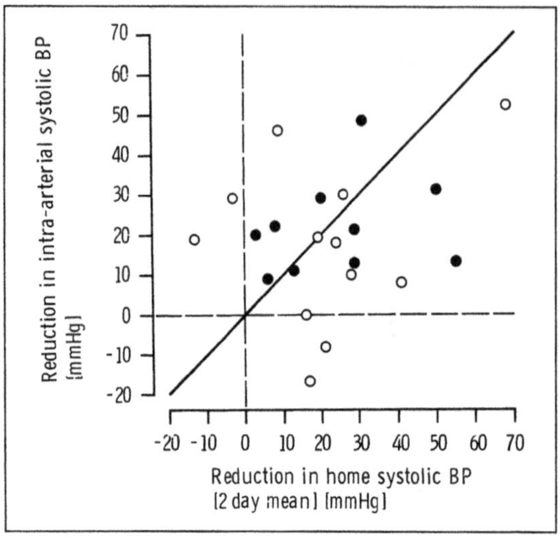

Fig. 6a. Scatter plot of systolic blood pressure changes recorded by home BP (2 day mean) vs Intra-arterial BP (mean daytime).

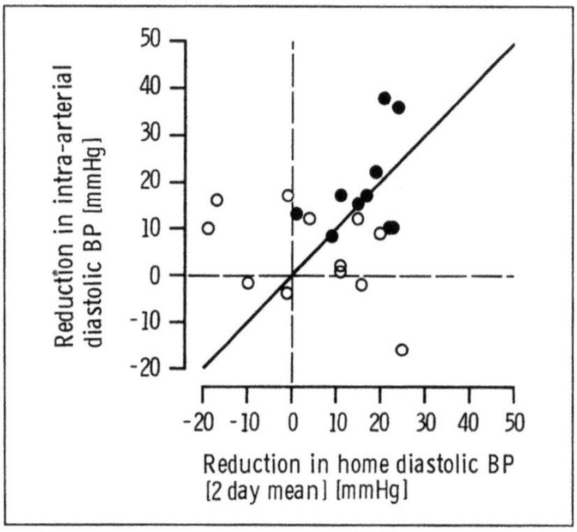

Fig. 6b. Scatter plot of diastolic blood pressure changes recorded by home BP (2 day mean) vs Intra-arterial BP (mean daytime).

ference in the relationship between self-recorded and clinic blood pressure measurements when compared to intra-arterial ambulatory blood pressures. There was good agreement of both indirect techniques as has been previously noted (5, 7, 8).

The Remler M2000 and Avionics 1978 pressurometer both showed a similar relationship to intra-arterial pressures when compared with self-recorded pressures. The comparison of Remler — Clinic BP showed less scatter than did the similar comparison of Avionics — Clinic BP. The Avionics Pressurometer when compared to intra-arterial blood pressure also over-estimated the diastolic pressure to a greater degree than the similar comparison for the Remler M2000.

These data show that indirect methods provide estimates of the intra-arterial pressure which may be inaccurate by as much as 50 mmHg. Of the three methods self-recorded pressures showed the closest agreement with standard indirect pressures indicating automated machines provide little advantage over self-recorded home blood pressure measurements. Self-recorded pressures recorded by patients on awakening and on going to bed (as used by epidemiologists (7)) do not relate well to mean daytime pressure and serial measurements are therefore advised. The reduction in self-recorded blood pressures during clinical trials agreed well with intra-arterial pressures as far as a group of patients was concerned but showed variable accuracy in each individual. This method is a useful tool for the assessment of the efficacy of anti-hypertensive agents in a group of patients. All indirect ambulatory methods are subject to the same inaccuracies as clinic (office) measurements. An accurate method for assessing blood pressure variability remains to be described.

References

1. Kirkendall WM, Burton AC, Epstein FH, Freis ED (1967) Recommendations for human blood pressure determination by sphygmomanometers. Circulation 36: 980—988.
2. Millar-Craig MW, Hawes D, Whittington J (1978) New system for recording ambulatory blood pressure in man. Med Biol Eng Comput 16: 727—731
3. Cashman PMM, Stott FD, Millar-Craig MW (1979) Hybrid system for fast data reduction on long term blood pressure recordings. Med Biol Eng Comput 17: 629—635
4. Bland MJ, Altman DG (1986) Statistical methods for assessing agreement between two methods of clinical measurement. Lancet 1: 307—310
5. Julius S, Ellis CN, Pascaul AV, Matice M, Hansson L, Hunyor SN, Sandler LN. Home blood pressure determination value in borderline ("labile") hypertension. J Am Med Assoc 229: 663—666, 1974
6. Laughlin KD, Fisher L, Sherrard DJ. Blood pressure reductions during self-recording of home blood pressure. Am Heart J 98: 629—634, 1979
7. Joossens JV, Brems-Heyns E, Claessens J (1976) In: Kesteloff W (ed) Commission of the European Communities Biological Sciences — Medical Research. Methodology and standardisation of non-invasive blood pressure measurement in epidemiological studies. Proceeding of a workshop in Leuven (Belgium), Commission of the European Communities, Directorate General "Research and Education"
8. Laughlin KD, Sherrard DJ, Fisher L (1980) Comparison of clinic and home blood pressure levels in essential hypertension and variables associated with clinic home differences. J Chron Dis 33: 197—206

Finapres, continuous noninvasive finger arterial pressure based on the method of Peñáz

K. H. Wesseling

TNO Biomedical Instrumentation, AMC, Amsterdam, The Netherlands

Twenty-one years ago, in 1967, Docent dr Jan Peñáz submitted a patent description of a method to measure indirectly the full arterial pressure waveform in a finger using a volume clamp technique, and at the 10th Conference on Medical and Biological Engineering at Dresden in 1973 (9), he actually demonstrated a device and published a one-page abstract on his new, important invention. In 1976 a small group of medical physicists of the TNO organization in The Netherlands began an R and D effort, first to copy the Peñáz device on the basis of his 1973 abstract, then to understand the physics and physiology of the method, and finally to construct a fully automatic device which could be used reliably and with confidence in the clinic.

The Peñáz technique

When the volume of an artery is fixed, clamped, at its unstressed but non-zero diameter, the transmural pressure, the pressure difference across the arterial wall is zero. At that state, regardless of the level of intraarterial pressure, the pressure inside and in the medium outside the artery are identical. Extraarterial pressure then is an indirect measure of intraarterial pressure. To clamp arteries in this way is not a new idea (5). However, clamping the arterial volume noninvasively can only be done by clamping the total finger volume and this is not possible to a sufficient accuracy in practice (11). Knowing the problems with earlier finger volume clamp techniques, Peñáz reasoned that the actual arterial volume could be measured photoelectrically and then be clamped at a constant level via an inflatable cuff by means of an electropneumatic servo system, regardless of the actual finger volume (9). An essential and major problem remaining is how to establish the actual arterial diameter or volume setpoint at which the artery is unstressed, at which transmural pressure is zero, and at which cuff pressure is identical to intraarterial pressure. A block diagram of the photoelectric arterial volume clamp method is shown in Fig. 1.

The Finapres instrument

It was found relatively early in the project at TNO, as soon as we had a primitive laboratory model working, that the operator of the instrument needed to be an expert to find the proper volume clamp level, or setpoint. The operator needed to be patient,

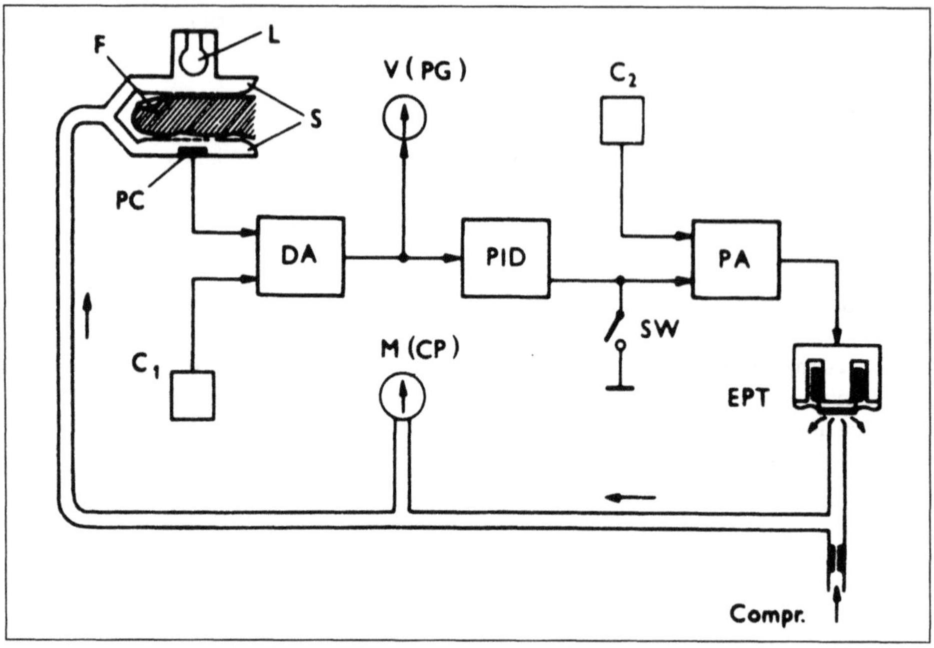

Fig. 1. Original block diagram of the method, drawn by Peňáz. The arrows in the diagram trace a servo control loop. A finger, F, is placed in cuff, S. The finger is transilluminated by a lamp, L, and observed by a photocell, PC. Changes in the photocell output are compared to the servo setpoint, C1, amplified in DA, PID and PA to drive a fast responding proportional valve, EPT. Cuff pressure is monitored by manometer M. The servoloop can be opened by closing switch, SW, and steady cuff pressure set with C2.

in addition, and approximate proof that the proper setpoint was found could only be obtained from comparison with an invasively obtained waveform at another site. In practice, our manually performed algorithm yielded satisfactory and repeatable *setpoints* by trained personnel in about 80% of a first series of hypertensive subjects. This was promising indeed, but insufficient for full scale application in the medical environment. We concluded that a clinically useful instrument had to be fully automatic, and had to include an intelligent algorithm to find the setpoint. Further, proof had to be found for the correctness of the setpoint arrived at by this or any other algorithm. The latter aspect of the development will not be discussed here.

We then went through the construction of a series of improved prototypes, each one extensively tested clinically, in different circumstances, on different patients.

Prototype 1 had an improved very high speed *servo system* including a novel, patented proportional valve of such small size that it could be mounted near the subjects finger and be connected to the cuff with only a short length of tubing.

Prototype 2 contained a microprocessor and a primitive algorithm to find a setpoint automatically. Therefore, full manual operation was retained.

Prototype 3 had an *infrared plethysmograph* using modulated light, which made it insensitive to ambient light. The plethysmograph included a patented method to compensate for temperature drift of its sensitivity. The setpoint algorithm soon became professional.

However, it was found that the volume clamp setpoint itself was not constant, but changed with the physiology of the finger circulation and the state of the patient. An initially primitive method was programmed to follow such physiologic changes in setpoint automatically.

Prototype 4 was a 50% smaller package. It contained two special purpose-built, patented expert systems to find the setpoint and to follow its changes. The systems in fact operated more precisely and reliably and faster than a human expert. The possibility of manual operation was discontinued in these instruments. After a continuous parallel development process of almost 6 years, the finger cuffs also reached a final form. As a series of 10 prototypes, model 4 was constructed and tested at major clinical sites in Germany, the USA, and the Netherlands mostly in the operating room.

Prototype 5 or rather model 5, is shown in Fig. 2. Its size is reduced by another 50%. It is fully self contained with a built-in air supply and *hardcopy output* via a *dot matrix printer/plotter.* The model 5 algorithms and expert systems, although not fundamentally different from those of prototype 4, are improved on numerous points. Its has single button start/stop operation. A further two buttons control the chart range and speed of the printer/plotter and two buttons control three forms of calibration. Model 5 also has a system for full electrical patient isolation. Five analog outputs are provided. One output

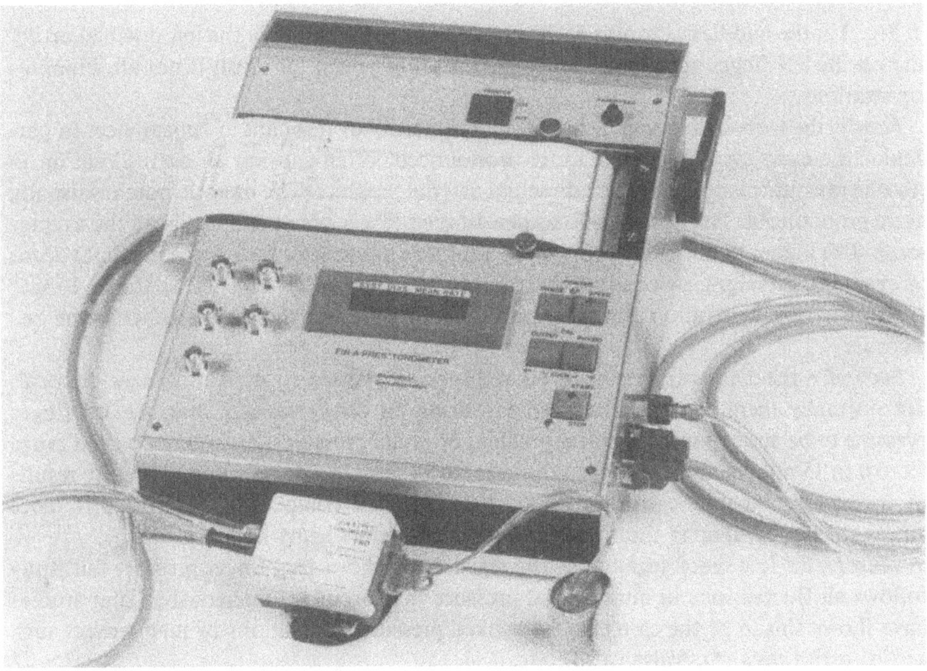

Fig. 2. The model 5 Finapres tonometer built by TNO Biomedical Instrumentation. The instrument is operated by a single START/STOP button. Three forms of calibration are selected by two CAL buttons. Two further buttons control the dot matrix printer/plotter on whose output chart, unfortunately, no waveform is yet visible. Five analog BNC connectors output the continuous waveform and the beat to beat systolic, diastolic and mean pressure levels and pulse rate. The small frontend box contains the valve, EPT, the plethysmographic preamplifiers and manometer M. The wrapable inflatable cuff has a built-in infrared LED, L, and photodiode, PC. It must be positioned with care in the way shown diagrammatically on the front-end box.

is the finger arterial pressure wave form. Four further outputs provide the beat-to-beat derived values of systolic, diastolic and mean pressure and of pulse rate. An RS 232C serial interface is optionally available. It allows full remote control of the instrument via a computer or PC in addition to outputting the beat-to-beat derived values. A series of these instruments have been built and copies are now under evaluation in Belgium, Finland, Germany, Great Britain, Italy and The Netherlands, and by ESA, in non-operating room situations. The instrument measures true *fin*ger *a*rterial *pres*sure and this can actually be proven in an indirect fashion. The instrument is therefore called FIN.A.PRES. This name is now a commercial trade mark*).

Although the operation of Finapres is automatic, requiring only the careful wrapping of a finger cuff and pressing the start/stop button, some knowledge of the properties and fundamental limitations of the method is desirable. Limitations of the method can be referred to a single basic fact: finger arterial pressure is not identical to aortic pressure. Finger pressure simply does not translate to more proximal arterial pressures, such as aortic, brachial or radial, in a one-to-one manner, even though deviations are usually small.

Some examples of Finapres results

In Fig. 3 in the middle two traces a 150 s registration of pressure in the left brachial artery and on the left finger are shown. The registration is typical for most, if not all, Finapres registrations.

Firstly, the waveform is somewhat more undulatory or resonant in appearance. In particular the early systolic peak is more pronounced, often causing an overestimation in systolic pressure compared to intrabrachial arterial pressure. The dicrotic notch is usually more pronounced. The upstroke is steeper. In fact, finger pressure dp/dt is on the average some 40% higher than brachial. In young adults we sometimes recorded a maximal dp/dt of over 4000 mmHg/s, twice as much as a normal dp/dt (max) in the left ventricle. Finger pressure in this registration also seems advanced in time, but this is an artifact of the pen recorder.

Secondly, the diastolic pressure levels in this particular registration are nearly identical, but normally there is a pressure gradient along an artery causing downstream finger pressure to be about 6 mmHg below brachial or radial pressures, on average, with a range from 0 to 15 mmHg and a standard deviation of 4 mmHg. These numbers are the results of invasive, comparative studies (2, 6, 10). One can compensate for this difference automatically by placing the finger about 10 cm below heart level.

Thirdly, the low speed segment of the registration shows that finger pressure faithfully follows all fluctuations in intraarterial pressure that occur spontaneously. Later studies have shown this to be the case also for evoked pressure fluctuations by manoeuvres such as tilt, orthostasis (4), Valsalva (3), etc.

The *photoplethysmogram*, pp, of the bottom trace in Fig. 3 shows the arterial volume pulsation remaining after the volume clamp. In other words, the volume clamp is not perfect, but typically shows a slight rest deviation or servo error. The scale is arbitrary

*) Of Ohmeda Monitoring Systems, Englewood, Colorado, USA, which sell the instrument as the Ohmeda Model 2300 Finapres™ BP Monitor.

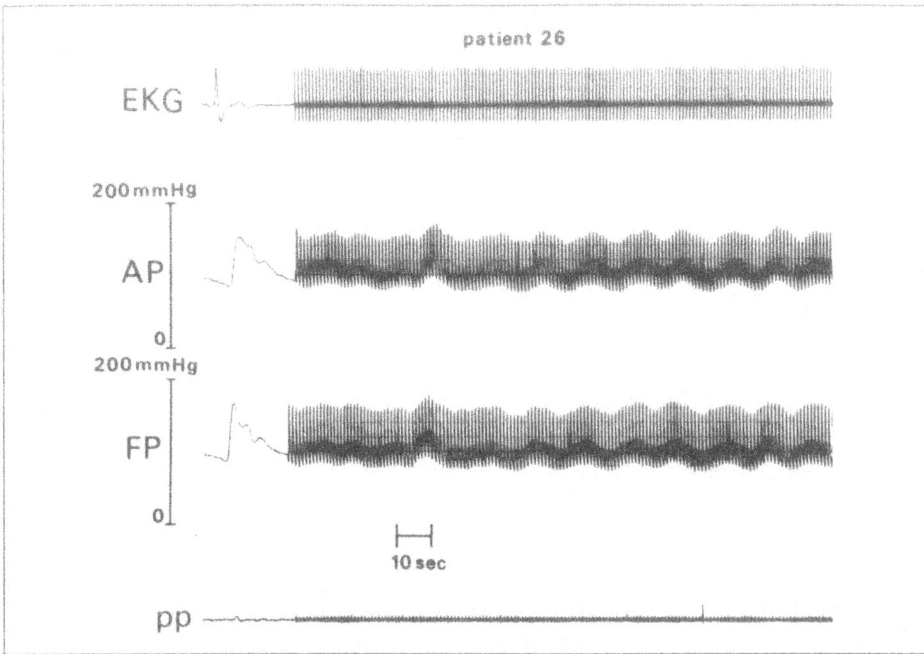

Fig. 3. An ECG and the intraarterial, AP, and finger pressure, FP, traces showing typical waveforms and fluctuations in pressure. pp is the small servo error signal remaining after the servoloop is closed.

but in this case pulsations are less than 5% of the open loop, unclamped, arterial plethysmogram. An open loop / closed loop ratio of 5 to 1 suffices in the majority of cases to obtain a negligible error in the determination of the systolic and diastolic levels of finger pressure. A ratio of 20 to 1 guarantees this in all cases.

Figure 4 compares in detail the intraarterial and finger systolic, mean and diastolic levels. The upper two traces are finger (upper) and intraarterial (next) systolic pressures determined beat-to-beat, low pass filtered at 0.5 Hz. Finger systolic pressure typically, overestimates intrabrachial pressure. The slight downdrift of 4 mmHg in 200 s is not typical for present day instruments, although up or downdrifts occur occasionally, due to slow relaxation or contraction of the finger arterial vascular smooth muscle. The same drift can be noted in the mean and diastolic traces. Close inspection of the traces reveals that each undulation, large or small, in each level is present in both finger and intrabrachial pressures. A *Fourier spectral estimate* based on three 200 s epochs of mean pressure, after baseline removal (1), is shown in the right panel. The larger spectrum is from finger pressure. Typically, finger spectral densities can be some 10% to 20% higher than brachial, and this is most pronounced in the spectral peak near 0.1 Hz. Thus it follows that within-subject differences in pressure are rather small if compared to direct arterial pressure.

Figure 5 is a further expression of this fact. In the left panel are some 20 comparisons of systolic and diastolic levels in a hypertensive subject taken on single, simultaneous waves 20 s apart over a 400 s epoch. The scatter is very small. In the right panel are shown such comparisons in 21 hypertensive subjects (6), in which individual patient scatter-

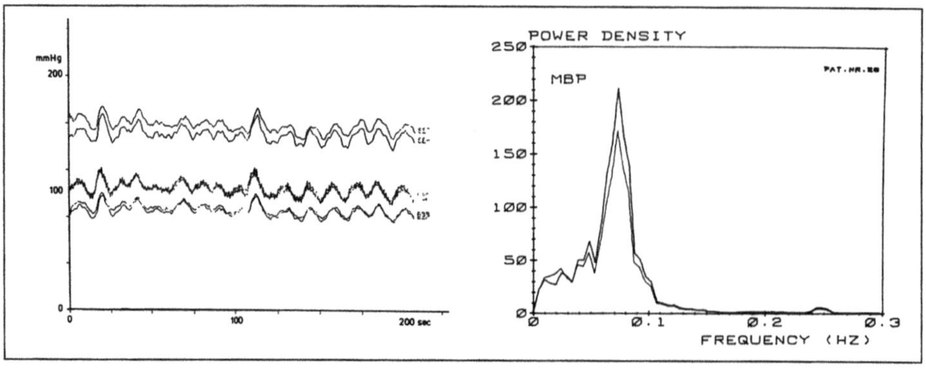

Fig. 4. Computer analysis of signals such as shown in Fig. 3. The systolic, mean and diastolic levels for arterial and finger pressure are plotted on the same scale in the left panel, showing close reproduction of the fluctuations. The panel on the right is the estimated power spectral density of mean pressure fluctuations obtained from three such epochs of 200 s duration. The finger spectral estimate is the larger of the two. Typically finger pressure fluctuations are 10% to 20% greater than intraarterial in this frequency range.

grams are averaged to a single value each for systolic and diastolic pressure. Scatter between patients, here, is clearly much larger than within patients. A two way ANOVA shows the variance ratio is 50 for systolic, 14 for diastolic, in this study. Thus, although variability of blood pressure in any one patient under constant conditions is clearly followed well, there are individual offsets in the estimation of the levels. Even though these differences do not seem larger than the errors of any other noninvasive method, and although they are operator independent — or objective — they may be clinically significant when interpreting finger pressure as "the" arterial pressure; then they become errors.

In using Finapres as a substitute for pressure at a more upstream site in the arterial system, two major effects are present:

1. The arterial system in the arm is nonhomogeneous. It shows reflections of the pulse wave at various sites along the arteries due to side branches and termination in the arterioles and due to a gradual taper of the arterial cross-sectional area and elastic modulus. This causes increasing distortion of the waveform towards peripheral which is most noticeable in an increased pulse pressure and in systolic pressure overshoot. The problem is that this effect is not fully predictable. It decreases with increasing age of the subject (7), with increasing level of the subjects blood pressure, i.e. it is less in hypertensive patients, and it decreases with increasing peripheral flow (14). Figure 6 is an illustration of the diminishing effect of hypertension on this distortion. The panel on the left is a registration in a hypertensive subject (blood pressure 200/90). The waveforms are practically identical, albeit with an emphasized dicrotic notch in the finger pressure tracing. Finger pulse amplitude is slightly less (by about 7%) than the brachial pulsation. In the basically normotensive subject recorded in the right panel (blood pressure 140/70) the finger pulse is more distorted and the pulse amplitude is enhanced (by about 25%) with respect to intrabrachial.

2. The arterial system in the arm has an internal resistance to flow. This causes a

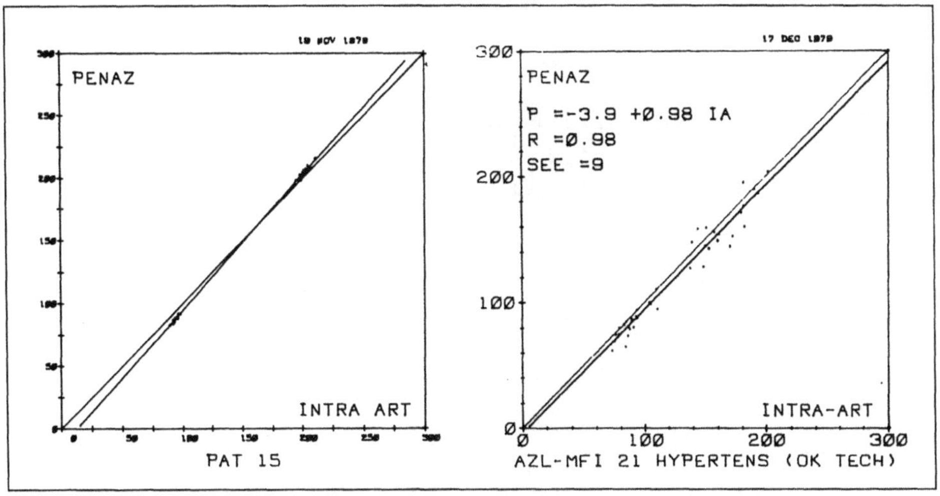

Fig. 5. Comparisons of finger pressure, PEÑÁZ, with intraarterial pressures in one hypertensive subject (left panel) and in 21 hypertensive subjects (right panel). To obtain the single point values in the right panel, all measurements such as shown on the left panel were averaged per patient, separately for systolic and diastolic. The within-subject variance over the 400-s observation period per patient, is obviously much smaller than between subjects.

pressure gradient along the arm arteries to exist which is greater when flow is increased and when the arterial diameter is decreased (Poiseuille's law). Most of the pressure drop occurs in the last 10 cm to the finger. On average, in normal conditions this causes a pressure difference between brachial or radial and finger pressure of 6 mmHg. However, under special circumstances such as occur during open heart surgery — low pump pressures, absence of pulsations and total body cooling may have caused contraction of the peripheral arterial and venous systems but blood flow is increased due to hemodilution and vasodilators administered — the pressure gradient can be so great that even pressures measured in the radial artery can no longer be trusted to reflect aortic pressures.

The effect of enhanced peripheral resistance is increased mean and pulse pressures as is illustrated in Fig. 7, recorded in an anesthetized patient undergoing gynaecological surgery. The upper trace is finger arterial pressure. The lower trace shows an infrared skin reflection plethysmogram taken on an adjacent finger. The amplitude of these pulsations is usually a linear, zero crossing measure of blood flow (8). An invasive blood pressure registration was not indicated in these patients, but finger pressures were verified with a Dinamap oscillometric measurement on the upper arm. For further details, see Wesseling et al. (14). In both cases of a sudden decrease in the plethysmogram, and thus in flow, a very clear, equally sudden increase in finger pressure is present. Note that both systolic and diastolic pressure levels rise, but systolic rises more than diastolic. Mean pressure, roughly at the level of the dicrotic notch in the finger pressure waveform, and pulse pressure are increased. It can also be noted very clearly that systolic pressure reaches preconstriction levels at the same time as the plethysmographic amplitude does. It was found in later animal studies that radial arterial pressure also shows this phenomenon, but to a lesser degree. Aortic pressure does not (Dorlas, unpublished communication). It is

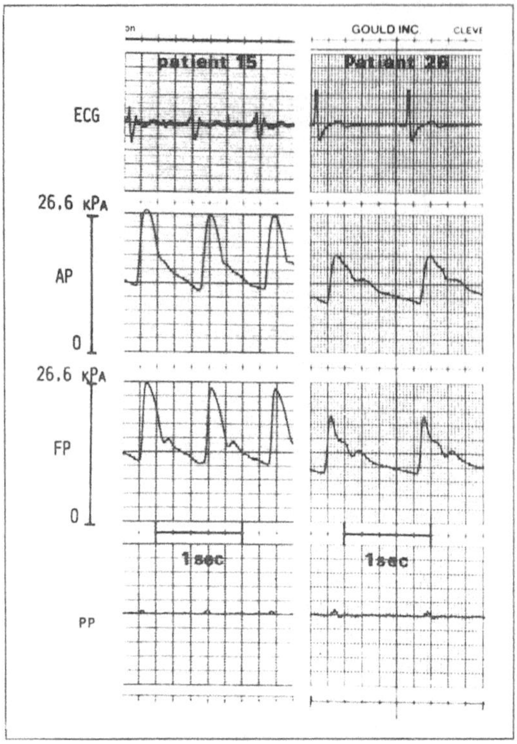

Fig. 6. Arterial, AP, and finger pressure, FP, waveforms in two subjects, one hypertensive (left panel), one normotensive (right panel). Typically, finger waveform reproduction of brachial pressures is more faithful in hypertensive subjects.

purely an effect of the altering hemodynamic conditions along the arm arteries. Changes in the pressure gradient thus produce a systematic difference which is unpredictable except when flow is simultaneously measured. The approximate peak-to-peak difference for mean pressure, from maximal flow to minimal flow, is about 10 mmHg.

The effect illustrated in Fig. 7 was already noted in 1980 (10) but an explanation was not available at the time. Figure 8 shows a clear example in a patient undergoing surgery for aortic valve replacement (AVR). The operation lasted almost 6 h, and a total of 133 measurements on mean pressure were taken, one every 160 s. The left panel in the figure reproduces the scattergram of left intraarterial (radial) pressure horizontally, and ipsilateral finger pressure vertically. Mean pressure in this patient varied from 18 to 138 mmHg, averaging 81 mmHg. The mean pressure difference between finger and radial artery was 4.2 $\pm$ 5.1 mmHg, ranging from -8 to +18 mmHg. The regression slope was 0.98 and the correlation coefficient 0.97. However, two clearly separated clusters can be seen, the lower one when finger mean pressure was almost on the line of identity, the upper cluster when finger pressure was about 10 mmHg higher than radial. In the interpretation of these figures it should be realized that the finger rested on the operating table about 10 cm (or an equivalent 7.5 mmHg) below heart level. Therefore, about 7 mmHg must be subtracted from the numbers. The right panel shows the time-course of these differences. The upper trace gives intraarterial pressure during the course of the operation. The lower trace shows the difference between finger and intraarterial pressure. Typically during the final period of the operation finger pressure is relatively high, sug-

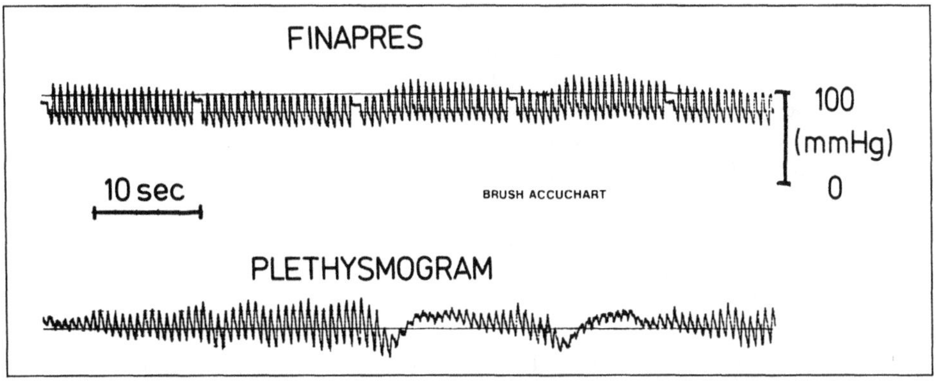

Fig. 7. Simultaneous registration of finger arterial pressure, FINAPRES, and a photoelectric skin reflection plethysmogram on an adjacent finger, PLETHYSMOGRAM, showing the coherence between the amplitude reduction in the plethysmogram and the increase in finger pressure.

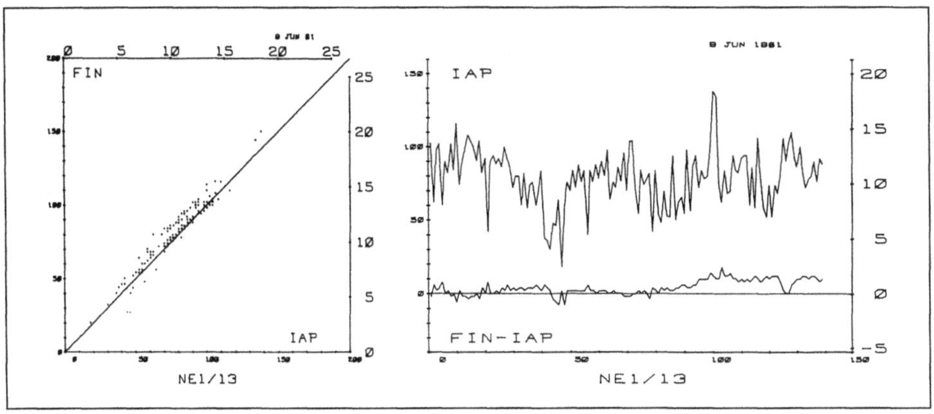

Fig. 8. Comparison of finger mean pressure, FIN, with intraradial, IAP, in a subject undergoing an AVR operation. Scales are in mm Hg and kPa. The left panel shows the scattergram with two distinct scatter groups. The right panel shows this to be an effect ordered in time.

gesting a low pressure gradient subsequent to a low peripheral flow state. Also note the lack of correlation between the difference trace and the absolute level of the pressure.

The excellent linearity of the Peñáz method, not only for mean pressure but also for systolic and diastolic is demonstrated in Fig. 9, recorded in the same study in a patient undergoing a coronary artery bypass graft (CABG) operation lasting 5 1/2 h. A total of 123 comparisons were made, with mean pressures ranging from 16 to 138 mmHg, average 67 mmHg. Average pressure difference was -0.2 $\pm$ 6.3 mmHg ranging from -14 to +14 mm Hg. The regression slope was 0.98 and the correlation coefficient 0.96. The left panel reproduces the mean pressure scattergram as before. At every fifth sample systolic/diastolic readings were also taken, i.e. at instants 800 s apart. Of course, no systolic and diastolic pressures were available when the patient was on total heart-lung bypass. Thus a total of 18 comparisons remained. The systolic average was 117 mmHg with pressures ranging from 54 to 184 mmHg, the average difference was -3.6 ± 7.7 mmHg, the regression slope was 0.97 and the correlation was also 0.97. For diastolic these values were average 54 mmHg, range 18 to 92, difference -2.7 ± 7.2 mmHg, slope 0.83, correlation coefficient 0.89. Thus over a very large pressure range, finger pressures bear an essentially linear relationship to upstream intraarterial pressures.

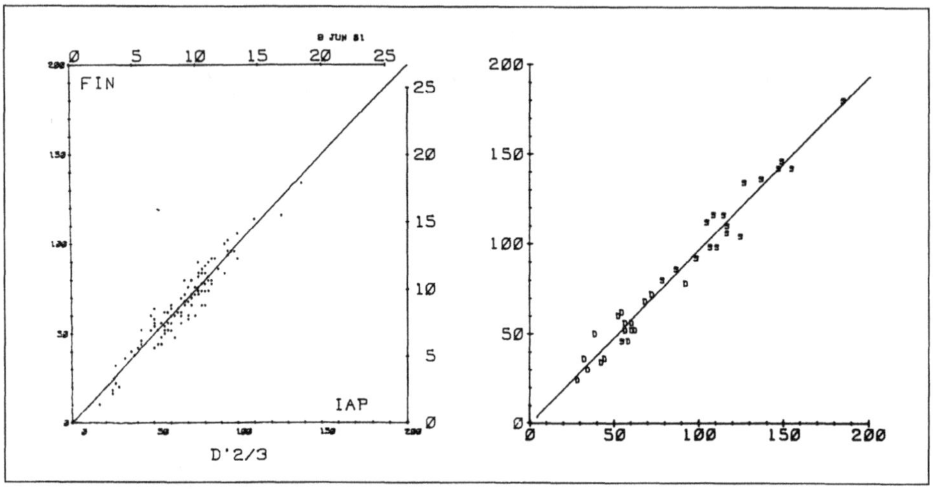

Fig. 9. Comparison of mean (left panel) and systolic and diastolic (right panel) finger with intraradial pressures in a subject undergoing a CABG operation. The linearity of Finapres over a wide range of pressures at each level is clearly demonstrated.

In patients with severe proximal arteriosclerotic lesions, however, a good linear relationship with small scatter is not obtained. In Fig. 10 comparisons are shown in a patient undergoing a left carotid-subclavian bypass operation. Intraarterial pressure was recorded on the right. Left finger pressure is plotted in the left panel of the figure vs right radial pressure. Right finger pressure is plotted right. Clearly, a large scatter in left mean pressure is shown, with a preponderance of finger pressures underestimating contralateral radial, due to the lesion. After the bypass is in place, full finger pressure is restored and comparisons are near the line of identity. In older patients in particular, one should be aware of the possibility of such lesions and, when feasible, measure finger pressure both left and right. With experience, hemodynamically significant lesions can be spotted from the long rise time of the finger pressure upstroke. Usually the right arm is the site of choice as it is also recommended for Riva-Rocci/Korotkoff measurements — although for other reasons. The costo-clavicular compression syndrome can cause similar finger pressure underestimates, and should be suspected in cases of erratic, suddenly increased or decreased finger pressures.

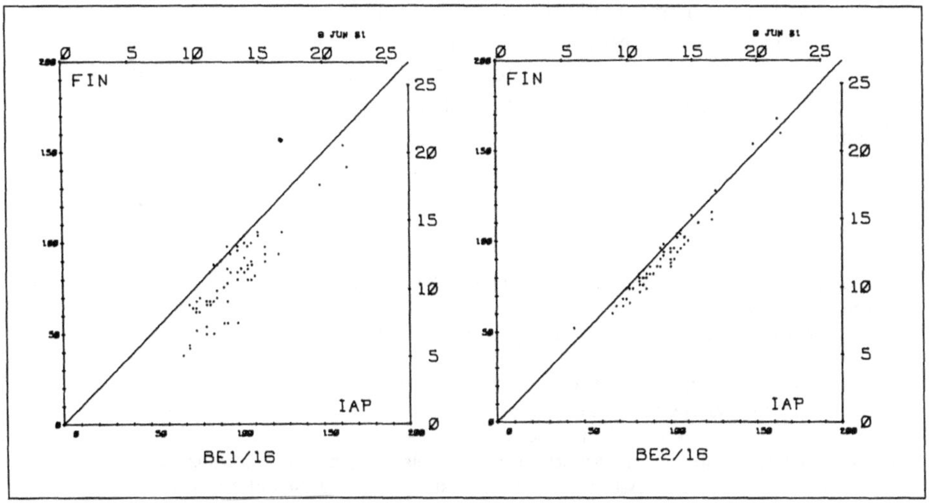

Fig. 10. Left and right finger pressures compared with right intraradial pressure in a subject with a subclavian artery lesion of hemodynamic significance. Left finger pressures are substantially below contralateral pressures until a carotid-subclavian bypass is in place.

Conclusion

The most important properties of finger pressure measurements with Finapres devices were mentioned, demonstrated by way of examples. They have to do with two aspects of the acral measurement site:

1. Reflections of the pulse wave occur in the arm arterial system causing the finger pressure waveform to be undulatory or resonant, with an enhanced dicrotic notch, an early systolic overshoot, increased pulse pressure, and steeper upstrokes than in the brachial artery. Reflection effects are stronger in the young, in normotensives, and at low peripheral flow states of the arm circulation.

2. Pressure gradients due to viscous flow in the narrow peripheral arteries cause decreased finger pressure levels compared to more upstream, plus enhanced fluctuation spectral density. Pressure differences average at about -6 mm Hg, range 0 to -15 mm Hg and, for an average person, can be compensated hydrostatically by placing the finger about 10 cm below heart level. The pressure difference increases with increasing peripheral flow.

Finapres produces clean waveforms, is relatively insensitive to motion artifact, measures true finger arterial pressure and is linear over a wide range of pressures. Proximal arteriosclerotic lesions of hemodynamic significance are seldomly seen. When present they are easily spotted as they are characterized by a slow pulse wave upstroke. Expert systems programmed to run on the built-in microprocessor establish a proper setpoint for the servoloop and adapt the setpoint to the changing physiology of the circulation under the cuff. In particular this is the case when the smooth muscle in the finger arterial wall changes its contractional state, and thereby arterial unstressed volume (12, 13). This system is called the Physio-cal system. It also corrects for changes in the color of the blood (oxygenation), for hemodilution and for washout of red blood cells in the microcirculatory compartment. Physio-cal further detects the moment when full arterial contraction is approaching and when it has occurred. It then signals the operator that finger pressures can no longer be interpreted in terms of arterial pressure. Without the Physio-cal system finger pressure measurements cannot be performed reliably and with confidence.

References

1. Bendat JS, Piersol AG (1971) Random data: Analysis and measurement procedures. Wiley Interscience, New York
2. van Egmond J, Hasenbos M, Crul JF (1985) Invasive vs noninvasive measurement of arterial pressure. Br J Anaesth 57: 434—444
3. Imholz BPM, van Montfrans GA, Settels JJ, van der Hoeven GMA, Wieling W, Karemaker JM. (1988) Continuous, noninvasive finger arterial pressure during the Valsalva manoeuvre compared to intrabrachial arterial pressure. Cardiovase Res 22; 390-397
4. van Lieshout JJ, Wieling W, van Montfrans GA, Settels JJ, Speelman JD, Endert E, Karemaker JM (1986) Acute dysautonomia associated with Hodgkin's disease. J Neurol Neurosurg Psychiatry 49: 830—832
5. Marey EJ (1878) La Methode Graphique. G Masson, Paris
6. Molhoek PG, Wesseling KH, Settels JJ, van Vollenhoven E, Weeda HWH, Arntzenius AC (1984) Evaluation of the Peñáz servoplethysmomanometer for the continuous, noninvasive measurement of finger blood pressure. Basic Res Cardiol 79: 598—609
7. O'Rourke MF (1970) Influence of ventricular ejection on the relationship between central aortic and brachial pressure pulse in man. Cardiovasc Res 4: 291—300
8. De Pater L, van den Berg JW, Bueno AA (1962) A very sensitive photoplethysmograph using scattered light and a photosensitive resistance. Acta Physiol Pharmacol Neerlandica 10: 378—390
9. Peñáz J (1973) Photoelectric measurement of blood pressure, volume and flow in the finger. Digest 10th Int Conf Med Biol Engng, Dresden, p 104
10. Smith NT, Wesseling KH, de Wit B (1985) Evaluation of two prototype devices producing noninvasive, pulsatile calibrated blood pressure from a finger. J Clin Monit 1: 17—29
11. Vendrik AJH, Vierhout RR (1959) Die unblutige Registrierung des Blutdrucks: Theoretische Betrachtungen. Pflügers Arch 268: 496—504
12. Wesseling KH (1984) Noninvasive continuous blood pressure waveform measurement by the method of Peñáz. Scripta Medica 57: 321—334
13. Wesseling KH, Peñáz J (1986) Indirect blood pressure measurement in the finger: Physiological background of a recent development. Scripta Medica 59: 203—205
14. Wesseling KH, Settels JJ, van der Hoeven GMA, Nijboer JA, Butijn MWT, Dorlas JC (1985) Effects of peripheral vasoconstriction on the measurement of blood pressure in a finger. Cardiovasc Res 19: 139—145

Diagnostic and therapeutic aspects of 24-h blood pressure measurement

W. Vetter[1], St. Hany[1], D. Edmonds[1], P. Walger[1], H. Vetter[2]

[1] Department of Internal Medicine, Zürich University Hospital, Zurich, Switzerland
[2] Medical Department, University of Bonn, Bonn, FRG

Introduction

Twenty-four-hour blood pressure measurement is being increasingly applied in the diagnosis and therapy of hypertension. Diagnostically, the method is mainly used to differentiate between normal and pathologically increased blood pressure values. At the same time, it is therapeutically valuable inasmuch as the multiple blood pressure measurements permit a more precise appraisal of the antihypertensive action profile of a given substance than do conventional procedures.

Diagnostic application

The diagnostic possibilities of 24-h blood pressure measurement extend from the determination of the degree of severity of a hypertension, or the differentiation of normotension/hypertension, to the chance discovery of a pheochromocytoma, which is sometimes associated with sudden increases of blood pressure and heart rate.
For differentiation of hypertensive and normotensive blood pressure values, the method yields a great number of results which, considered separately and/or together, permit an assessment of the degree of severity of hypertension. It must be noted in this connection that, worldwide, the so-called normal range has not yet been definitively established.
In interpreting the measurement data, it is advisable to first consider the mean values of the entire measurement period as well as those during the day and the night. Pathological results of individual measurements exert little influence on this type of analysis. Table 1 gives the mean values (24 h, day, night) published by various investigators (2—13). This shows that all examined groups of patients and healthy normal persons had markedly lower systolic and diastolic values during the night than during the day. Furthermore, though hypertensive patients do show higher mean values than normal persons, the difference from the healthy subjects is confined to a few millimeters of mercury. This applies particularly to cases with only a slight increase in blood pressure.
These remarks make it clear that analysis of the discussed mean values only permit partial statement, and other parameters must therefore also be taken into consideration. Precedence is taken here by computer-assisted analysis of the percentage comprised by individual pathological blood pressure values in the total of all measurements. The percentages commonly referred to are those of values exceeding 160 or 140 mmHg systolically and 95 or 90 mmHg diastolically. It should be taken into account that the greater fluctuations of the systolic blood pressure values render the assessment of their percentage increases more difficult than for the diastolic pressure. Here too, the normal ranges

Table 1. Diurnal, nocturnal and total mean values normotensives and hypertensives

Examined collective	Number Patients (n)	Total	Mean Values Day	Night	Literature
1) Normotension					
— Men and women	34		121/75[1]		(3)
	29	120/75	126/79	107/67	(8)
	101	117/73			(9)
— Men	34	122/76	128/80	107/67	(6)
	149	116/72	121/77	106/65	(5)
— Women	50	104/73	109/77	95/64	(5)
2) Hypertension					
— "Labile" hypertension	25	126/85			(12)
	25	130/84	136/88	119/78	(13)
— Borderline hypertension	34	130/85	136/89	122/79	(13)
	10		152/88	127/74	(11)
— Mild hypertension	8		124/84	110/72	
— Moderately severe hypertension	18		132/94	112/79	(2)
— Severe hypertension	8		164/104	145/90	
— Untreated hypertension	245	139/87			(7)
	14	150/97[2]			(4)
	29	140/92	145/96	132/86	(8)
	26	165/96			(10)
	22	144/92	150/95	133/85	(13)

[1] Mean value of two days
[2] Mean value of three days

are in the process of being established worldwide. Table 2 shows the values observed by Drayer and Weber in normotensives and hypertensives. Analysis of individual measurements yields little information as a rule, but does occasionally permit the recognition of blood pressure peaks such as may, for example, occur in patients with a pheochromocytoma [1, 14]. However, the registration of such sudden blood pressure fluctuations does not appear to be pathognomonic for a pheochromocytoma.

The 24-h blood pressure curve follows a typical circadian rhythm. It is common practice today to combine the numerous individual measurements registered during the day in hourly mean values. The documentation of one or more patients is thus more clearly represented.

Analysis of such curve courses is also interesting inasmuch as our experience has shown that, in contrast to essential hypertensives, patients with a secondary blood pressure rise display a flattening of the 24-h blood pressure curve [1]. The extent to which these results are of diagnostic significance must be clarified by further investigations.

Finally, analysis of the 24-h curve makes it possible in some cases to recognize situational blood pressure increases such as those that are typical for the so-called practice hypertension (Fig. 1).

Table 2. Percentage of pathological blood pressure values in normotensives and hypertensives during a 24-h measuring period

	systolic values > 140 mmHg %	diastolic values > 90 mmHg %
Normotensives		
— Drayer and Weber [8] (n = 29)	12	14
Hypertensives		
— Drayer and Weber [8] (n = 29)	46	56

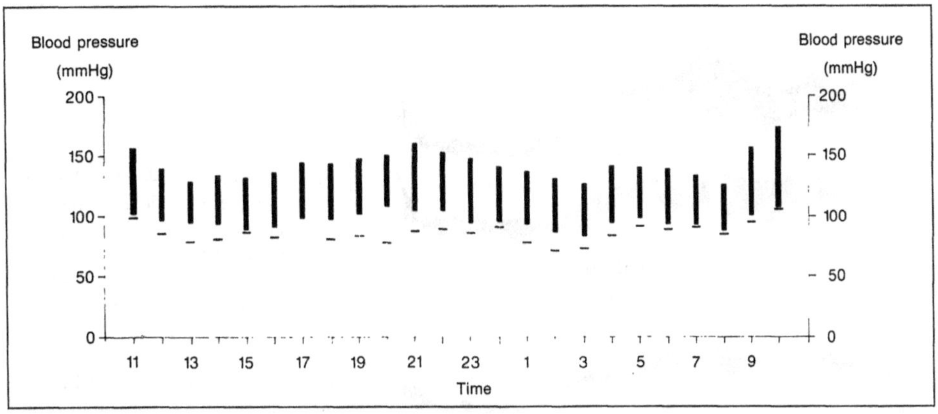

Fig. 1. 24-h blood pressure measurement (hourly mean value) in "practice hypertension". Clearly recognizable are the increased values (red columns) on placement and removal of the device in the clinic. Heart rate = black bars; (according to (9)).

Therapeutic application

Since the assessment of an effect improves with an increase of measurements, it is clear that continuous 24-h blood pressure measurement represents an ideal method for appraising the therapeutic effect of an antihypertensive substance.

In principle, it is possible to employ continuous blood pressure measurement both in acute therapy and chronic antihypertensive treatment, but its main area of application is in the analysis of long-term therapies. Here, the spectrum of application extends from a dose optimization in patients with severe hypertension to the evaluation of action principles of new antihypertensives or new modes of application [15].

Figure 2 shows the effect of a single daily dose of 240 mg of verapamil RR on systolic and diastolic mean hourly values in 27 patients with essential hypertension [16]. The

24-h blood pressure profiles were obtained before and after a 4-week application of verapamil. The results show that, in the total collective, a marked blood pressure reduction was observed during the day, while only a slight effect was detectable during the night. Comparable results were published by Gould et al. [17], though they used intraarterial blood pressure measurements.

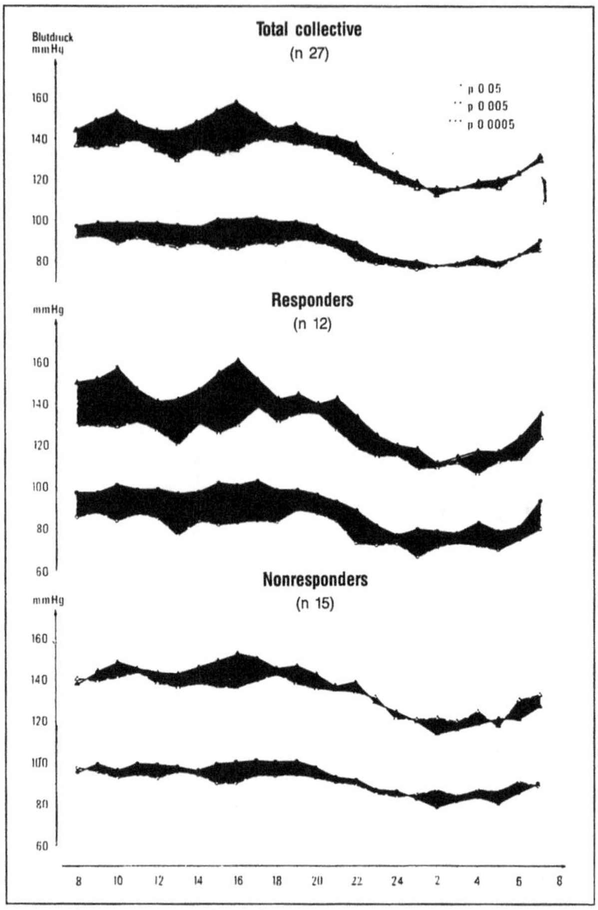

Fig. 2. Effect of a 4-week therapy with a single daily dose of 240 mg of verapamil RR on the systolic and diastolic 24-h blood pressure of 27 essential hypertensives (total collective). Separately presented are patients with a more than 10% reduction of the daily diastolic mean value (responders) and those with a less than 10% reduction (non-responders). This clearly shows the different degree of blood pressure reduction in responders and non-responders. Significant differences between the hourly mean values are marked by asterisks, (according to [19]).

Subdivision of the patient collective into cases with a good blood pressure response (responders) and those with a poor one (non-responders) did, however, reveal the former to show a marked antihypertensive effect even during the nocturnal hours (Fig. 2). These results also illustrate the difficulties involved in assessing the antihypertensive effect of a given substance by analysis of total collectives, which are, of course, always composed of responders and non-responders, though the proportions may vary.
Among the newer forms of therapy, a special role is played by the transdermal therapeutic systems (TTS) [18, 19]. The first successful antihypertensive TTS was a clonidine-

TTS developed some years ago [20]. Though a good antihypertensive effect was achieved even with low circulating clonidine levels, a relatively frequent skin allergy proved to be therapy-limiting [21].
We recently described for the first time a beta-blocker-containing transdermal system (mepindolol-TTS, Pharmed and Smith/Kline Deuelsberg, Göttingen, FRG) [22]. The 24-h blood pressure measurements performed in patients treated with mepindolol-TTS revealed it to have a marked 24-h effect (Fig. 3). However, further studies are necessary for a definitive assessment of its applicability, which can be significantly limited, especially because of local skin allergies.

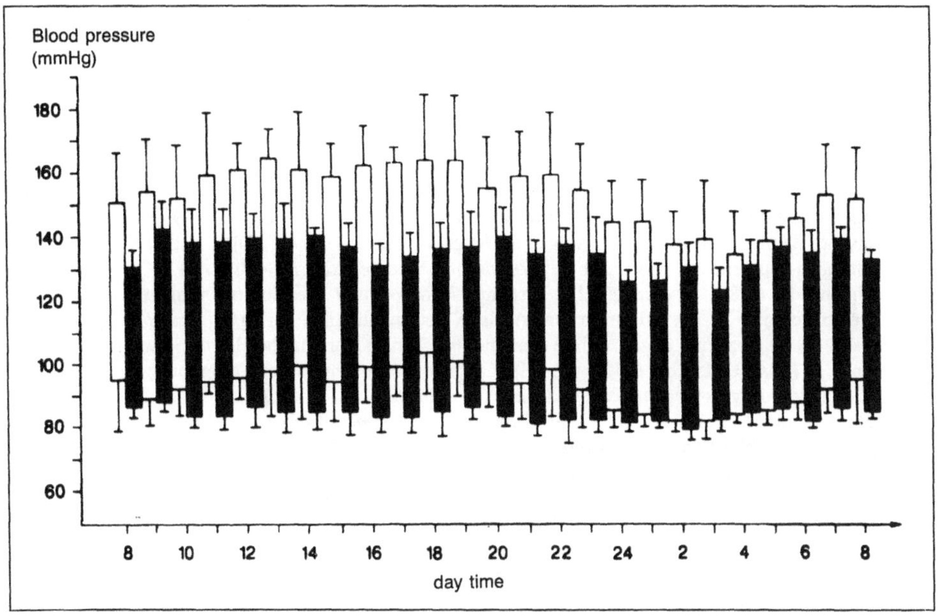

Fig. 3. 24-h blood pressure profiles in essential hypertensives (n = 5) prior to therapy (light columns) and after three weeks of transdermal beta-blocker therapy (dark columns). The figure shows the systolic and diastolic mean hourly values (± standard deviation). A marked reduction of the systolic and diastolic blood pressure values is recognizable during the entire 24-h period (according to [18]).

Conclusion

Twenty-four-hour blood pressure measurement is increasingly applied in the diagnostics of hypertension for differentiating between normal and pathologically increased blood pressure. Furthermore, the procedure frequently makes it possible to recognize situational blood pressure rises, e. g., those characteristic for "practice hypertension". Therapeutically, the method is mainly applied for investigating the action profile of antihypertensive substances.

References

1. Drayer JIM, Weber MA (1985) Definition of normalcy in wholeday ambulatory blood pressure monitoring. Clin Exp Hypertens 7: 195—204
2. Drayer JIM, Weber MA, Chard ER (1983) Non-invasive automated blood pressure monitoring in ambulatory normotensive men. In: Weber MA, Drayer JIM (eds) Ambulatory Blood Pressure Monitoring. Steinkopff Verlag, Darmstadt; Springer Verlag, New York, p 129—135
3. Edmonds D, Vetter H, Walger P, Vetter W (1986) Verapamil 240 mg — effective blood pressure reduction with a single daily dose? J Hypertension 4 (suppl 5) 455—457
4. Fitzgerald DJ, O'Malley K, O'Brien ET (1983) Reproducibility of ambulatory blood pressure recordings. In (2) Springer Verlag New York, p 71—74
5. Frielingsdorf J, Stricker M, Hany St, Foerster C-Ch, Vetter W (1985) 24-Stunden-Blutdruckmessung bei Hypertonien verschiedener Schweregrade. Schweiz Rundschau Med (Praxis) 74: 1260—1265
6. Gould BA, Hornung RS, Kieso HA, Altmann DG, Cashman PMM, Raftery EB (1984) Evaluation of the Remler M2000 blood pressure recorder. Comparison with intraarterial blood pressure recordings both at hospital and at home. Hypertension 6: 209—215
7. Gould BA, Mann St, Kieso H, Subramanian VB, Raftery EB (1982) The 24-hour ambulatory blood pressure profile with verapamil. Circulation 65, 22—27
8. Groth H, Vetter H, Knüsel J, Foerster E, Siegenthaler W, Vetter W (1984) Transdermal clonidine application: Long-term results in essential hypertension. Klin Wschr 62, 925—930
9. Hany St, Baumgart P, Bättig B, Walger P, Vetter W, Vetter H (1987) Diagnostische Aspekte der 24-Stunden-Blutdruckmessung. Schweiz Rundschau Med (Praxis) 76: 480—484
10. Heilmann K (1982) Therapeutische Systeme. Konzept und Realisation programmierter Arzneiverabreichung. 2., überarb. u. erweit. Auflage, Ferdinand Enke Verlag Stuttgart
11. Hess H (1984) Arzneiformen und ihre Anwendung. Verlag Hans Huber Bern, Stuttgart, Wien
12. Irving JB, Brash HM, Kerr F, Kirby BJ (1976) The value of ambulatory monitoring in border-line and established hypertension. Postgrad med J 52 (Suppl 7): 137—139
13. Jacot des Combes B, Pochet M, Waeber B, Brunner HR (1984) Ambulatory blood pressure recordings. Reproducibility and unpredictability. Hypertension 6: 110—114
14. Nomura A, Yasuda H, Kato K, Shimono H, Murakami T, Minami M, Takechi S (1985) Direct blood pressure monitoring in patients with pheochromocytoma. Jpn H J 26: 845—849
15. Pickering TG, Harshfield GA, Kleinert HD, Blank S, Laragh JH (1982) Blood pressure during normal daily activities, sleep and exercise. J Am Med Ass 247: 992—996
16. Reeves RA, Johnson AM, Shapiro AP, Traub YM, Jacob R (1983) Ambulatory blood pressure monitoring: methods to assess severity of hypertension, variability and sleep changes. In: (2)
17. Shaw JE, Urquhart J (1981) Transdermal drug administration — a nuisance becomes an opportunity. Br Med J 283: 875—876
18. Spieker C, Vetter W, Hany St, Liedtke R, Vetter H (1987) Transdermaler Betablocker: Wirkung auf 24-Stunden-Blutdruckprofile bei Hypertoniepatienten. Schweiz Rundschau Med (Praxis) 76: 467—468
19. Vetter W, Schmid-Zumstein A, Bättig B, Oertel R, Hany S, Edmonds D, Baumgart P, Vetter H (1987) 24-Stunden-Blutdruckmessung: therapeutische und prognostische Bedeutung. Schweiz Rundschau Med (Praxis) 76: 462—466
20. Waeber B, Jacot des Combes B, Porchet M, Biolaz J, Schaller M-D. Brunner HR (1984) Ambulatory blood pressure recording to identify hypertensive patients who truly need therapy. J Chron Dis 37: 55—57
21. Wallace JM jr, Thornton WE, Kennedy HL, Pickering TG, Harshfield GA, Frohlich ED, Messerli FH, Gifford RW jr, Bolen K (1983) Ambulatory blood pressure in 199 normal subjects, a collaborative study. In: (2)
22. Weber MA, Drayer JIM, Chard ER (1983) Blood pressure fluctuation and amplitude in normal human subjects. In: (2)

Circadian Variation of blood pressure in postoperative coarctation patients*

J. Sehested, F. Hermansen, A. Bloch and C. Mais

Department of Thoracic and Cardiovascular Surgery, Aarhus Kommunehospital, Aarhus C and Department of Clinical Physiology, Rigshospitalet, Copenhagen O, Denmark

Introduction

Coarctation of the aorta is a congenital lesion causing hypertension in the upper part of the body and hypo- or normotension in the lower part.
In general, reconstructive surgery is followed by a drop in pressure in the upper part, towards normal levels, although a host of hemodynamic abnormalities often persist, even years after operation. These abnormalities include a higher peripheral resistance in the upper extremities compared to the normal resistance found in the lower extremities [2, 3]. Due probably to changes in the precoarctational vascular bed, the baroreceptor function is altered, reset to a higher level and shows a reduced sensitivity [1, 4].
The vasomotor wave activity is reduced in both vascular beds [5], and the blood pressure response to physical exercise is exaggerated [6].
The long term influence of these abnormalities upon the circadian blood pressure profile has not been evaluated until now.

Material and methods

Intra-arterial blood pressures, over a period of 18 to 22 h, were recorded in 11 coarctation patients 6 to 8 years after surgery.
Table 1 gives a clinical summary of the patients. None of them received any drugs during the study. Informed consent was obtained from all patients.
The simultaneous pressure recordings in the right brachial and right femoral arteries were done by radiotelemetry and stored on magnetic tape for later analysis. A detailed description of the telemetry system has been published previously [5].

Results and discussion

Figure 1 shows the distribution of hourly mean values of systolic and diastolic brachial pressures in 11 postoperative coarctation patients and in two normal controls.
Apart from the elevated level in the patients, these show a normal blood pressure pattern, and a nocturnal pressure drop of the same magnitude as that seen in normal subjects.

* This study was supported by the Danish Heart Association

Table 1. Clinical summary of 11 postoperative coarctation patients

Patient No.	Sex	Age at study (years)	Preoperative Time to study (years)	Preoperative Brachial pressure (mmHg)	Preoperative Systolic gradient (mmHg)	Postoperative Brachial pressure (mmHg)	Postoperative Overall systolic gradient (+/—)	Vasomotor wave activity (mmHg/min)	Number of vasomotor (waves/min)
1	F	17	7.7	128/85	17	119/68	+	49.4	8.0
2	M	26	6.4	175/100	90	142/83	+	77.0	6.0
3	M	27	6.7	187/95	67	177/103	+	41.2	8.3
4	F	39	6.6	145/85	15	139/85	+	43.2	8.3
5	M	17	6.7	150/90	45	168/73	+	97.8	7.3
6	M	27	8.5	184/94	54	167/94	+	104.9	5.0
7	M	22	7.7	176/88	86	152/88	—	58.7	7.7
8	F	48	8.5	120/73	28	145/71	—	43.8	7.7
9	F	41	7.1	210/90	90	139/72	—	43.3	8.7
10	F	20	7.8	138/88	66	133/88	—	82.3	8.3
11	M	21	7.5	130/67	22	117/74	—	101.4	7.3

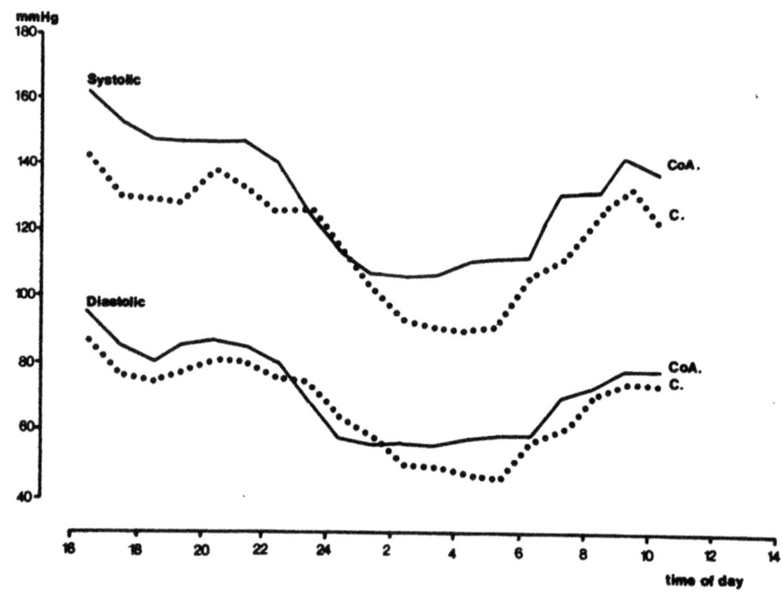

Fig. 1. Mean systolic and diastolic brachial pressures in 11 postoperative coarctation patients (CoA) and in two normal controls (C).

Figure 2 shows the systolic brachial blood pressure profile of those of the 11 patients having an overall positive brachial to femoral systolic pressure gradient, and the profile of those who do not have a gradient. A positive brachial to femoral pressure gradient normally indicates residual or recurrent coarctation.

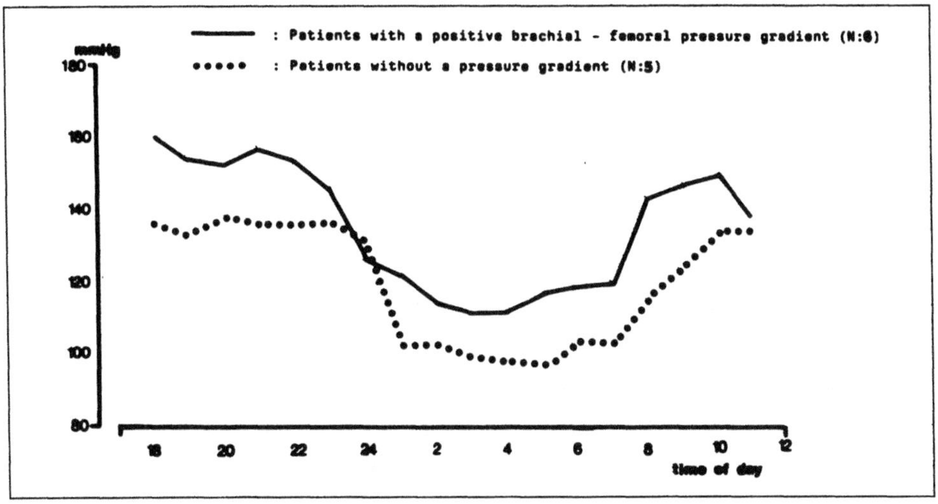

Fig. 2. Mean systolic brachial pressures in 11 postoperative coarctation patients with and without a systolic pressure gradient.

The presence or absence of a stenosis in the two groups of patients was verified by CT-scans of the thoracic aorta.

A higher blood pressure level, as expected, is seen in the patients with a stenosis. Otherwise, the two pressure profiles are virtually identical. The differences in nocturnal pressure drop and morning pressure rise are due to differences in the periods of sleep. The normal, gradual rise in pressure in the early morning hours in both groups of patients is noteworthy.

While the relatively slow pressure variations of circadian rhythmicity appear to be normal in postoperative coarctation patients, irrespective of the presence of a stenosis or not, this is not so regarding the much faster variations of the vasomotor waves.

Figure 3 gives the results of a study of vasomotor wave activity during active orthostasis, in a larger group of postoperative coarctation patients compared with a normal control series.

The number of vasomotor waves are the same in patients and controls, but the amplitudes are significantly reduced in the patients.

In the two groups mentioned above, no difference was found in the vasomotor wave activity being reduced in both to 65.9 mmHg/min in the no-gradient group and 68.9 mmHg/min in the group with a pressure gradient.

The number of vasomotor waves was normal in both groups, 7.9 waves/min and 7.2 waves/min, respectively.

In conclusion, long-term blood pressure recording in postoperative coarctation patients has shown a normal circadian rhythmicity, while the short term variations of vasomotor wave activity are significantly reduced.

This might further support the concept of different mechanisms behind fast and slow variations in blood pressure.

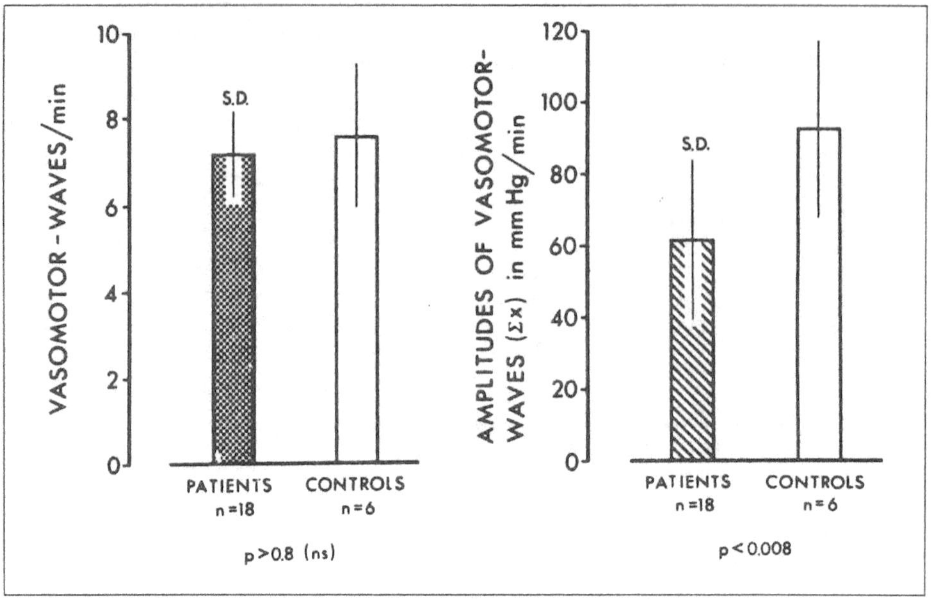

Fig. 3. Vasomotor waves per minute and vasomotor wave activity, i.e., summarized systolic pressure amplitudes in mmHg per minute in 18 postoperative coarctation patients and in six normal controls.

References

1. Beekman RH, Katz BP, Moorehead-Steffens C, Rocchini AP (1983) Altered baroreceptor function in children with systolic hypertension after coarctation repair. Am J Cardiol 52: 112—117
2. Gidding SS, Rocchini AP, Moorehead C, Schork MA, Rosenthal A (1985) Increased forearm vascular reactivity in patients with hypertension after repair of coarctation. Circulation 71: 495—499
3. Šamánek M, — etc. Goetzová J, Fiserová J, Škovránek J (1976) Differences in muscle vblood flow in upper and lower extremities of patients after correction of coarctation of the aorta. Circulation 54: 377—381
4. Sehested J, Baandrup U, Mikkelsen E (1982) Different reactivity and structure of the prestenotic and poststenotic aorta in human coarctation. Circulation 65: 1060—1065
5. Sehested J, Schultze G (1982) Vasomotor wave and blood pressure response to erect posture after operation for aortic coarctation. Br Heart J 48: 357—363
6. Sehested J, Kornerup HJ, Pedersen EB, Christensen NJ (1983) Effects of exercise on plasma renin, aldosterone and catecholamines before and after surgery for aortic coarctation. Eur Heart J 4: 52—58

Spontaneity and reactivity of autonomic control systems in patients with end-stage renal disease: a new integrative approach*

H.-H. Abel[1], G. Schultze[2], D. Klüßendorf[1], W. Meyer-Sabellek[3], J. Sehested[4], H.P. Koepchen[1]

[1] Institut für Physiologie, Freie Universität Berlin, Berlin, FRG
[2] Nephrologische Abteilung, Humboldt-Krankenhaus, Berlin, Berlin, FRG
[3] Medizinische Klinik und Poliklinik, Klinikum Steglitz, Freie Universität Berlin, Berlin, FRG
[4] Deutsches Herzzentrum Berlin, Berlin, FRG

Introduction

Autonomic control systems are involved in the regulation of a great number of organismic functions to provide maintenance of the milieu intérieur. An adequate adaptation of the organism to changing external and internal environmental conditions is attained by mechanisms of homeostatis and adaptation to physical work. Pathophysiological processes are in general accompanied by disturbances of autonomic control systems. Using clinical tests, the type and severity of these dysregulations can be described only phenomenologically, since in man certain limits restrict the analysis of mechanisms on which these disturbances are based.

Corresponding to the methodological approach of reflex research for the analysis of somatomotricity [96], also for the investigation of autonomic control systems, reflex tests have predominantly been applied. Thereby the response to a given stimulus is studied. Spontaneity, on the other hand, has been investigated relatively seldomly in both research fields; in the field of motricity, for instance, von Holst studied the spontaneous forms of coordination of rhythmic motor patterns [56]. The analysis of spontaneous patterns is particularly important for respiratory and circulatory control systems, since spontaneous fluctuations of autonomic acitivities are permanently existent and especially pronounced at rest. On the other hand, a characteristic phenomenon of various pathological processes is a change in spontaneous rhythmicity of autonomic control systems. Moreover, it has become evident that the spontaneous rhythmic activity of cardiorespiratory control systems follows the same principles as those found by von Holst in spontaneous limb movements [63]. The significance of the analysis of rhythmic patterns in the behavior of autonomic control systems for the characterization of pathophysiological states was demonstrated in extensive studies by Zwiener [112]. Modern recording and evaluation techniques have improved the ability to continuously assess the time structure of spontaneous autonomic patterns by means of non-invasive methods [3, 65]. These recently developed techniques have been applied to the

* This project has been supported by Hospital Medizin-Technik, Nürnberg, FRG. The evaluation procedure was developed partly in cooperation with the Hospital for Sport Injuries at Hellersen (supporter: Sporthilfe e. V.).

characterization of disturbances in autonomic control in patients with end-stage renal disease (ESRD). A further aim was to investigate the reliability of this analytic procedure in comparison with customary autonomic reflex tests.

Uremia is a very inhomogenous and complex pathophysiological process accompanied by disturbed autonomic regulations. The autonomic dysfunction is indicated by a decreased sensitivity of the baroreceptor reflex [84], reduced bradycardia in the Valsalva maneuver [99], and in the diving reflex [110], orthostatic hypotension [27], and a reduced blood pressure increase during isometric handgrip [36].

The results of these clinical autonomic tests, which are based on the analysis of reflex reactions, are confirmed by studies on the spontaneous behavior of autonomic control systems. The reduced dynamics of cardiovascular control at rest are evident from the decrease in heart rate variability [25, 34] and heart rate rhythmicity in various spectral components [7, 15].

In the present investigations in patients with ESRD, the changes in the dynamics of autonomic control systems have been studied in a short-term range and correlations with results of the 24-h blood pressure monitoring are provided. To achieve this, the influence of the central nervous activity on the relations between variability, rhythmicity, and tone in different autonomic efferents was analyzed. Furthermore, the results of autonomic tests and those of heart rate pattern analysis were compared with regard to the judgement of specific alteration of parasympathetic cardiac innervation. Finally, the reliability of the differentiating heart rate pattern analysis will be discussed.

Methods

Various study protocols have been performed for the analysis of mechanisms, temporal dynamics and individual degree of the autonomic insufficiency (Table 1). Neurovegetative indicators have been selected with the aim to assess specific innervation patterns of autonomic control systems (Table 2). During the investigations in the laboratory, the continuously recorded data were digitized in an on-line procedure (max. 16 analogue and

Table 1. Study design

1. Spontaneous behavior under conditions of low central nervous activity (relaxed at rest, listening to soft indifferent back-ground music, duration: 45 min).
2. Cognitive-motivational strain (Raven test under time and efficiency control, duration: 15 min).
3. Autonomic test procedures
3.1 Baroreceptor sensitivity (angiotensin II, dose: 0.04 μg/kg BW)
3.2 Vagal blockade (atropine, dose: 0.02 mg/kg BW)
3.3 Voluntary slow respiration (external rhythm: T = 10 s, tidal volume not controlled, duration: 70 s)
4. Heart rate pattern monitoring (computer-aided continuous analysis of cardiac interbeat intervals, duration: 5–6 h).
5. Ambulatory, indirect 24-h blood pressure monitoring.

Table 2. Neurovegetative indicators

1. ECG (sympathetic and parasympathetic cardiomotor innervation).
2. Photo-electrical finger plethysmogram (regional sympathetic, vasomotor innervation).
3. Arterial blood pressure measured directly/indirectly (integrated indicator of nervous and humoral cardiovascular control).
4. Pneumogram (peripheral representation of the central neuronal mechanisms underlying respiration).

event channels) and fed into an LSI11/23 computer. When measurements were performed in the hospital, analogue data were stored on a 14-channel recorder (EMI). Blood pressure was measured directly in the arterio-venous fistula which was temporarily occluded. Automatic 24-h measurements of the indirect blood pressure were carried out with three different devices (PAR, Del Mar Avionics, ICR-Squibb) [80].

The ECG signal was transformed into a beat-to-beat interval signal (RR-interval signal), and mean value and standard deviation were calculated. Computing power spectra, the duration of the evaluation period determines the frequencies comprised in a spectrum. When the immediate temporal changes in certain frequencies are of interest, conflicts arise in the definition of evaluation periods. In order to include also low frequencies in the analysis of fluctuations of the RR-interval signal with a period of T = 80 s, consecutive 4-min evaluation periods were used. The temporal variability of rhythms in the range of T = 25 s to 2 s was assessed in 1-min and 2-min sections, respectively. Figure 1 shows a typical RR-interval power spectrum of a 1-min evaluation section of a healthy

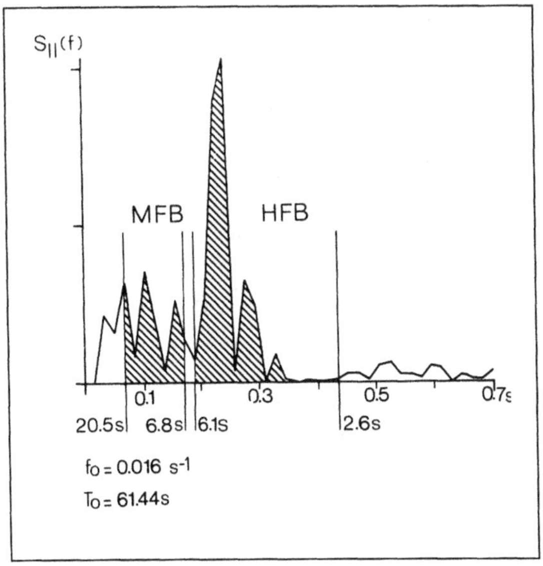

Fig. 1. Analysis of rhythmicity of heart beat intervals. Heart rate power spectrum of a healthy subject, calculated from a 61.44 s section of the interbeat interval signal (RR-interval signal). Largest peak at 0.25 Hz (T = 4.0 s) represents the heart rate modulation in the range of respiration ("respiratory sinus arrhythmia", RSA). Calculation of slower rhythmicity superimposed upon the RR-interval signal of two frequency bands by integration of the corresponding segments of the power spectrum (hatched areas): a) area of high-frequency band (HFB), f: 0.164 to 0.385 Hz, T: 6.1 to 2.6 s, and b) area of mid-frequency band (MFB), f: 0.049 to 0.147 Hz, T: 20.5 to 6.8 s.

subject. The large peak at 0.25 Hz (T = 4.0 s) corresponds to the modulation of heart rate in the range of respiration ("respiratory sinus arrhythmia", RSA). A smaller peak at 0.1 Hz indicates a simultaneously existing 10 s cardiovascular rhythm, which can be interpreted as the action of the baroreceptor reflex during a 10 s blood pressure rhythm and/or an intrinsic rhythm of central heart rate control mechanisms in the same frequency range [40]. To simplify the evaluation of serial RR-interval spectra, areas of two frequency bands were analyzed, which were calculated by integration of corresponding sections of the power spectrum (area of high-frequency band, HFB, 0.164 to 0.385 Hz, period duration: 6.1 to 2.6 s; area of mid-frequency band, MFB, 0.049 to 0.147 Hz, period duration: 20.5 to 6.8 s). These two frequency ranges were selected because of the existence of two characteristic peaks. Since the extent of rhythmicity in the HFB is closely correlated to the parasympathetic cardiomotor innervation [32, 37, 60] and, on the other hand, the rhythmicity in the MFB is considered to be an indicator of the modulation of sympathetic cardiomotor innervation [33, 75], the analysis of the frequency bands may provide a criterion for the contribution of parasympathetic and sympathetic heart rate control.

The pneumogram resulting from summation of synchronously recorded alterations of the thoracic and abdominal circumference was automatically evaluated breath-by-breath (Fig. 2). Partial components of one single breath (inspiratory time, mean inspiratory flow, expiratory time) are indicators of partial mechanisms of a central neuronal network involved in the rhythmogenesis of respiration and modulated by a great number of central and peripheral influences [1, 6, 35, 57, 66, 88]. By means of a differentiated analysis of respiratory partial components, detailed information can be obtained about the dynamic organization of central control systems in the same way as by means of a differentiated analysis of heart beat intervals.

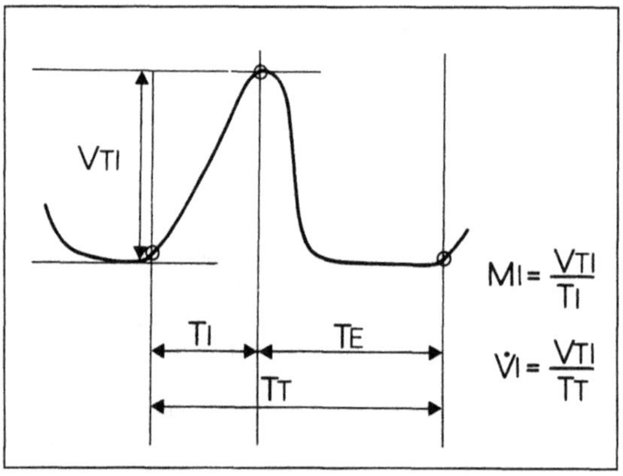

Fig. 2. Analysis of respiratory partial components. Evaluation scheme of the calculation of partial components of a respiratory cycle. TI: inspiratory time, TE: expiratory time, TT: total respiratory cycle time, VTI: inspiratory tidal volume, MI: mean inspiratory flow (calculated as quotient VTI over TI), VI: ventilation per respiratory cycle (calculated as quotient VTI over TT).

In the course of automatic indirect blood pressure measurement, systolic and diastolic blood pressure and heart rate where recorded during the day in 15-min intervals and during the night in 30-min intervals. Maxima, minima, mean value, SD, and time-course of the parameters were calculated for the entire period of 24 h and separately for day and night periods.

In this investigation 38 patients with ESRD and maintenance hemodialysis have been studied. There was no selection regarding renal disease, age, sex and degree of rehabilitation. Not all patients were included in the entire experimental protocol.

Results

A – Spontaneous variability and rhythmicity

Heart rate: In humans as well as in animals the mean RR-interval and RR-interval variability are positively correlated. As this correlation can also be demonstrated by the techniques applied by us [4], it seems to be useful for the comparability of different subjects to relate variability and rhythmicity to the mean RR-interval. In order to study the mutual relations between mean RR-interval (mean-RR), RR-interval variability (SD-RR) and RR-interval rhythmicity in both frequency bands (HFB, MFB) at rest, these parameters were calculated from consecutive 1-min periods, which were sensitive for the analysis of temporal variations. The relation between mean-RR and SD-RR, which is positive in healthy subjects, is altered in a characteristic manner in the patients (Fig. 3). The SD-RR/mean-RR correlation has a diminished slope and is shifted towards lower

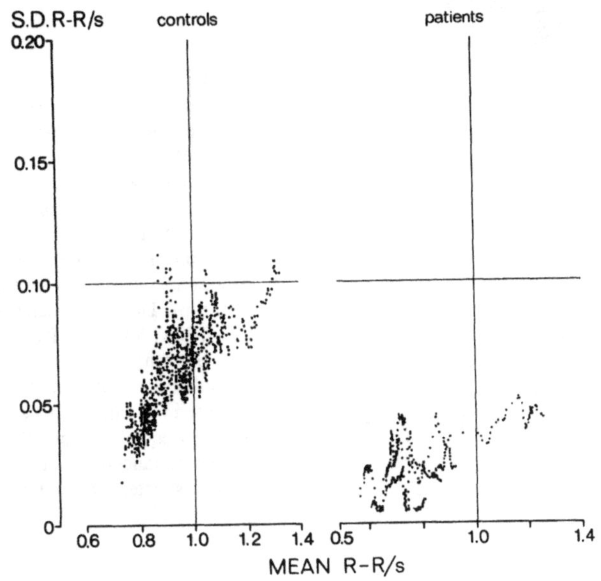

Fig. 3. Spontaneous heart rate variability. Left: in control subjects (n = 21): positive relation between mean cardiac interbeat interval (mean-RR) and standard deviation (SD-RR) during physical rest, smoothed with Hanning filter. Right: the same characteristic is flattened in hemodialysis patients (n = 14) and shifted towards lower values of variability. Larger deviation of SD-RR values at a lower mean-RR range (0.7 s) in comparison with healthy subjects.

values of variability. The RR-interval variability which is enhanced in the controls in the range of a mean-RR of 1.0 s, appears in the patients at shorter mean-RR. To enable both the estimation of the primarily parasympathetic and the primarily sympathetic contribution to heart rate rhythmicity within the 1-min total variability, the degree of rhythmicity of the analyzed frequency bands was brought into relation with the mean RR-interval (Fig. 4). In healthy subjects the area of HFB increases with augmentation of the mean-RR. With a mean-RR of 1.0 s a more than proportional increase of HFB rhythmicity occurs. The area of MFB has also a maximum of rhythmicity in the range of a mean-RR of 1.0 s, but decreases, however, with shorter and longer mean-RRs. Thus, rhythmicity in both frequency bands depends in a characteristic manner on the mean-RR and has a common resonance-like augmentation of amplitude at a mean heart rate of 60/min. In patients the relations are in general shifted in parallel towards shorter mean-RRs, so that now the spontaneous resonance maximum appears at a heart rate around 90/min.

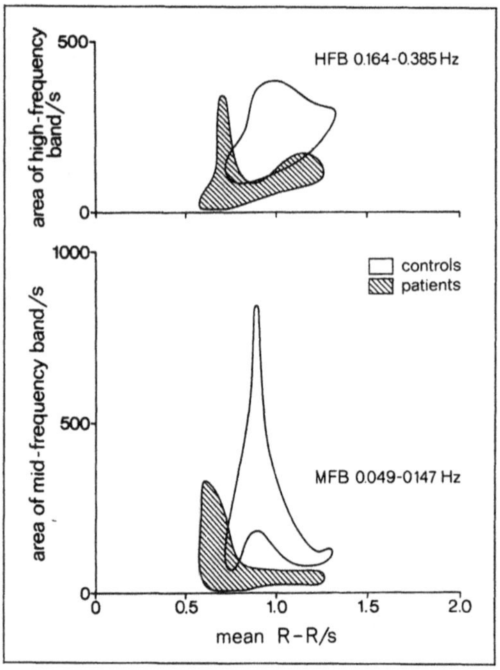

Fig. 4. Spontaneous heart rate rhythmicity. Relation between mean cardiac interbeat interval (mean-RR) and area of high-frequency band (HFB) and area of mid-frequency band (MFB) during physical rest, smoothed with Hanning filter. Control subjects (n = 21): increase in rhythmicity in the HFB with prolongation of mean-RR with over-proportional increase in the mean-RR range of 1.0 s (open area, top). Distinctly increased rhythmicity in the MFB with a mean-RR range of 1.0 s (open area, bottom).
Hemodialysis patients (n = 14): distinct decrease in spontaneous heart rate rhythmicity in both frequency bands (hatched area). Shift of the resonance-like maximum of rhythmicity towards shorter RR-intervals.

Vasomotricity: In addition to marked alterations of rhythmicity in the autonomic cardiomotor innervation, the patients show also a changed modulation of cutaneous vasomotor activity. For example, a 13.5-min section of the finger plethysmogram was used to determine the frequency of period durations ($5.0 < T < 60.0$ s) which are superimposed on the pulse-synchronous oscillations of finger volume as slower fluctuations (Fig. 5A). In healthy subjects, period durations between 5 and 25 s with a maximum around T = 15 s were found. In patients the spectrum is extended to longer period durations which occur without any characteristic maximum. The frequency distribution of the amplitudes of pulse-synchronous finger volume oscillations calculated after high-pass filtering (0.3 Hz) of the plethysmogram shows a distinct reduction of variability (Fig. 5B).

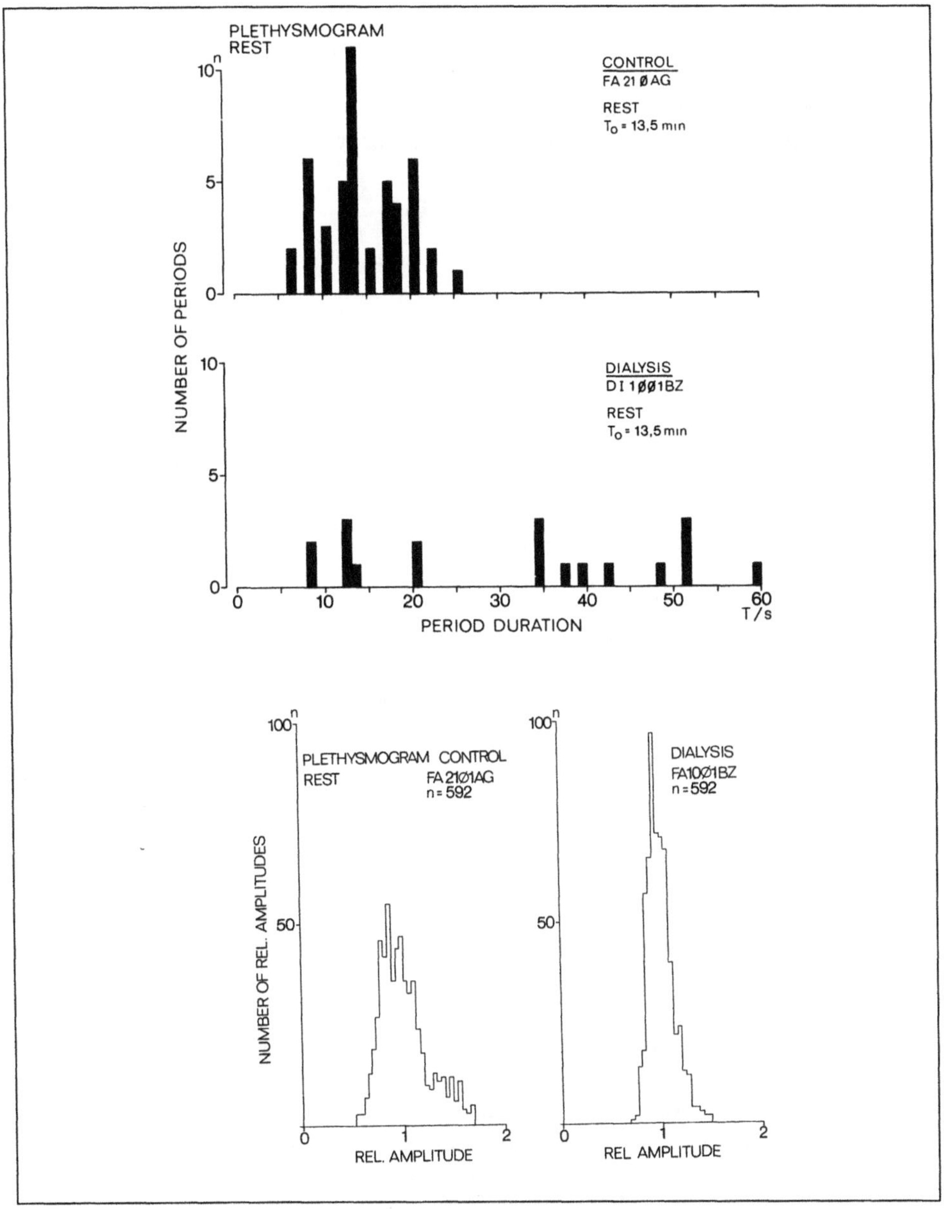

Fig. 5. Spontaneous vasomotricity.

A: Frequency distribution of the period durations (5.0 < T < 60.0 s) of the photo-electrically recorded finger plethysmogram calculated from two 13.5 min sections during physical rest. In the dialysis patient (bottom), longer period durations appear without occurrence of a characteristic frequency maximum as in the healthy subject (top).

B: Frequency distribution of the relative amplitudes of pulse synchronous finger volume changes, calculated from the two 13.5 min sections. The dialysis patient (right) has a clear restriction of variability of pulse-synchronous vascular activity in comparison with the healthy subject (left).

Respiration: In contrast to the general reduction of variability of cardiovascular parameters, an increase in the variability of respiratory partial components was observed in patients (Fig. 6). As a measure of variability, the SD related to the intraindividually calculated mean value was used. The enhancement of variability is very distinct in the primary partial components inspiratory time, expiratory time, and mean inspiratory flow.

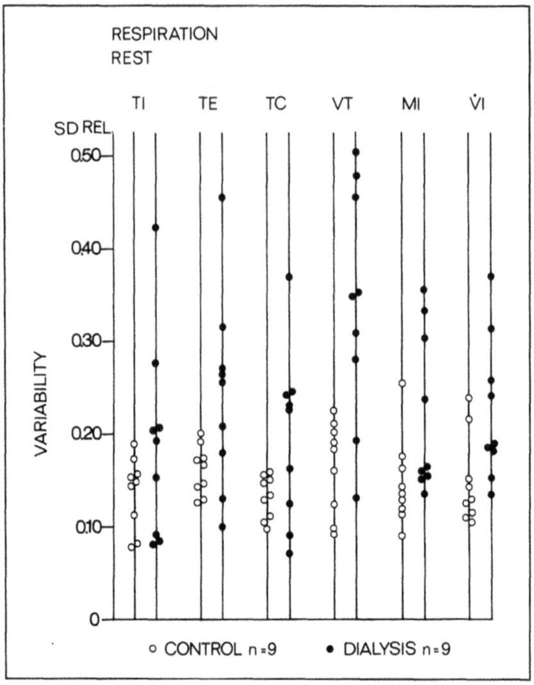

Fig. 6. Spontaneous respiratory variability. Calculation of the variability of respiratory partial components as standard deviation related to the intraindividual mean value. In general, the dialysis patients (closed circles) show a distinctly increased variability in all parameters compared with healthy subjects (open circles).

B – Reactivity (Relations between tone and rhythm)

Heart rate: Figure 7 represents individual time courses of mean-RR, SD-RR, area of HFB, area of MFB and the quotient of both (area MFB: area of HFB) calculated from 1-min sections in two subjects before, during, and after the Raven test. In the healthy subject (control), mean-RR and the degree of rhythmicity in both frequency bands during rest (PRE) fluctuate markedly from minute to minute. The rhythmicities in the HFB and MFB are partly independent of each other. During cognitive-motivational stress (Raven test) an initial diminution of the mean-RR, decrease in heart rate fluctuations in the frequency range of respiration (area of HFB) and increase in rhythmicity in the mid-frequency band (area of MFB) occur. In the further course of the Raven test, mean-RR returns towards the PRE-value, whereas the rhythmicity in both frequency bands shows temporarily a strong deviation from the mean-RR course. These dynamics in the relation between mean-RR and HFB- and MFB-rhythmicity, i.e., the specific time-dependent relation between these parameters, become even more distinct in the subsequent resting phase (POST). Although mean-RR has reached the PRE-value again, rhythmicity in the

HFB is still reduced. In the patient, a clear decrease in spontaneous rhythmicity occurs. There is a larger dissociation between the course of mean-RR and the rhythmicity in the frequency bands. With a similar course of mean-RR, changes in heart rate rhythmicity do not occur during the Raven test.

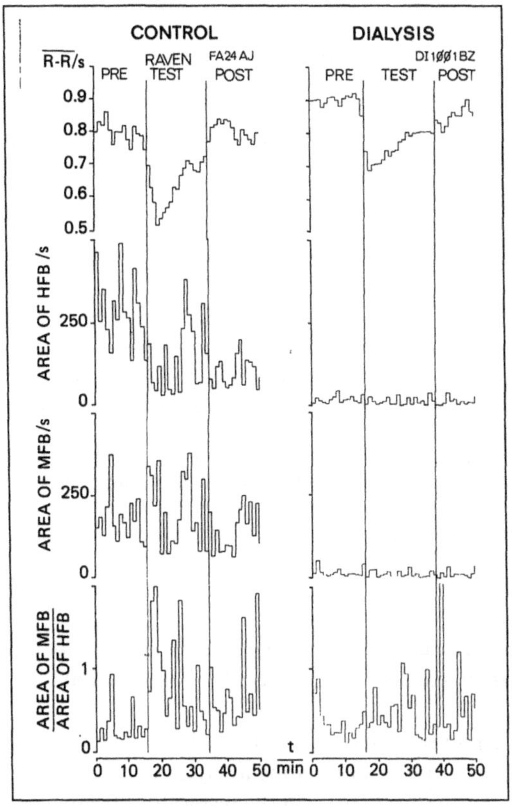

Fig. 7. Reactive heart rate rhythmicity. Individual time courses of mean cardiac interbeat interval (mean-RR), area of high-frequency band (HFB), area of mid-frequency band (MFB) and the quotient of the frequency bands (area of MFB over area of HFB) during rest (PRE), cognitive-motivational strain (RAVEN TEST) and recovery period (POST). The values were calculated from consecutive 61.44 s sections.
Control (left): distinct variability of parameters at rest. At the beginning of the Raven test distinct decrease in mean-RR and area of HFB with increase in rhythmicity in the MFB (increase of the quotient of the frequency bands). In the POST phase a striking outlasting of the diminished rhythmicity in the HFB, whereas mean-RR is already restored.
Dialysis patient (right): strong decrease in rhythmicity in both frequency bands. No reactive behavior of the frequency band rhythmicities with similar time course of mean-RR.

Vasomotricity: The analysis of the amplitude of pulse-synchronous oscillations of finger volume in the healthy subject exhibits a distinct, spontaneous variability of the consecutively calculated 1-min mean values and a marked vasoconstriction during the Raven test, in particular at the beginning (Fig. 8). In the patient, the variability of mean values is diminished during rest and mental strain. Apart from a small initial vasoconstriction, the reaction of digital cutaneous vasomotricity is almost entirely absent during the Raven test.

C – Indicators of parasympathetic innervation

In five well rehabilitated and cooperative patients with no signs of cardiovascular complications and not being under cardiovascular medication, neurovegetative functions at rest, reactions to autonomic tests, and circadian changes in blood pressure were studied in order to provide information on interindividual differences in the extent of the

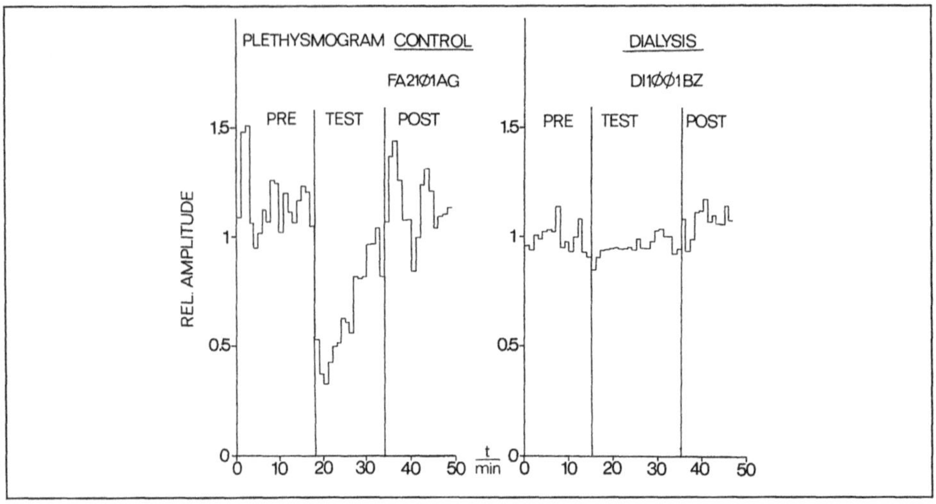

Fig. 8. Reactive vasomotricity. Individual time courses of the relative 61.44 s mean values of pulse synchronous finger volume changes referring to the PRE mean value, at rest (PRE), cognitive-motivational strain (RAVEN TEST) and recovery period (POST).
Control (left): distinct variability of pulse synchronous finger volume amplitude at rest. At the beginning of the Raven test distinct decrease of the parameter and return towards initial value already during the test. Dialysis patient (right): diminution of spontaneous variability at rest. During the Raven test only an initial, slight decrease in pulse synchronous finger volume amplitude and further restriction of variability with unchanged mean value in the course of the test.

parasympathetic part of the autonomic insufficiency. Figure 9A-D shows the results of two patients with distinct differences in their parasympathetic cardiac innervation.

Rest: The RR-interval power spectrum of 2-min sections of patient A shows a clear peak in the HFB which corresponds to the so-called respiratory sinus arrhythmia (Fig. 9A). Due to resonance phenomena, the respiratory heart rate peak in the respiratory frequency range usually increases with a decrease in respiratory frequency [10]. In patient B, however, this heart rate peak is diminished, although he has a slower respiratory rhythm. In addition to the HFB, this decrease in rhythmicity also affects the MFB.

Atropine: In patient A, intravenous application of 0.02 mg/kg atropine leads to a decrease in mean-RR from 0.829 s to 0.667 s (Δ%: —19.6) and of S.D.-RR from 20.25 ms to 7.04 ms (Δ%: —65.3), in comparison to a merely small decrease of mean-RR from 0.775 s to 0.710 s (Δ%: —8.4) and unchanged S.D.-RR (from 7.54 ms to 7.60 ms, Δ%: + 0.9) in patient B (Fig. 9B).

Deep respiration: It is known that with voluntary deceleration of respiratory frequency, the respiratory sinus arrhythmia increases and has its maximum at about six respiratory cycles per minute. During voluntary slow respiration heart rate oscillations correlated to respiration (6 cycles/min) were measured as respiratory sinus arrhythmia (RSA) before and after application of atropine. RSA was calculated as the mean difference between the longest and shortest RR-interval during each respiratory cycle in percent of the mean-

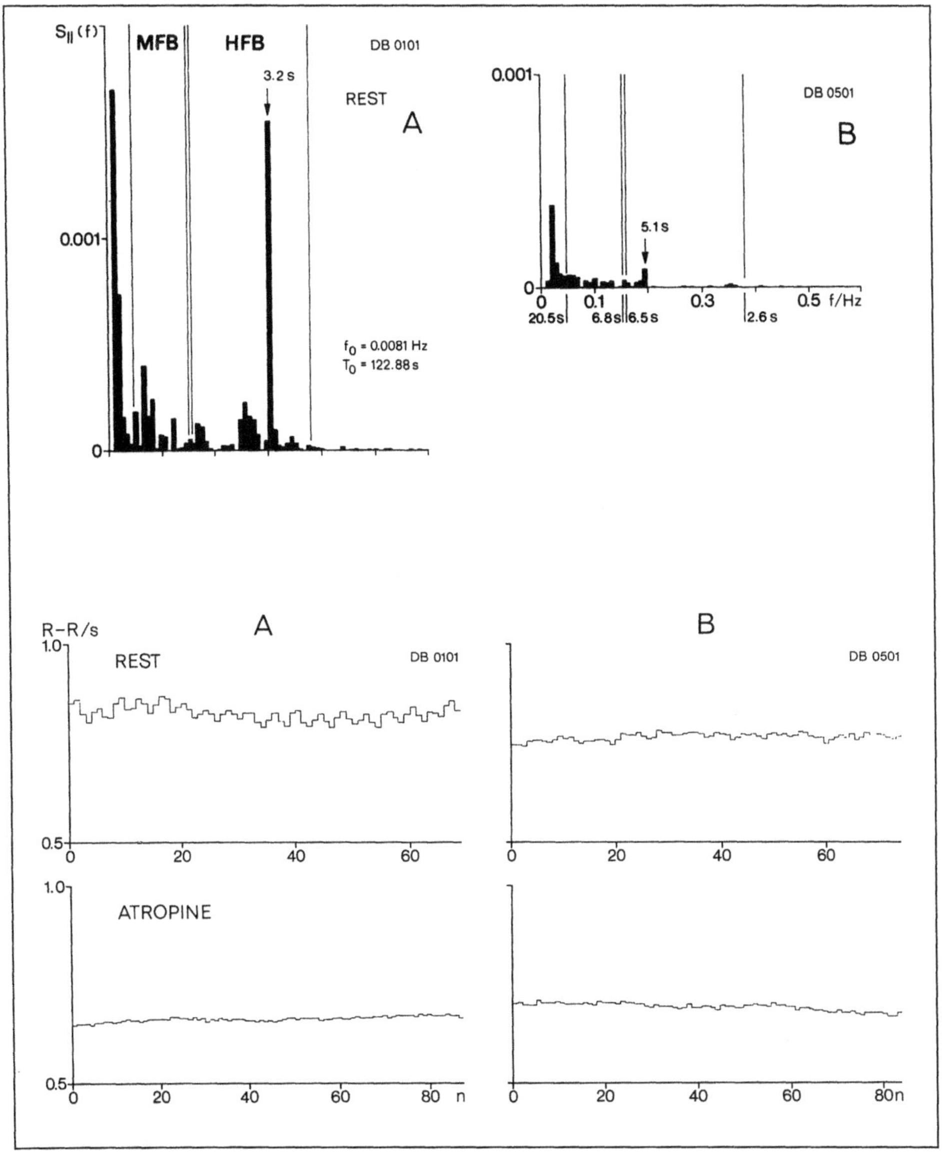

Fig. 9. Reactions to autonomic tests. Comparison of two hemodialysis patients (patient A and patient B) with autonomic insufficiency, which is less distinct in patient A.
A: Heart rate power spectra at physical rest calculated from 122.88 s sections of the cardiac interbeat interval signal. Arrows indicate the highest peak corresponding to the momentary respiratory frequency in the power spectrum of the pneumogram (patient A: T = 3.2 s, patient B: T = 5.1 s). Patient A (top) has a higher rhythmicity in both heart rate ranges than patient B (bottom).
B: Spontaneous course of consecutive RR intervals before (top) and after application of atropine (0.02 mg/kg BW) (bottom). Abscissa: number of RR intervals. Patient A (left) has a lower heart rate more strongly modulated by respiratory rhythm (RSA) than patient B (right). Typical disappearance of RSA with heart rate increase after application of atropine.

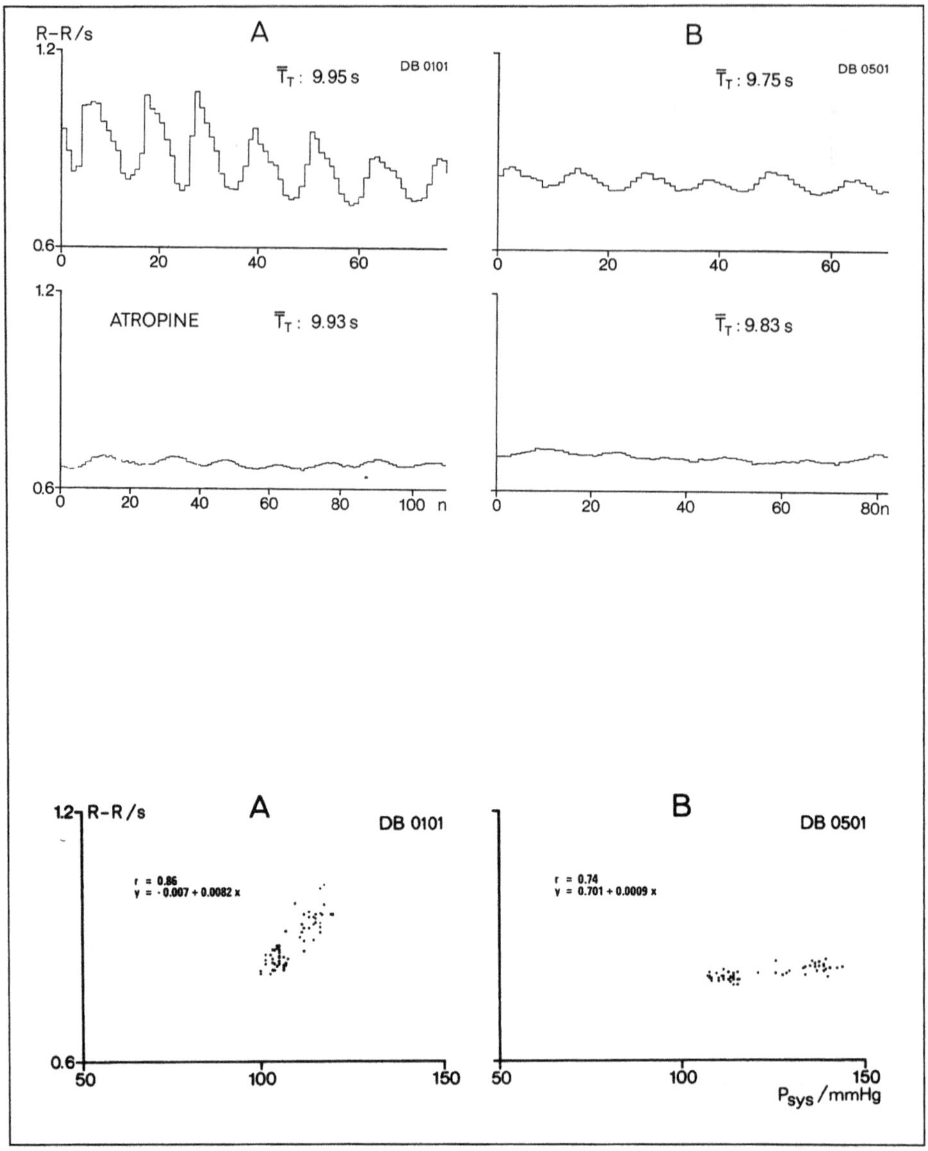

Fig. 9.

C: Course of consecutive RR intervals during voluntary slow respiration before (top) and after application of atropine (0.02 mg/kg BW) (bottom). External respiratory frequency: 6/min. Abscissa: number of RR intervals. Patient A (left) has a higher RSA in the resonance area than patient B (right), which is less completely suppressible after application of atropine.

D: Relation between systolic pressure and consecutive RR-interval during bolus injection of angiotensin II (0.04 μg/kg BW). This relation has a higher slope in patient A (left) than in patient B (right).

RR ((mean-RR max. – mean-RR min.): mean-RR * 100). Patient A showed a reduction of RSA from 23.5% to 3.4%, whereas in patient B the already reduced RSA decreased from 6.6% to 0.5% (Fig. 9C).

Angiotensin II: Heart rate changes occurring after bolus application of a pressor dose of Angiotensin II (0.04 μg/kg BW) were plotted against systolic blood pressure. Data were then submitted to a regression analysis (Fig. 9D). In patient A the slope is distinctly steeper (B = 8.2 ms/mmHg) than in patient B (B = 0.9 ms/mmHg).

Circadian variability of blood pressure and heart rate: In patients with different severity of autonomic insufficiency, systolic (Psys) and diastolic blood pressure (Pdia) and heart rate (HR) were measured indirectly throughout 24 h (Fig. 10A). In patient B, who has a more distinct autonomic insufficiency, the typical reduction of blood pressure and heart rate during the night period is less pronounced in comparison with patient C (day vs night in patient B: Psys 143.1 ± 14.0/146.5 ± 8.6 mmHg, Pdia 83.1 ± 10.0/81.2 ± 7.6 mmHg, HR 95.6 ± 11.7/80.1 ± 3.5 min.$^{-1}$; in patient C: Psys 159.5 ± 18.0/150.0

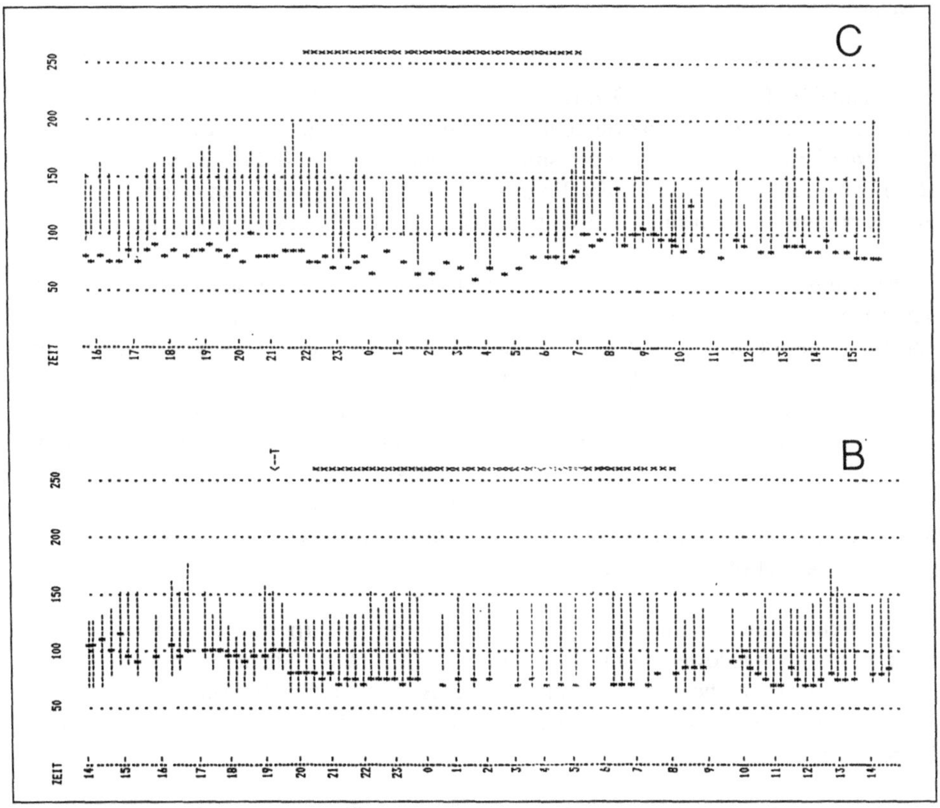

Fig. 10. Diurnal blood pressure and heart rate. Comparison of two hemodialysis patients (patient C and patient B) with autonomic insufficiency, which is less pronounced in patient C.
A: Time course of systolic and diastolic pressure (vertical lines) and heart rate (***). Sleep phases are marked at the upper border of the figure (xxx). Patient C: top, patient B: bottom.

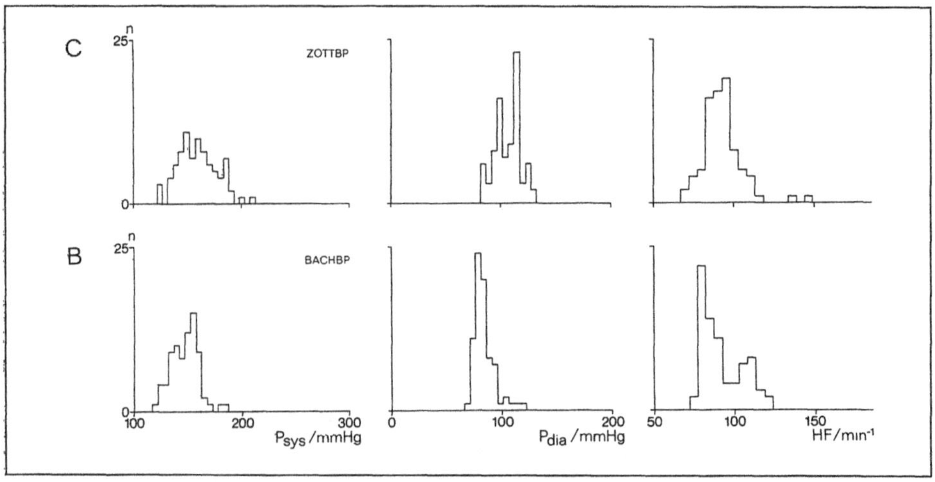

Fig. 10.
B: Frequency distribution of the systolic and diastolic pressure and heart rate values (Psys, Pdia, HR) monitored over 24 h. Patient C: top, patient B: bottom.

± 15.8 mmHg, Pdia 105.5 ± 9.7/103.2 ±14.1 mmHg, HR 94.4 ± 11.3/81.6 ± 6.8 $min.^{-1}$). The comparison of variation coefficients for Psys, Pdia, and HR results in a lower value only for the systolic blood pressure in patient B (patient B: Psys 8.5%, Pdia 11.0%, HR 13.5%; patient C: Psys 11.4%, Pdia 10.7%, HR 12.9%). The frequency distribution of this parameter accordingly shows a smaller basis of the histograms (Fig. 10B).

Heart rate pattern monitoring: The results of autonomic tests in hemodialysis patients had shown interindividual differences in the reactivity of the cardiovascular control system. Therefore, it was of interest to study heart rate control by analysis of the pattern of heart rate during hemodialysis treatment. To achieve this, a cross-over study was done in 10 non-selected patients. Each patient participated in two consecutive hemodialysis treatments carried out with different dialyzer membranes (cuprammonium cellulose, CAC, Lundia 5N, Gambro vs polyacrylonitrile, PAN, Biospal 2400, Hospal). Mean value (mean-RR) and standard deviation (S.D.-RR) were calculated from the RR-intervalsignal of consecutive 2-min sections. The time courses of mean-RR and S.D.-RR were compared by application of the *t*-test (Table 3).

The patterns of mean values were different in five patients ($p < 0.2$); in four cases the mean heart rate was lower with utilization of the PAN membrane in hemodialysis (Table 3A). The courses of heart rate variability likewise exhibited differences in five patients ($p < 0.2$), in four cases the heart rate variability was enhanced with application of the PAN membrane.

In comparison to patient B (DL02), who had a more distinct autonomic insufficiency, patient A (DL07) had a lower heart rate at both test sessions. Both patients had a lower mean heart rate during hemodialysis with PAN. On the other hand, patient A (DL07) had a higher heart rate variability only with the PAN membrane.

Table 3. Time courses of heart rate during hemodialysis treatment. Comparison of heart rate pattern at two therapeutic sessions during which different membranes were used (Biospal 2400, Hospal, and Lundia 5N, Gambro) with the *t*-test.

Table 3 A. Mean value of mean RR-intervals calculated consecutively of 2 min test sections at both sessions.

	PAN			CAC			t-Test
Pat.	n	mean/ms	S.D./ms	n	mean/ms	S.D./ms	P ≦
DL01	107	761,3	33,4	110	721,5	36,1	0,0001
DL02	111	644,1	59,6	99	618,7	59,9	0,01
DL03	102	589,8	26,5	104	589,7	17,5	
DL04	118	665,3	23,9	122	667,8	31,6	
DL05	36	767,1	47,9	67	697,4	51,1	0,0001
DL06	97	575,2	52,6	119	583,1	70,3	
DL07	114	671,8	30,0	111	640,1	36,4	0,0001
DL08	100	674,3	61,4	67	681,4	43,1	
DL10	127	697,1	33,3	126	703,9	36,6	0,2

Table 3 B. Standard deviations of mean RR-intervals calculated consecutively of 2 min test sections at both sessions.

	PAN			CAC			t-Test
Pat.	n	mean/ms	S.D./ms	n	mean/ms	S.D./ms	P ≦
DL01	107	24,0	7,8	110	22,6	8,3	
DL02	111	10,4	5,1	99	10,6	6,1	
DL03	102	14,4	6,6	104	13,1	6,2	0,1
DL04	118	31,6	12,8	122	29,6	10,0	0,2
DL05	36	24,9	6,4	67	21,9	10,7	0,2
DL06	97	29,5	13,2	119	31,1	12,8	
DL07	114	15,3	4,9	111	11,9	3,8	0,0001
DL08	100	12,4	5,9	67	13,9	9,4	
DL10	127	21,2	7,1	126	24,3	10,8	0,01

D – Differentiating heart rate pattern analysis

In 14 patients it was studied whether the analysis of patterns of variability and rhythmicity of heart rate can be used for the description of clinical states (Fig. 11). The correlations between mean-RR and S.D.-RR, mean-RR and area of HFB, mean-RR and area of MFB demonstrate that immediately after the end of hemodialysis no relation between sympathetically mediated modulation of the RR-interval signal (area of MFB) and mean RR-interval (group 2) exists, that heart rate rhythmicity in both frequency bands increases in the dialysis-free interval (group 3), and that variability and rhythmicity are particularly diminished with an additional diabetes mellitus (group 4).

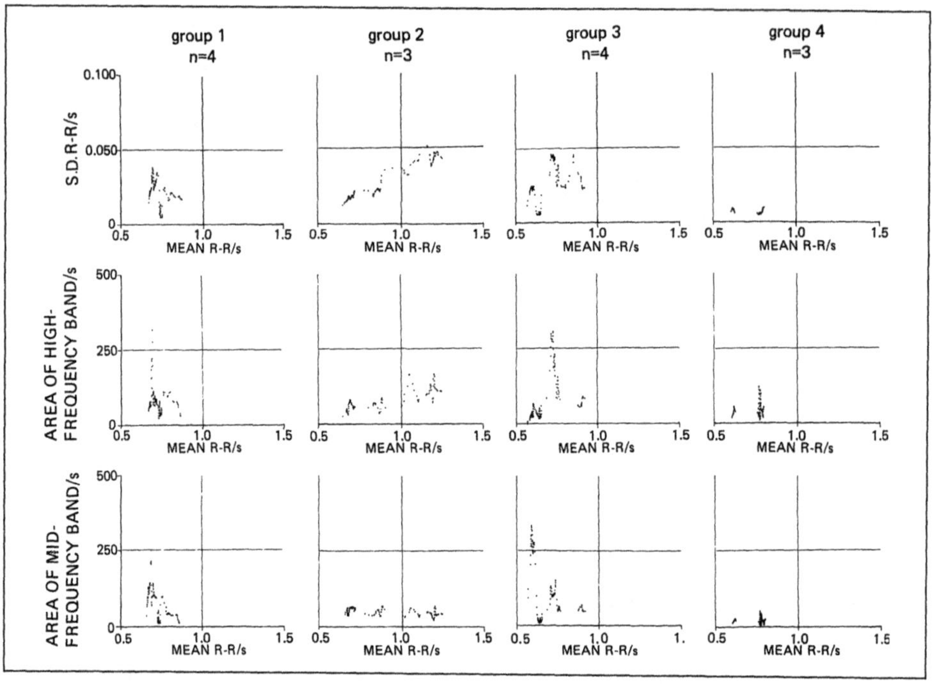

Fig. 11. Differentiating heart rate pattern analysis. From top to bottom: relation between mean cardiac interbeat interval (mean-RR) and standard deviation (S.D.-RR), mean-RR and area of high-frequency band, mean-RR and area of mid-frequency band. Group 1: pre-dialysis. Group 2: 3 h after dialysis treatment. Group 3: dialysis-free interval. Group 4: with additional diabetes mellitus 3 h after dialysis treatment.

Discussion

Heart rate control

The analysis of the relation between mean heart rate and its variability has its origin in the work of Schlomka and Reindell. They detected not only the enhancement of heart rate fluctuations related to respiration ("respiratory sinus arrhythmia," RSA) when mean heart rate decreases, but demonstrated also the age-dependent diminution in RSA [90]. In animal experiments, Koepchen and Thurau first described a close quantitative relationship between mean heart beat interval and variability after elimination of respiratory mechanisms, i.e., with purely central coupling [67]. The coupling of cardiac rhythm to respiratory innervation is caused by peripheral feedback loops via arterial baroreceptors (cf. [107]), receptors from the low-pressure system (cf. [79]) and lung stretch receptors [11, 44]. On the other hand, central nervous mechanisms are involved, like the respiratory phase-dependent modulation of the baroreceptor reflex [31, 68] and the spontaneous rhythmicity of neurones in the reticular formation firing in relation to respiratory rhythm [39, 59].

Alteration of cardiac vagal innervation constitutes a highly sensitive measure of the degree and progression of the pathophysiological state of various diseases. A reduction of the age-dependent heart rate variability was described in cases of autonomic diabetic neuropathy [43] and ESRD [25].

Our observation that there is a larger decrease in the variability of RR-intervals at longer mean RR-intervals in patients with ESRD shows that under these pathological conditions the deviations of heart rate variability are even more distinct at slow heart rate.

The analysis of lower frequencies superimposed upon the cardiac interbeat intervals can be utilized for the differentiation of control systems converging on efferent cardiac innervation. As a rule, the power spectra calculated from the cardiac interbeat interval signal of resting healthy subjects show three main spectral components which are usually assumed to reflect the spontaneous fluctuations in the behavior of control systems: oscillations in the cardiorespiratory coordination and in the control systems of blood pressure regulation and temperature regulation [9, 33, 89].

The spectral components investigated (HFB, MFB) are involved in different ways in the RR-interval variability depending on the mean RR-interval. At long RR-intervals, the variability is represented by heart rate rhythmicity, which is almost entirely of vagal origin and is related to respiration. At a mean heart rate around 60/min, the temporal modulations of sympathetic and para-sympathetic cardiac innervation have a resonance-like maximum, which can be extremely elevated, e.g., in endurance-trained athletes [4]. The maximum of variability and rhythmicity appearing at a frequency range of 60/min can be explained as a synchronization of central oscillators, the existence of which has been proposed by investigations on the rhythmicity of reticular brainstem neurones [71]. Under mental stress, the dynamics of heart rate control change in a characteristic manner. While under resting conditions a coordination between the cardiovascular and the respiratory system occurs preferentially in the respiratory frequency range (HFB, RSA) and the coordination between both systems under cognitive-motivational strain is shifted towards a lower frequency range (MFB) [2]. In contrast, the rhythmicity in the HFB and MFB decreased with increasing difficulty of tasks of another type of mental stress [82].

Already at rest, but particularly with an increased state of central nervous activity, a different behavior of mean RR-interval and RR-interval rhythmicity is found in healthy subjects [64]. This dissociation becomes particularly clear in patients on maintenance hemodialysis during the Raven test where changes in mean heart rate occur without related changes in heart rate rhythmicity. This supports our hypothesis that separate mechanisms exist, for the generation of mean activity determining the mean value and, on the other hand, for the generation of temporal modulation determining the time structure. The amplitude of rhythmicity does not primarily depend on the basic activity. This seems to apply especially for the respiration-dependent, vagally mediated heart rate fluctuations: during alterations of central nervous activity the change of rhythmicity in the HFB is a more sensitive indicator than deviations of mean heart rate.

The increase in heart rate at rest in patients with ESRD is explained by enhanced adrenergic activity [18, 73, 78] and a decrease in vagal tone [108]. The cardiac effect of an adequate dose of atropine consists chiefly in a simultaneous increase in heart rate and decrease in heart rate variability, so that the values of healthy subjects lie in the lower left part of the correlation between mean RR-interval and RR-interval variability (Fig. 3). However, since, in patients this correlation is not only shifted towards shorter RR-intervals but also has a reduced slope, a change in the central characteristics of mechanisms generating vagal innervation has to be assumed. The reaction of mean heart rate to mental strain, which is hardly altered in comparison with the healthy subjects, occurs on a cardiac autonomic innervation level with a relatively small portion of parasympathetic innervation [25, 109]. This is manifested by the higher mean heart rate in patients. It suggests itself to attribute the reduction in variability to a similar change in mean heart rate, at least in part. Of course, an attenuation of the efferent parasympathetic innervation or its afferent control due to a generalized neuropathy could also be involved [48, 74, 83]. Changes in central organization [76] or in excitation transfer in the pacemaker tissue are likewise conceivable. A systematic analysis of these single components has not been performed. After renal transplantation, the mechanisms generating the tonic component [46], as well as those generating the rhythmic component, seem to normalize [34].

Vasomotricity

The regulation of vascular tone is determined by membrane properties of vascular smooth musculature [97, 100], by endothelial mechanisms [26], by the biochemical environment and by an abundance of sensory afferents [95]. On the other hand, an effective influence on vasomotricity is exerted also by neuronal networks at the brainstem level, in the limbic system and at the cortical level [70]. The rhythmic phenomena of vasomotricity are brought about by an interaction between the rhythmic vascular innervation and the intrinsic rhythmicity of vascular smooth musculature [94, 97]. Thus, a structure arranged longitudinally on the neuraxis is established for the integration of cardiovascular innervation patterns. This longitudinal organization explains the mental, emotional and reflex influences, the interaction of which affects the overall reaction of vasomotricity in healthy and diseased humans [22, 51, 81].

In hemodialysis patients, the cutaneous vasomotricity exhibits a change in spontaneous rhythmic patterns. Lower frequencies supervene, and the frequency maximum in the higher-frequency range is lacking. Whether common central or peripheral mechanisms underlie this distinct reduction of vascular rhythms and heart rate modulations at the frequency range corresponding approximately to the MFB requires further investigations. The vasomotor reactivity as reflected in the pulse synchronous volume amplitude of the finger plethysmogram is also diminished at rest. This can be estimated from a decrease in the range of variation of the finger pulse amplitude. Similar to "cold stress" [8], vascular reactivity is diminished under "mental stress". The assessment of the disturbance of sympathetic innervation is controversial. In the pre-dialysis stage, a sympathetic disturbance is believed to prevail [27], which, in contrast to the parasympathetic one, is reversible in the course of dialysis treatment [46]. The methodological approach of the customary autonomic tests permits only an inadequate differentiation of various sympathetic efferents. Skin and muscle sympathetic innervation, however, exhibit differentiated patterns under physiological conditions [104, 105]. As patients under "mental stress" show heart rate acceleration in the normal range, the altered reactivity of their vasomotricity could be due either to a weaker reactivity of the sympathetic innervation patterns [103] or of the effector organ [17]. Our analysis of spontaneous cutaneous vasomotor rhythmicity likewise shows distinct by attenuated reactivity. Again, it is not clear whether the change has to be attributed to an alteration of the innervation pattern or to an alteration of the reactivity of vascular smooth musculature or to both.

Respiration

Among autonomic control systems, respiration holds an intermediate position, because it is also considered to be part of the somatomotor system on account of its motor efferents, motor effectors, and its susceptibility of voluntary control. The rhythmogenesis of respiration originates from the interaction of inspiratory, post-inspiratory and expiratory neurone populations in a complexly structured neuronal network which is part of the reticular formation of the brainstem [35, 88]. The activity of this network, and thus the resulting respiration, is influenced by the instantaneous central nervous activity [24], by afferents affecting not only respiration, e.g., chemoreceptors [30, 50, 69], by affective behavior [49] and somatomotor behavior during physical work [29], and also in the scope of specialized cortical functions, e.g., speaking and singing [86].

The respiratory parameters calculated from the single breath (inspiratory time, mean inspiratory flow, expiratory time) indicate the activity of neuronal mechanisms involved in respiratory rhythmogenesis [1, 35, 66, 88]. This kind of indirect analysis allows the differentiation of, e.g., the interaction of afferent feedback (CO_2) and central autonomic innervation during cognitive-motivational or motor behavior concerned with speaking [5]. Central respiration-generating structures are subject to modulations [41, 54] which manifest as rhythmicity of respiratory parameters and which are caused by oscillatory influences on the activity of mechanisms concerned with the respiratory rhythmogenesis in a lower frequency range.

Under the pathophysiological conditions of ESRD, the spontaneous variability in the respiratory control system increases in the interval between dialysis sessions in contrast to the reduction of spontaneous rhythmicity in the cardiovascular control system. During dialysis an increase in variability of respiratory parameters likewise occurs depending on the composition of the dialysate [16]. An uremic peripheral neuropathy will hardly explain this finding, since in the autonomic nervous system a peripheral neuropathy is supposed to cause a reduction of cardiovascular variability and rhythmicity. Thus, it is suggested that the increased variability of respiratory parameters is due to central nervous disturbances.

Tests of autonomic control

The interest in the function of autonomic control systems in patients with ESRD originates in findings indicating an autonomic neuropathy [99] existing in parallel with a peripheral sensomotor neuropathy [12], in hypertension [23] frequently concomitant with dialysis-induced hypotension [61], and in changes in baroreceptor function [77]. Generally, in the uremic dysfunction of autonomic control systems, the afferent pathway, the central control mechanism, and the efferent side represented by sympathetic and parasympathetic innervation can be affected in different combinations and degrees. Based on a more detailed analysis by means of clinical autonomic tests [102], however, a primary disturbance at the afferent side is suggested [27, 73, 108], though certainly the efferent side is likewise concerned to a various extent in this autonomic dysfunction [25]. The autonomic tests usually applied for the characterization of parasympathetic functions – voluntary slow respiration [108], diving reflex [110] and Valsalva maneuver [99] – indicate in most predialysis patients a beginning or an already manifest parasympathetic abnormality, which can be improved depending on the type of dialysis treatment [111] and after successful transplantation [34]. The results of tests of sympathetic function – mental stress, cold pressure, isometric handgrip, and orthostasis [28] – however, suggest an infrequent and less pronounced sympathetic dysfunction in predialysis patients which is reversible during the dialysis treatment [18, 46, 110]. Nevertheless, such a strict classification into tests of sympathetic and parasympathetic functions seems to be an over-interpretation since in many of these tests both parts of the autonomic innervation are involved.

The results from heart rate pattern analysis during physical rest are compared with those of autonomic tests in order to examine the reliability of this indirect non-invasive method with regard to autonomic insufficiency. An indirect measure of the momentary state of parasympathetic innervation, which can be calculated from the course of heart beat intervals, is the degree of rhythmicity in the so-called respiratory frequency band (HFB) or "respiratory sinus arrhythmia" (RSA) [33, 37, 60]. Administration of atropine suppresses heart rate rhythmicity in this frequency band [9]. With spirometrically recorded spontaneous respiration, the degree of rhythmicity is moreover dependent on the momentary respiratory frequency and depth [52]. These results could be confirmed with pneumographically recorded spontaneous respiration [4]. This method avoids the occurrence of reflex alterations in the respiratory pattern with spirometric recordings [13, 53]. On the other hand, the degree of rhythmicity in the HFB depends on the mean heart beat interval [67, 90], on the extent of mental stress [58], on physical fitness [4, 91], on age [47, 90] and on the general state of health, e.g., for diabetes mellitus [43] or ESRD [25].

With voluntary deceleration of respiratory frequency, the amplitude of RSA reaches a maximum around six breaths per minute which also depends on the amount of the tidal volume [10, 52], whereby phase shifts can occur between respiration and respiratory heart rate fluctuations [10]. As mentioned above, various central and peripheral mechanisms are involved in the occurrence of RSA. With deceleration of respiratory frequency, the respiratory rhythm moves from the high-frequency band (HFB), in which it is usually found, to the mid-frequency band (MFB). When the slowed respiratory rhythm coincides with a 10 s rhythm occurring also in circulatory and brainstem rhythmicity, a resonance-like augmentation of heart rate fluctuations appears. During slow rhythmic respiration, the marked respiratory-synchronous heart rate oscillations have to be attributed not only to parasympathetic, but also to sympathetic cardiomotor innervation. This is evident from maintained but attenuated heart rate fluctuations after parasympathetic blockade (Fig. 9C).

The baroreceptor reflexes buffer deviations of arterial blood pressure, the mean value of which is determined by the state of central nervous excitation as well as by peripheral reflectory influences. As far as reflex heart rate changes are concerned, the characteristics of this homeostatic blood pressure control can be analyzed pharmacologically [98]. In comparison with orthostatic tests, this procedure has the advantage that blood pressure alterations relatively independent of other interfering influences can be induced. The slope of the relation between systolic blood pressure and RR-interval, i.e., the sensitivity of the baroreceptor heart rate reflex is susceptible to modulations in both directions. During inspiration [31, 68], during progressive physical work [20], and with increasing age [42], a decrease in the slope of this relation occurs which can also be shifted without a change in slope, as in hypercapnia [19]. The reflex heart rate decelerations occurring with artificially evoked blood pressure increases are mediated preferentially via the parasympathetic innervation [85]. The baroreceptor reflex, which is relayed primarily at the brainstem level, is also modulated by anterior limbic brain structures [55, 62] and hypothalamic regions [38]. After parasympathetic blockade, these modulations are no longer detectable. In pathological processes related to hypertension [21, 101] or ESRD [72, 106], the heart rate alteration in relation to arterial blood pressure changes is diminished.

The results of testing heart rate control which have shown a different degree of autonomic dysfunction in two exemplary patients, are in good agreement with the results of the non-invasive heart rate pattern analysis. The stronger rhythmicity in the high-frequency band, where the respiratory rhythm is normally found, and the stronger "respiratory sinus arrhythmia" (which can be largely blocked by administration of atropine) during slower respiration in patient A lead to the conclusion of a lesser decrease in parasympathetic heart rate modulation as well as a higher sensitivity of the baroreceptor heart rate reflex in patient A in contrast to patient B.

Heart rate pattern analysis

This continuous evaluation of indicators of heart rate variability and rhythmicity and their correlation to the mean RR-interval permit a judgement of the mutual interaction of sympathetic and parasympathetic cardiac innervation. These correlations are influenced among other factors by respiration and the state of physical training [4] and by pathological processes [7]. This type of heart rate analysis can primarily achieve a phenomenological discrimination of different physiological and pathophysiological states, since a large number of central nervous and peripheral mechanisms exert their influence with temporally varying importance on these effector mechanisms controlling heart rate. Thus, narrow limitations are set to the application of this non-invasive method to analyze the underlying mechanisms. In spite of these methodological restrictions, the high sensitivity of rhythmicity parameters to alterations of internal and external conditions presents an interesting aspect. Changes in heart rate rhythmicity can be utilized as a nonspecific "early warning symptom" reflecting the integrated position of effector mechanisms of heart rate control.

Circadian variability of blood pressure and heart rate

Direct long-term measurements of arterial blood pressure [14, 87] reveal periodic changes even in the short-term range (3 s up to 20 min), exhibiting a close correlation between blood pressure and heart rate [92]. By means of indirect automatic measurement with intervals of 15 to 30 min, however, only behavioral or diurnal blood pressure changes can be assessed. Mean values and variability parameters, on the other hand, are determined in accordance with each other by both methods. With regard to systolic and diastolic pressure and heart rate the variation coefficients throughout 24 h in normotensive persons was 11.0%/15.8%/20.1% and in patients with a medium degree of essential hypertension 10.3%/11.9%/16.6% [45, 93], whereas in hemodialysis patients blood pressure was more variable (22.1%/20.0%) and heart rate less (14.3%) variable. During the night, systolic and diastolic blood pressure and heart rate decreased in all normotensive (N) and hypertensive (H) persons (N: –6.4/–3.5 mmHG/–8.8 bpm; H: –15.0/–9.4 mmHG/–11.2 bpm). In dialysis patients, these parameters were partly higher during the night (mean value and range for Psys –3.8 mmHG (–15 to +3), for Pdia –4.2 mmHG (–20 to +8) and for heart rate –2.0/min (–16 to +16)). The observed deviations correspond to the severity of the autonomic dysfunction.

Acknowledgement

The authors are indebted to Mrs. H. Semmler for technical assistance, Mr. J. Petsch for development and production of data acquisition electronics, Mr. D. Winzer for the preparation of the figures, Mr. P. Holzner for the photographs, and Mrs. E. Gaebel for translation and typing of the manuscript.

References

1. Abel H-H, Klüßendorf D, Koepchen HP (1985) Interaction of behavioural and chemical drive in ventilation and respiratory pattern during and after mental load in human subjects. Pflügers Arch 405: R 50

2. Abel H-H, Klüßendorf D, Koepchen HP (1987) Correlated low frequency oscillations in respiratory and cardiovascular control. Pflügers Arch 408: R 66
3. Abel H-H, Klüßendorf D, Koepchen HP (1987) New approach of analysing the neurovegetative state in man. In Innovative Monitoring in Anaesthesia, ed by Droh R, Spintge R, Springer (im Druck)
4. Abel H-H, Krause R, Klüßendorf D, Koepchen HP, with the technical assistance of Semmler H (1987) Changed relations between cardiorespiratory parameters and heart rate variability in endurance-trained individuals at rest. In: Hildebrandt G, Moog R, Raschke F (eds) Chronobiology & Chronomedicine. Basic Research and Applications. Peter Lang, Frankfurt am Main, Bern, New York, Paris pp 187–192
5. Abel H-H, Mottau B, Klüßendorf D, Koepchen HP (1987) Differential influence of respiratory drives on central partial mechanisms of respiratory rhythmogenesis in man. Pflügers Arch 408 (Supp.): S 34
6. Abel H-H, Mottau B, Klüßendorf D, Koepchen HP (1987) Pattern of different components of the respiratory cycle and autonomic parameters during speech. In Respiratory Muscles and Their Neuromotor Control, ed by Sieck GC, Gandevia SC, Cameron WE. Alan R Liss Inc, New York pp 109–113
7. Abel H-H, Schultze G, Molzahn M, Koepchen HP (1986) Muster spontaner Herzfrequenzvariabilität bei Urämie und Dialyse. Nieren- und Hochdruckkrankh 15: 365
8. Aizawa Y, Yuasa Y, Ohmori T, Taziri M, Hirasawa Y (1977) Diminished vascular reactivity to a cold stress in azotemic patients. J Dialysis 1: 781–792
9. Akselrod S, Gordon D, Ubel FA, Shannon DC, Barger AC, Cohen RJ (1981) Power spectrum analysis of heart rate fluctuation: a quantitative probe of beat-to-beat cardiovascular control. Science 213: 220–222
10. Angelone A, Coulter NA Jr (1964) Respiratory sinus arrhythmia: a frequency dependent phenomenon. J Appl Physiol 19: 479–482
11. Anrep GV, Pascual W, Rössler R (1936) Respiratory variations of the heart rate. I – The reflex mechanism of the respiratory arrhythmia. Proc Roy Soc Lond (B) 119: 191–217
12. Asbury AK, Victor M, Adams RD (1963) Uremic polyneuropathy. Arch Neurol 8: 413–420
13. Askanazi J, Silverberg PA, Foster RJ, Hyman AI, Milic-Emili J, Kinney JM (1980) Effects of respiratory apparatus on breathing pattern. J Appl Physiol 48: 577–580
14. Athanassiadis D, Draper GJ, Honour AJ, Cranston WI (1969) Variability of automatic blood pressure measurements over 24 hour periods. Clin Sci 36: 147–156
15. Axelrod S, Lishner M, Oz O, Bernheim J, Ravid M (1987) Spectral analysis of fluctuations in heart rate: an objective evaluation of autonomic nervous control in chronic renal failure. Nephron 45: 202–206
16. Backer WA de, Heyrman RM, Wittesaele WM, Waeleghem JP van, Vermeire PA, Broe ME de (im Druck) Ventilation and breathing patterns during hemodialysis induced CO_2 unloading. Am Rev Resp Dis
17. Botey A, Gaya J, Montoliu J, Torras A, Rivera F, Lopez-Pedret J, Revert L (1981) Postsynaptic adrenergic unresponsiveness in hypotensive haemodialysis patients. Proc Eur Dial Transplant Ass 18: 586–590
18. Brecht HM, Ernst W, Koch KM (1976) Plasma noradrenalin levels in regular haemodialysis patients. Dial Transpl Nephrol 12: 281–289
19. Bristow JD, Brown EB Jr, Cunningham DJC, Goode RC, Howson MG, Sleight P (1971) The effects of hypercapnia, hypoxia and ventilation on the baroreflex regulation of the pulse interval. J Physiol (Lond) 216: 281–302
20. Bristow JD, Brown EB Jr, Cunningham DJC, Howson MG, Peterson ES, Pickering TG, Sleight P (1971) Effect of bicycling on the baroreflex regulation of pulse interval. Circ Res 28: 582–502
21. Bristow JD, Honour AJ, Pickering GW, Sleight P, Smyth HS (1969) Diminished baroreflex sensitivity in high blood pressure. Circulation 39: 48–54
22. Brod J (1970) Psychological influences on the cardiovascular system. In Modern Trends in Psychosomatic Medicine 2, ed by Hill OW. Buttherworths
23. Brown JJ, Duesterdieck G, Frager R, Lever AF, Robertson JJ, Tree M, Weir RJ (1971) Hypertension and chronic renal failure. Brit Med Bull 27: 128–135
24. Bülow K (1963) Respiration and wakefulness in man. Acta Physiol Scand 59: Suppl 209
25. Burgess ED (1982) Cardiac vagal denervation in hemodialysis patients. Nephron 30: 228–230

26. Busse R (1986) Regulation des Gefäßtonus: Rolle endothelialer Mechanismen. Physiologie aktuell 2: 179–200
27. Campese VM, Romoff MS, Levitan D, Lane K, Massry SG (1981) Mechanisms of autonomic nervous system dysfunction in uremia. Kidney Int 20: 246–253
28. Clarke BF, Ewing DJ, Campbell IW (1979) Diabetic autonomic neuropathy. Diabetologia 17: 195–212
29. Comroe JH Jr (1944) The hyperpnea of muscular exercise. Physiol Rev 24: 319–339
30. Dell P (1952) Corrélations entre le système végétatif et le système de la vie de relation mesencephale et cortex cérébral. J Physiol (Paris) 44: 471–557
31. Eckberg DL, Orshan CR (1977) Respiratory and baroreceptor reflex interactions in man. J Clin Invest 59: 780–785
32. Eckoldt K (1984) Verfahren und Ergebnisse der quantitativen automatischen Analyse der Herzfrequenz und deren Spontanvariabilität. Dt. Gesundh-Wesen 39: 856–863
33. Eckoldt K (1985) Herzfrequenzvariabilität und deren spektrale Komponenten bei unterschiedlichen autonomen Funktionszuständen. Ergeb exp Med 46: 106–116
34. Endre ZH, Perl SI, Kraegen EW, Charlesworth JA, Macdonald GJ (1982) Reduced cardiac beat-to-beat variation in chronic renal failure: a ubiquitous marker of autonomic neuropathy. Clin Sci 62: 561–562
35. Euler C von (1983) On the central pattern generator for the basic breathing rhythmicity. J Appl Physiol 55: 1647–1659
36. Ewing DJ, Winney R (1975) Autonomic function in patients with chronic renal failure on intermittent haemodialysis. Nephron 15: 424–429
37. Fouad FM, Tarazi RC, Ferrario CM, Fighaly S, Alicandri C (1984) Assessment of parasympathetic control of heart rate by a noninvasive method. Am J Physiol 246: H838–H842
38. Gebber GL, Snyder DW (1970) Hypothalamic control of baroreceptor reflexes. Am J Physiol 218: 124–131
39. Gilbey MP, Jordan D, Richter DW, Spyer KM (1984) Synaptic mechanisms involved in the inspiratory modulation of vagal cardio-inhibitory neurones in the cat. J Physiol (Lond) 356: 65–78
40. Golenhofen K, Hildebrandt G (1958) Die Beziehungen des Blutdruckrhythmus zu Atmung und peripherer Durchblutung. Pflügers Arch 267: 27–45
41. Goodman L (1964) Oscillatory behavior of ventilation in resting man. IEEE BME-13 82–93
42. Gribbin B, Pickering TG, Sleight P, Peto R (1971) Effect of age and high blood pressure on baroreflex sensitivity in man. Circ Res 29: 424–431
43. Gunderson HJG, Neubauer B (1977) A long-term diabetic autonomic nervous abnormality. Reduced variations in resting heart rate measured by a simple and sensitive method. Diabetologia 13: 137–140
44. Hainsworth R (1974) Circulatory responses from lung inflation in anesthetized dogs. Am J Physiol 226: 247–255
45. Hauff A, Schultze G (1981) Assessment of circadian rhythm of blood pressure and heart rate in ambulatory patients. Biotelemetry Patient Monitg 8: 106–112
46. Heidbreder E, Schafferhans K, Heidland A (1985) Disturbances of peripheral and autonomic nervous system in chronic renal failure: effects of hemodialysis and transplantation. Clin Nephrol 22: 222–228
47. Hellman JB, Stacy RW (1976) Variation of respiratory sinus arrhythmia with age. J Appl Physiol 41: 734–738
48. Hennessy WJ, Siemsen AW (1968) Autonomic neuropathy in chronic renal failure. Clin Res 16: 385–390
49. Hess WR (1949) Das Zwischenhirn. Syndrome, Lokalisationen, Funktionen. Benno Schwabe & Co Verlag, Basel
50. Heymans C, Neil E (1958) Reflexogenic areas of the cardiovascular system. J & A Chruchill Ltd, London
51. Hilton SM (1982) The defence-arousal system and its relevance for circulatory and respiratory control. J exp Biol 100: 159–174
52. Hirsch JA, Bishop B (1981) Respiratory sinus arrhythmia in humans: how breathing pattern modulates heart rate. Am J Physiol 241: H620–H629
53. Hirsch JA, Bishop B (1982) Human breathing patterns on mouthpiece or face mask during air, CO_2, or low O_2. J Appl Physiol 53: 1281–1290

54. Hlastala MP, Wranne B, Lenfant CJ (1973) Cyclical variations in FRC and other respiratory variables in resting man. J Appl Physiol 34: 670–676
55. Hockman CH, Talesnik J, Livingston KE (1969) Central nervous system modulation of baroceptor reflexes. Am J Phyisol 217: 1681–1689
56. Holst E von (1939) Die relative Koordination als Phänomen und als Methode zentralnervöser Funktionsanalyse. Erg Physiol 42: 228–306
57. Hugelin A (1986) Forebrain and midbrain influence on respiration. In Handbook of Physiology, Section 3: The Respiratory System, vol II: Control of Breathing, Part 1, ed by Fishman AP, Cherniack NS, Widdicombe JG, Geiger SR. American Physiological Society, Bethesda pp 69–91
58. Hyndman BW, Gregory JR (1975) Spectral analysis of sinus arrhythmia during mental loading. Ergonomics 18: 255–270
59. Joels N, Samueloff M (1956) The activity of the medullary centres in diffusion respiration. J Physiol (Lond) 133: 360–372
60. Katona PG, Jih F (1975) Respiratory sinus arrhythmia: noninvasive measure of parasympathetic cardiac control. J Appl Physiol 39: 801–805
61. Kersh ES, Kronfield SJ, Under A, Popper RW, Cantor S, Cohn K (1974) Autonomic insufficiency in uremia as a cause of hemodialysis-induced hypotension. New Engl J Med 290: 650–653
62. Klevans LR, Gebber GL (1970) Facilitatory forebrain influence on cardiac component of baroreceptor reflexes. Am J Physiol 219: 1235–1241
63. Koepchen HP (1962) Die Blutdruckrhythmik. Dr Dietrich Steinkopff Verlag, Darmstadt
64. Koepchen HP, Abel H-H, Klüßendorf D (1985) Heart-rate dynamics in healthy humans before, during and after a mental test. Pflügers Arch 405: R50
65. Koepchen HP, Abel H-H, Klüßendorf D (1987) Physiological concepts of cardiovascular and respiratory control: theoretical basis and applicability in man. In Innovative Monitoring in Anaesthesia, ed by Droh R, Spintge R, Springer (im Druck)
66. Koepchen HP, Abel H-H, Klüßendorf D, Lazar H (1988) Differentiation between partial components of respiratory rhythmogenesis in animal experiments and in man. In Funktionsanalyse biologischer Systeme 18, ed by Grote J. Gustav-Fischer-Verlag, Stuttgart, New York (pp 141—148)
67. Koepchen HP, Thurau K (1959) Über die Entstehungsbedingungen der atemsynchronen Schwankungen des Vagustonus (Respiratorische Arrhythmie). Pflügers Arch 269: 10–30
68. Koepchen HP, Wagner P-H, Lux HD (1961) Über die Zusammenhänge zwischen zentraler Erregbarkeit, reflektorischem Tonus und Atemrhythmus bei der nervösen Steuerung der Herzfrequenz. Pflügers Arch 273: 443–465
69. Korner PI (1971) Integrative neural cardiovascular control. Physiol Rev 51: 312–367
70. Korner PI (1979) Central nervous control of autonomic cardiovascular function. In Handbook of Physiology, Section 2: The Cardiovascular System, vol I: The Heart, ed by Berne RM, Sperelakis N, Geiger SR. American Physiological Society, Bethesda pp 691–739
71. Langhorst P, Lambertz M, Schulz G (1981) Central control and interactions affecting sympathetic and parasympathetic activity. J Auton Nerv Syst 4: 149–163
72. Lazarus JM, Hampers CL, Lowrie EG, Merrill JP (1973) Baroreceptor activity in normotensive and hypertensive uremic patients. Circulation 47: 1015–1021
73. Lilley JJ, Golden J, Stone RA (1976) Adrenergic regulation of blood pressure in chronic renal failure. J Clin Invest 57: 1190–1200
74. Mallamaci F, Zoccali C, Ciccarelli M, Briggs DJ (1986) Autonomic function in uraemic patients treated by haemodialysis or CAPD and in transplant patients. Clin Nephrol 25: 175–180
75. Malliani A, Lombardi F, Pagani M, Cerutti S (1986) The problem of approaching the sympathetic and vagal „tone''. J Auton Nerv Syst Suppl 191–196
76. Marsh JT, Brown WS, Wolcott D, Landsverk J, Nissenson AR (1986) Electrophysiological indices of CNS function in hemodialysis and CAPD. Kidney Int 30: 957–963
77. McCubbin JW, Green JH, Page IH (1956) Baroceptor function in chronic renal hypertension. Circ Res 4: 205–210
78. McGrath BP, Ledingham JGG, Benedict CR (1978) Catecholamines in peripheral venous plasma in patients on chronic haemodialysis. Clin Sci Molec Med 55: 89–96
79. Melcher A (1976) Respiratory sinus arrhythmia in man. A study in heart rate regulating mechanisms. Acta Physiol Scand Suppl 435
80. Meyer-Sabellek W, Schulte K-L, Distler A, Gotzen R (1987) Technische Aspekte der ambulanten,

automatischen, nichtinvasiven 24-Stunden-Blutdruckmessung. Schweiz Rundschau Med (PRAXIS) 76: 443-449

81. Monnier M (1968) Functions of the Nervous System, vol 1: General Physiology. Autonomic Functions. Elsevier Publishing Company, Amsterdam, London, New York
82. Mulder G, Mulder LJM (1981) Information processing and cardiovascular control. Psychophysiology 18: 392-402
83. Nielson VK (1973) The peripheral nerve function in chronic renal failure. V. Sensory and motor conduction velocity. Acta Med Scand 194: 445-454
84. Pickering TG, Gribbin B, Oliver DO (1972) Baroreflex sensitivity in patients on long-term haemodialysis. Clin Sci 43: 645-657
85. Pickering TG, Gribbin B, Petersen ES, Cunningham DJC, Sleight P (1972) Effects of autonomic blockade on the baroreflex in man at rest and during exercise. Circ Res 30: 177-185
86. Proctor DF (1980) Breathing, Speech, and Song. Springer-Verlag, Wien, New York
87. Richardson DW, Honour AJ, Fenton GW, Stott FH, Pickering GW (1964) Variation in arterial pressure throughout the day and night. Clin Sci 26: 445-460
88. Richter DW (1982) Generation and maintenance of the respiratory rhythm. J exp Biol 100: 93-107
89. Rompelman O (1980) The assessment of fluctuations in heart-rate. In The Study of Heart-Rate Variability, ed by Kitney RI, Rompelman O. Clarendon Press, Oxford pp 59-77
90. Schlomka G (1937) Untersuchungen über die physiologische Unregelmäßigkeit des Herzschlages. III. Mitteilung. Über die Abhängigkeit der respiratorischen (Ruhe-)Arrhythmie von der Schlagfrequenz und vom Lebensalter. Z Kreislaufforschg 29: 510-524
91. Schlomka G, Reindell H (1936) Untersuchungen über die physiologische Unregelmäßigkeit des Herzschlages. Z Kreislaufforschg 28: 473-492
92. Schultze G, Hauff A, Hullmeine D, Isichei E (1978) Frequency distribution of the 24 hour blood pressure and heart rate. In Biotelemetry IV, Proceedings of the Fourth International Symposium on Biotelemetry, ed by Klewe HJ, Kimmich HP. Döring-Cruck, Braunschweig pp 145-148
93. Schultze G, Hauff A, Hullmeine D, Isichei E, Dißmann Th (1978) Economic digital analysis in long term arterial blood pressure telemetry. In ISAM 1977, Proceedings of the Second International Symposium on Ambulatory Monitoring, ed by Stott FD, Raftery EB, Sleight P, Goulding L. Academic Press, London pp 173-183
94. Seller H, Langhorst P, Polster J, Koepchen HP (1967) Zeitliche Eigenschaften der Vasomotorik. II. Erscheinungsformen und Entstehung spontaner und nervös induzierter Gefäßrhythmen. Pflügers Arch 296: 110-132
95. Shepherd JT (1983) Circulation to skeletal muscle. In Handbook of Physiology, Section 2: The Cardiovascular System, vol III: Peripheral Circulation and Organ Blood Flow, part 1, ed by Shepherd JT, Abboud FM, Geiger SR. American Physiological Society. Bethesda pp 319-370
96. Sherrington CS (1906) The integrative action of the nervous system. Yale University Press, New Haven (1947[2]), Nachdruck 1961
97. Siegel G (1986) Membranphysiologische Grundlagen der peripheren Gefäßregulation. Physiologie aktuell 1: 31-52
98. Smyth HS, Sleight P, Pickering GW (1969) Reflex regulation of arterial pressure during sleep in man. A quantitative method of assessing baroreflex sensitivity. Circ Res 24: 109-121
99. Soriano G, Eisinger RP (1972) Abnormal response to the Valsalva manoeuvre in patients on chronic haemodialysis. Nephron 9: 251-256
100. Speden RN (1970) Excitation of vascular smooth muscle. In Smooth Muscle, ed by Bülbring E, Brading AF, Jones AW, Tomita T. Edward Arnold Ltd, London pp 558-588
101. Takeshita A, Tanaka S, Kuroiwa A, Nakamura M (1975) Reduced baroreceptor sensitivity in borderline hypertension. Circulation 51: 738-742
102. Thomson PD, Melmen KL (1968) Clinical assessment of autonomic function. Anesthesiology 29: 724-731
103. Wallin BG, Delius W, Hagbarth KE (1973) Comparison of sympathetic nerve activity in normotensive and hypertensive subjects. Circ Res 33: 9-21
104. Wallin BG, Delius W, Hagbarth KE (1974) Regional control of sympathetic outflow in human skin and muscle nerves. In Central Rhythmic and Regulation. Circulation, Respiration, Extrapyramidal Motor System, ed by Umbach W, Koepchen HP. Hippokrates Verlag, Stuttgart pp 190-195
105. Wallin BG, Sundlöf G, Delius W (1975) The effect of carotid sinus nerve stimulation on muscle and skin nerve sympathetic activity in man. Pflügers Arch 358: 101-110

106. Wehle B, Bevegard S, Castenfors J, Davidsson S, Lindblad LE (1983) Carotid baroreflexes during hemodialysis. Clin Nephrol 29: 236–242
107. Wesseling KH, Settels JJ (1985) Baromodulation explains short-term blood pressure variability. In Psychophysiology of Cardiovascular Control. Models, Methods, and Data, ed by Orlebeke JF, Mulder G, van Doornen LJP. Plenum Press, New York, London pp 69–97
108. Zoccali C, Ciccarelli M, Maggiore Q (1982) Defective reflex control of heart rate in dialysis patients: evidence for an afferent autonomic lesion. Clin Sci 63: 285–292
109. Zoccali C, Ciccarelli M, Mallamaci F, Maggiore Q (1986) Parasympathetic function in haemodialysis patients. Nephron 44: 351–354
110. Zuccalà A, Degli Esposti E, Sturani A, Chiarini C, Santoro A, Catizone L, Zucchelli P (1978) Autonomic function in hemodialyzed patients. Int J Artif Organs 1: 76–82
111. Zucchelli P, Sturani A, Degli Esposti E, Chiarini C, Santoro A, Zuccalà A (1983) Hemodialysis, in contrast to CAPD, improves parasympathetic function in ESRD patients. Trans Am Soc Artif Intern Organs 29: 617–622
112. Zwiener U (1976) Pathophysiologie neurovegetativer Regelungen und Rhythmen. Systemstudien und biokybernetische Ansätze zu klinischen Funktionstests. VEB Gustav Fischer Verlag, Jena

Reversed circadian variation of blood pressure in heart transplant patients?*

J. Sehested[1], W. Meyer-Sabellek[2] and R. Hetzer[1]

[1]Deutsches Herzzentrum Berlin, Berlin, FRG
[2]Medizinische Klinik und Poliklinik, Klinikum Steglitz, Freie Universität Berlin, Berlin, F.R.G.

Introduction

In patients undergoing orthotopic heart transplantation, part of the recipient atrium, as well as the sinus node, remains in the patient. The atria of the donor heart, with its sinus node, is connected to the recipient atria, and the pulmonary arteries and the aortas are anastomosed.

This leaves the patient with a completely denervated pair of ventricles and a pair of partly denervated atria.

Although the baroreceptor-sinus node reflex-arch of the recipient atrium is known to remain intact for years [1, 5], no evidence so far clearly indicates that reinnervation of the donor heart takes place in man [1, 3, 5].

This means that the pumping action of the heart is based on the Frank-Starling law and the intrinsic, autonomous action of the heart alone. Adjustment of cardiac function to the various demands of the body is now brought about, generally speaking, by two means: alterations in the peripheral resistance, and alterations in circulating, vasoactive hormones.

Apart from providing the opportunity to study human cardiovascular physiology following cardiac denervation, heart transplant patients present with the problem of hypertension of uncertain origin. Since the introduction of cyclosporine A for the control of rejection, hypertension has been considered an important side effect in these patients [2].

In cardiac transplant patients not receiving cyclosporine as part of the postoperative treatment, hypertension is rarely observed [2].

As this de novo hypertension is seen to develop rather quickly, often within the first couple of months following transplantation, 24-h blood pressure measurements were made shortly after the patients had left the intensive care unit and had become ambulatory.

Material and Methods

Twelve consecutive heart transplant patients, operated on at Deutsche Herzzentrum Berlin, were observed. Table 1 shows a clinical summary of the patients. The majority of patients were studied within the first 2 weeks after transplantation. Only one patient

* This study was supported by the Danish Heart Association

Table 1. Clinical summary of 12 heart transplanted patients

Patient No.	Sex	Age at transplant (years)	Time after Tx (weeks)	Day BP (mm Hg)	Day Mean heart rate (bpm)	Night BP (mm Hg)	Night Mean heart rate (bpm)	Anti-hypertensive therapy
1	M	38	3	122/78	91	137/91	79	—
2	M	52	2	129/67	77	150/69	71	—
3	M	50	2	103/67	98	108/73	92	diur.
4	F	43	1	122/77	90	152/87	89	diur., capt.
5	M	51	4	102/68	90	101/63	77	diur.
6	M	31	2	119/81	106	121/87	101	nif., capt.
7	M	45	2	102/59	77	114/69	67	diur.
8	M	60	2	116/74	93	125/80	89	diur.
9	M	53	3	103/58	72	109/59	72	capt.
10	M	22	1	137/49	89	140/55	84	diur., nif., capt.
11	M	16	2	117/65	85	123/71	77	—
12	M	26	2	117/61	89	134/77	79	—

Diur. = diuretics, capt. = captopril, nif. = nifedipine.

was studied as late as 4 weeks after surgery. The mean age of the patients was 41 years, the youngest being 16, the oldest 60 years of age.

With the exception of one patient (No. 5), who showed very little variation, blood pressure increased in all patients at night. A decrease in heart rate at night, however, was seen in all but one patient (No. 9).

Half of the patients received diuretics, either alone or combined with ACE-inhibitors and nifedipine. These two drugs were given without diuretics in two patients. All patients received cyclosporine A, azathioprine and prednisolone for immunosuppression.

Blood pressure and heart rate were measured every 15 min during the day and every half hour at night. These data were obtained by a self-inflating, portable cuff instrument (Spacelabs, Squibb) and processed to give hourly mean values for systolic and diastolic pressures and heart rates.

Results and discussion

Figure 1 shows the combined 24-h profiles of mean systolic and diastolic pressures and heart rates in the 12 patients.

It is obvious that the normal drop in pressure at night is absent, despite a decrease in heart rate. In fact, the pressure curves suggest that a fall in pressure has been substituted by a pressure increase.

The findings in these newly heart-transplanted patients are thus comparable to those reported in groups of patients investigated several weeks, even years, after heart transplantation [4, 6].

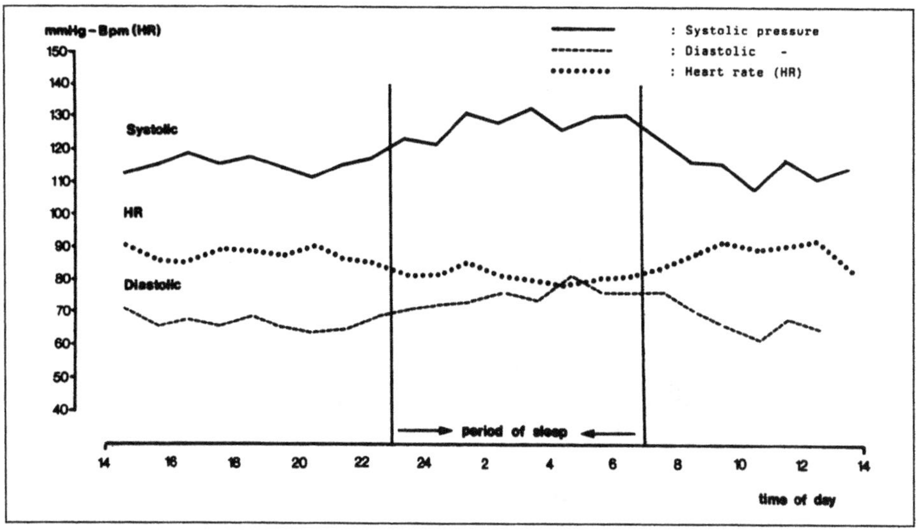

Fig. 1. Variations in systolic and diastolic pressures and heart rate in 12 orthotopic cardiac transplant patients.

The reason for this nocturnal abnormality in blood pressure is not clear. Five possible explanations might be considered:

An abnormal blood pressure profile might be present even before heart transplantation: three patients were investigated before transplantation, and in none of these did pressure increase at night. They showed either a severely blunted pressure drop at night or no variation at all. Figure 2 shows the pressures and heart rates in a patient before and after surgery. The pressure curves are quite different, while the heart rate curves are similar, both showing a drop during the hours of sleep.

It has been speculated whether or not coronary bypass patients, for instance, maintain a normal day — night variability in blood pressure, because such patients may experience a degree of cardiac denervation following surgery [4]. A normal nocturnal fall in blood pressure, however, was found in all three coronary bypass patients, studied within 2 weeks after surgery. The patients had 2,3 and 3 grafts, respectively (Fig. 3).

The disturbed circadian rhythmicity might be caused by the immunosuppressive medication, in particular cyclosporine A, believed to be responsible for the development of hypertension. The ruling out of this possibility involves a comparison with cardiac transplant patients on azathioprine and corticosteroids alone, as well as with other types of transplantation patients, receiving cyclosporine. This remains to be done.

Furthermore, little or nothing is known about circadian variations in circulating vasoactive hormones in heart transplant patients. At present, one cannot exclude the possibility of an abnormal hormonal pattern being involved in the nocturnal blood pressure increase.

A fifth hypothesis explains increased nocturnal blood pressure as the result of a "mismatch" between the function of the denervated heart and the peripheral vascular tree [4, 6]. In the supine position at night, cardiac output is increased by the increase in

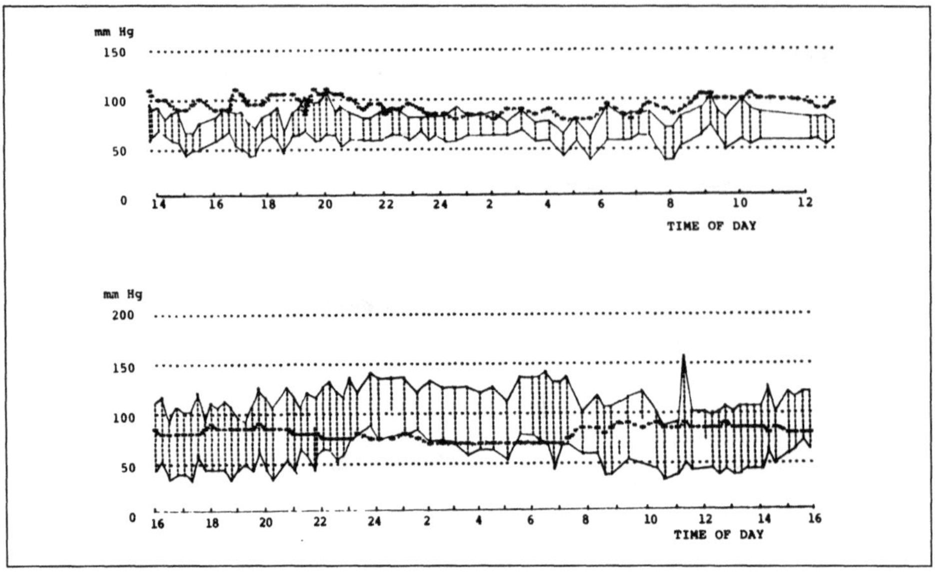

Fig. 2. Variations in blood pressure and heart rate in a patient with dilated cardiomyopathy: Before (upper panel) and 2 weeks after heart transplantation (lower panel).

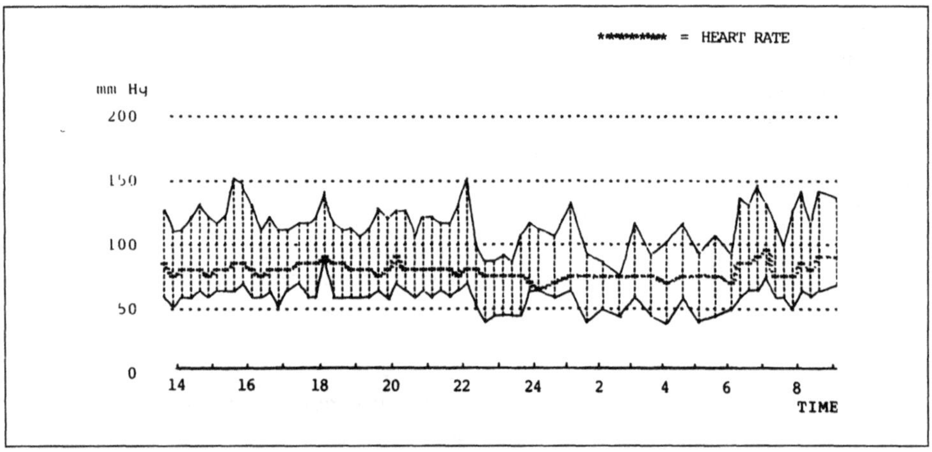

Fig. 3. Circadian variation of blood pressure and heart rate 2 weeks after a 3-graft coronary bypass operation. The patient awoke at midnight and walked around before going to sleep again at 01.00 hours.

venous return. This counteracts the blood pressure lowering effect of a reduced sympathetic drive on the heart and blood vessels at night. The assumed reduction of circulating catecholamines accounts for the drop in heart rate. According to this hypothesis, a circadian rhythmicity is preserved, but "masked" by an increased cardiac output. This would imply, furthermore, that if cardiac output is kept constant, pressure will show a circadian variation.

This, however, was not so in one patient, who has been living with an artificial heart implanted for nearly 4 months. During a period of 16 days, the pump frequency was kept constant at a rate of 90 beats per min and with a constant cardiac output of 7.2 l per min. The patient was dialysed six times because of acute renal failure; data from these 6 days have been omitted.

Figure 4 shows the hourly mean values of systolic and diastolic pressures, central venous pressure and calculated peripheral resistance over a period of 10 days: there is no indication of either a nocturnal drop or rise in pressure in this patient, in whom cardiac output was adjusted *not* to offset any variation in peripheral resistance. (These data were obtained with the kind collaboration of Prof. E. S. Bücherl and Dr. E. Hennig, Klinikum Charlottenburg der FU, Berlin).

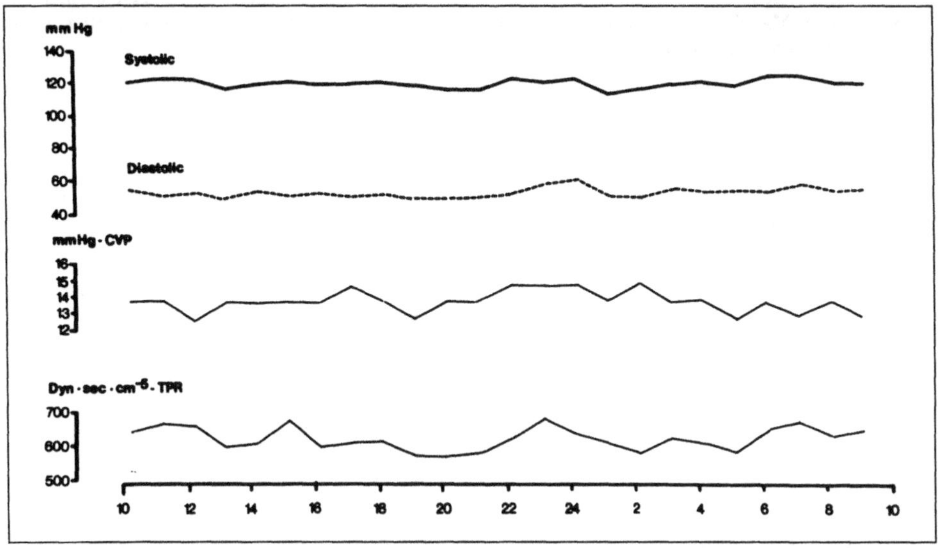

Fig. 4. Mean values over 10 days of arterial and central venous (CVP) pressures and calculated peripheral resistance (TPR) in one patient with a Berliner artificial heart.

In conclusion, following orthotopic heart transplantation, patients experience a reversed, circadian-like variation of blood pressure. The reason for this is still unclear, but is probably related to the lack of efferent, as well as of afferent, neural connections between the central nervous system and the heart.

A number of patients showing normal blood pressures during the day, become hypertensive at night necessitating medical treatment. 24-h blood pressure recordings in heart transplant patients, especially in those receiving cyclosporine A, should thus be emphasized as an important part of the follow-up of these patients.

References

1. Cannom DS, Rider AK, Stinson EB, Harrison DC (1975) Electrophysiologic studies in denervated transplanted human heart. Am J Cardiol 36: 859—866
2. Greenberg ML, Uretsky BF, Reddy PS, Bernstein RL, Griffith BP, Hardesty RL, Thompson ME, Bahnson HT (1985) Long-term hemodynamic follow-up of cardiac transplant patients treated with cyclosporine and prednisone. Circulation 71: 487—494
3. Mason JW, Stinson EB, Harrison DC (1976) Autonomic nervous system and arrhythmias: Studies in the transplanted denervated human heart. Caridology 61: 75—87
4. Reeves RA, Shapiro AP, Thompson ME, Johnsen AM (1986) Loss of nocturnal decline in blood pressure after cardiac transplantation. Circulation 73: 401—408
5. Stinson EB, Schroeder JS, Griepp RB, Shumway NE, Dong E (1972) Observations on behavior of recipient atria after cardiac transplantation in man. Am J Cardiol 39: 615—622
6. Wenting GJ, Meiracker AH, Simoons ML, Bos E, Ritseman v Eck HJ, Man in't Veld AJ, Weimar W, Schalekamp MADH (1987) Circadian variation of heart rate but not of blood pressure after heart transplantation. Transplant Proc 19: 2554—2555

Variability of arterial blood pressure in normal and in hypertensive pregnancy

T. Öney[1], W. Meyer-Sabellek[2], H. Weitzel[1]

[1] Abt. für Gynökologie und Geburtshilfe, Klinikum Steglitz, Freie Universität Berlin, Berlin, FRG

[2] Medizinische Klinik und Poliklinik, Klinikum Steglitz, Berlin, Berlin, FRG

The measurement of arterial blood pressure has traditionally been an important part of prenatal care. Beside the detection of a significant hypotension, the major aim of regular blood pressure controls is the early diagnosis of hypertensive complications of pregnancy, especially severe cases of preeclampsia, and the prevention of eclamptic convulsions. Although there has been a marked reduction in fatal courses of preeclampsia and eclampsia since the establishment of standardized and effective therapeutic measures, maternal mortality is nevertheless considerably affected by hypertensive complications during pregnancy [1—3]. In addition, the severe forms of preeclampsia are an important cause of prematurity and perinatal mortality. Clinical experience has shown that in a large number of patients with severe preeclampsia prenatal care had been either insufficient (e.g., long intervals between prenatal visits in the third trimester) or the significance of a major rise in blood pressure was misjudged or had not been sufficiently treated. Considering that hypertension is a major symptom of preeclampsia, an exact knowledge of the changes in arterial blood pressure during pregnancy is an important prerequisite of modern prenatal care.

It has been known for decades that the blood pressure pattern in normal and in hypertensive patients is subject to marked circadian fluctuations [4, 5]. The changes in systemic blood pressure dependent on the time of day in healthy pregnant women, as well as in women with hypertensive complications, however, have only been documented in the past 15 years ([6—10]; Fig. 1).

In normal pregnancies there are considerable hemodynamic and endocrinological changes in connection with the physiological adaptation processes that are important for the regulation of blood pressure [3]. The blood pressure during pregnancy also stays within normal limits because of extensive regulatory mechanisms. Based on a prospective study in primiparous women, Schwarz, using standardized procedures, was able to show in 1964 that diastolic blood pressure decreased during the early weeks of pregnancy and then, up to the time of birth, increased continually beyond its initial (prepregnancy) value [11]. On the other hand, systolic blood pressure remained largely constant over the course of pregnancy. Page and Christianson (1976), using the evaluation of blood pressure values obtained in approximately 15,000 pregnant women, were able to show that mean arterial pressure (MAP) decreases continually in the first and at the beginning of the 2nd trimester, reaches its lowest value in the 22nd week of pregnancy, then rises again until delivery [12].

This peculiarity in the course of MAP has to be taken into consideration especially in the care of pregnant women with preexistent hypertension. Thus, mainly in women with less pronounced hypertension, this results in a normalization of blood pressure values

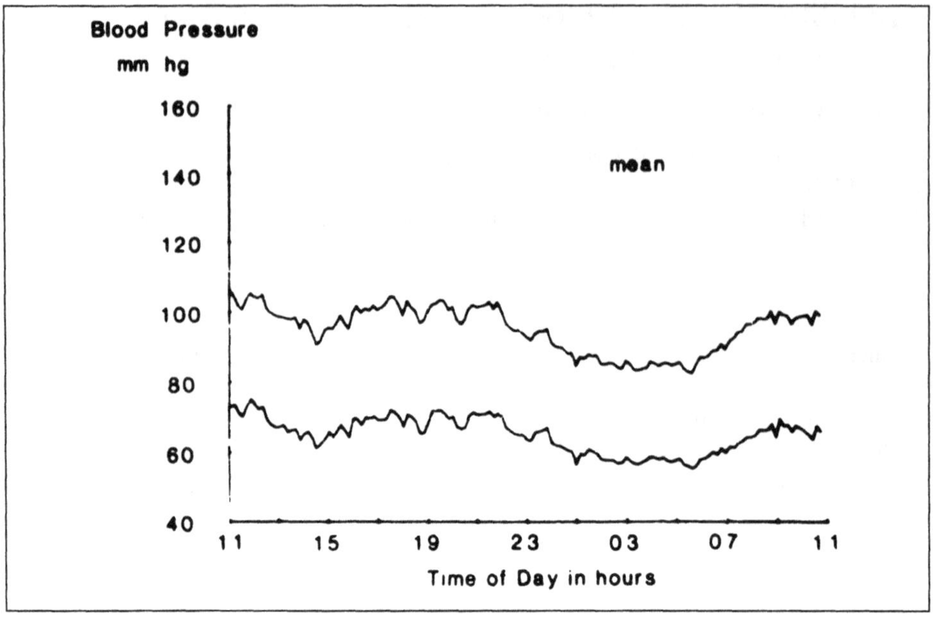

Fig. 1. Circadian rhythm of the mean systolic and diastolic blood pressure in 16 normotensive pregnant women (9)

in the second trimester. These patients must be provided with intensive prenatal care so that a renewed rise in blood pressure in the further course of pregnancy can be recognized in time. Contrary to formerly existing opinions, it has been demonstrated in the past few years with the help of prospective studies that an antihypertensive therapy during pregnancy, even if there is mild hypertension, has a favorable effect on the fetal prognosis or prevents superimposed preeclampsia [13:, 14]. Moreover, determination of MAP in the second trimester (MAP-II value) can be used as a simple method for early detection of hypertensive complications in the further course of pregnancy. We were able to show in a recent study that pregnant women with an MAP-II value of 90 mm Hg or more have a significantly higher incidence of preeclampsia than women with lower MAP-II values [3]. The methodological problems involved in indirect blood pressure measurement are generally known [15]. An exact determination of arterial blood pressure during pregnancy is additionally complicated by the effect the posture has on systolic and particularly diastolic blood pressure [3]. Thus, compression of the inferior vena cava in the supine position may lead to erroneously low values (so-called supine hypotensive syndrome). In the left lateral position usually preferred by pregnant women, on the other hand, the blood pressure is markedly higher in the right (upper) than in the left (lower) arm due to the hydrostatic effect.

In 1971, Seligman, using the indirect method by Richardson, was able to demonstrate for the first time in healthy pregnant women, examined under rigid confinement to bed, that the circadian rhythm of blood pressure is also maintained during normal pregnancy, and that, just as in nonpregnant women, there is a nocturnal decrease in blood pressure during the sleep phase [6]. The nocturnal decrease in blood pressure was even greater in patients with preexistent essential hypertension. Patients with preeclampsia, on the other hand, had a markedly lower decrease of mean blood pressure values during the night. Further investigations by Redman et al. using ultrasound technique (Roche Arteriosonde monitor) and under standardized conditions (rigid confinement to bed, measurement of Korotkoff's sounds phase IV), as well as by Dame et al. using intraarterial blood pressure measurement, confirmed the nocturnal decrease in blood pressure in pregnant women in the second and third trimester [7, 8]. In contrast to the results obtained by Seligman, nocturnal blood pressure peaks or a reversal of the blood pressure decrease after midnight were observed by Dame et al. in two out of five and by Redman et al. in 10 out of 17 patients with severe preeclampsia. In other words, the highest systolic and diastolic blood pressure values were measured during the night and the lowest between 0800 and 1600 hours (Fig. 2).

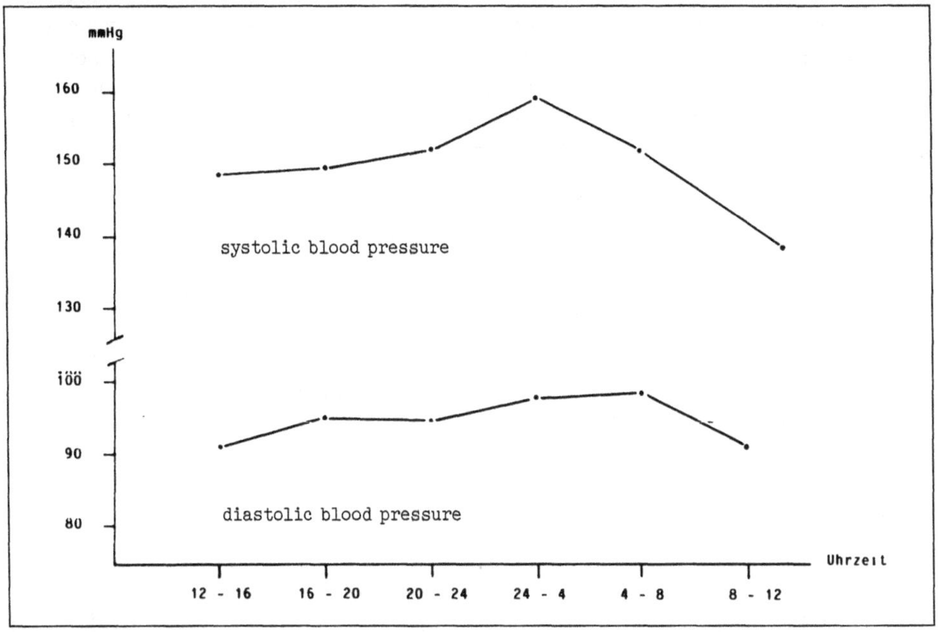

Fig. 2. Mean systolic and diastolic blood pressure in 17 patients with severe preeclampsia showing the reversal of the circadian rhythm (7)

Furthermore, Redman et al. were able to demonstrate in healthy pregnant women and in patients with preexistent hypertension that, if the 24-h blood pressure profiles of the 36th and the 28th week of pregnancy were compared, healthy pregnant women with intact circadian rhythms showed a slight but significant increase in the mean systolic blood pressure values in the late afternoon hours and during the night [7]. On the other hand, in women with preexistent hypertension, the rise in mean systolic blood pressure values had rather shifted to the night hours, and above all to the sleep phase. These patients on the average exhibited a higher increase of the mean diastolic blood pressure values during the entire 24-h measurement period than normotensive patients whose relative diastolic blood pressure increase was likewise concentrated in the night hours.

Murnaghan et al. were later able to check these findings with the help of an intraarterial method. In contrast to the findings obtained by Seligman, the nocturnal blood pressure decrease was no more pronounced in pregnant women with essential hypertension than in normotensive pregnant women. The 24-h blood pressure profile was not influenced by an antihypertensive treatment. Yet it was striking that seven out of ten pregnant women with essential hypertension had on average normotensive values during the intraarterial measurement. In another ten patients with preeclampsia, the nocturnal blood pressure decrease was markedly lower than in normotensive pregnant women or in patients with essential hypertension.

Recently, Sawyer et al. using a DINAMAP apparatus established 24-h blood pressure profiles in each of the 15 pregnant women with a normal course of pregnancy, with preexistent essential hypertension and with mild preeclampsia [10]. The results obtained by the investigators were comparable to those shown in other reports. The decrease in systolic blood pressure was most pronounced in pregnant women with essential hypertension during the sleep phase. Although the mean diastolic blood pressure decreased during the night it was not possible to show a significant difference between the groups. The circadian rhythm was abolished in another two patients with severe preeclampsia. These patients also exhibited the greatest short-term fluctuations in blood pressure values (Fig. 3).

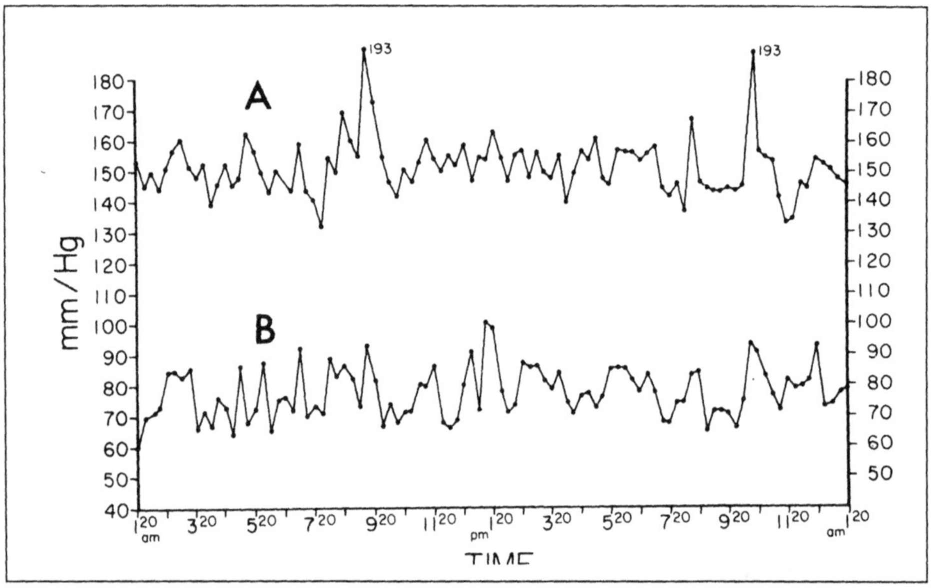

Fig. 3. Loss of the circadian rhythm in a patient with severe preeclampsia: (A) systolic blood pressure; (B) diastolic blood pressure (10)

Preliminary results of our own investigations with an automatic device for non-invasive blood pressure measurement (Pressure Master, ICR Squipp) also demonstrated, in four women with mild preeclampsia, a clear circadian rhythm with a decrease in systolic and diastolic blood pressure during the sleep phase (Fig. 4).

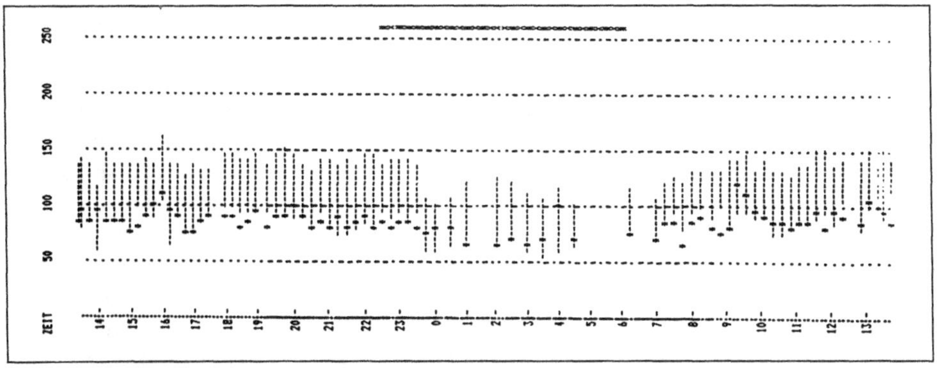

Fig. 4. Circadian rhythm of the arterial blood pressure in a patient with mild preeclampsia

Discussion

Although the investigations performed so far on the variability of arterial blood pressure are not unified with respect to the method of blood pressure measurement as well as the standardization of measurement conditions in pregnant women and must therefore be considered critically, some conclusions can nevertheless be derived.

In normal pregnancies, in pregnant women with preexistent hypertension and mild preeclampsia, the circadian rhythm of blood pressure with a nocturnal decrease in blood pressure is maintained, especially during the sleep phase [6—10]. However, in patients with mild preeclampsia the nocturnal decrease in blood pressure can be markedly less pronounced [6—9]. Women with severe preeclampsia have a reversal of the circadian rhythm or nocturnal blood pressure peaks, or have a persistent increase in blood pressure during the entire sleep phase as well [7, 8, 10]. In healthy pregnant women towards the end of pregnancy there is, compared to the 2nd trimester, a slight physiological increase in systolic and diastolic blood pressure with accentuation of the blood pressure increase in the late afternoon hours and during the night [7].

The causes of this relative increase in blood pressure towards the end of normal pregnancy and the abolition or reversal of the circadian rhythm in severe preeclampsia remain unclear. Diurnal changes of the cardiac output and the peripheral vascular resistance or the vascular response with respect to endogenous vasopressor functions can be discussed as the possible mechanisms involved. In normal pregnancies, even as early as the 10th week there is a marked decrease of vascular responsiveness to the pressor effect of exogenously administered vasopressor substances, such as angiotensin II (A II; [16, 17]). Women with preeclampsia, on the other hand, manifest several weeks before the first clinical symptoms a marked decrease in this pregnancy-specific refractoriness to A II [17]. Women with preeclampsia have a similar or even higher vascular reactivity to A II than nonpregnant women [18].

Even though a circadian rhythm of angiotensin sensitivity is not known in normal or pathological pregnancies, it is nevertheless possible that the blood pressure behavior in patients with preeclampsia is either regulated directly via a central mechanism and by circulating vacoptessor substances or indirectly by an increase in vascular responsiveness.

A disturbed dopaminergic control was postulated by Stumpe et al. to be the possible cause of essential hypertension [19]. They successfully treated men with essential hypertension and mild hyperprolactinemia with the synthetic dopamine agonist bromocriptine. Recently, Lehtovirta et al. reported a significantly higher mean prolactin serum concentration in 20 women on hormonal contraceptives than in normotensive women who were also taking oral contraceptives [20]. The authors assumed an alteration of the dopaminergic transmission to be the cause of increased prolactin secretion. Our own investigations showed that the vascular responsiveness to AII in healthy pregnant women between the 28th and 32nd week of pregnancy can be decreased by oral administration of 1000 mg L-Dopa [20]. Although the exact causes of this attenuation of the blood pressure reaction are not clear, it seems reasonable to assume that we are dealing here with the depressive effect of L-Dopa on the activity of the sympathetic nervous system via a central mechanism. This assumption was indirectly confirmed since it is possible to demonstrate that the angiotensin sensitivity of healthy pregnant subjects was significantly increased after the administration of 10 mg metoclopramid i.v. [3]. These results suggest that a higher mechanism, like a reduced dopaminergic activity of the central nervous system, is involved in the pathogenesis of hypertensive complications in pregnancy. With regard to the results presented so far, the following two consequences can be deduced for clinical practice.

1. Patients with severe preeclampsia are more susceptible to a hypertensive crisis at night, especially after midnight, than during the day and must be monitored accordingly.
2. The antihypertensive treatment must be adapted to the demands of the reversed circadian rhythm.

References

1. Chesley LC (1978) Hypertensive disorders in pregnancy. Appleton Century Crofts, New York
2. Pritchard JA, Pritchard SA (1975) Standardized treatment of 154 consecutive cases of eclampsia. Am J Obstet Gynaecol 123: 543
3. Öney T, Kaulhausen H (1983) Früherkennung und Prävention von hypertensiven Komplikationen in der Schwangerschaft. Springer, Berlin
4. Bevan AT, Honour AJ, Stott FH (1969) Direct arterial pressure recording in unrestricted man. Clin Sci 36: 329
5. Richardson DW, Honour AJ, Fenton GW (1964) Variation in arterial pressure throughout the day and night. Clin Sci 26: 445
6. Seligman, SA (1971) Diurnal blood-pressure variation in pregnancy. J Obstet Gynaecol Brit Commonw 78: 417
7. Redman CWG, Beilin LJ, Bonnar J (1976) Variability of blood pressure in normal and abnormal pregnancy. In: Lindheimer MD, Katz AI, Zuspan FP (eds) Hypertension in pregnancy. Wiley, New York, pp 53—60
8. Dame WR, Bachour G, Böttcher HD, Beller FK (1977) Direkte kontinuierliche Blutdruckmessung bei normalen und präeklamptischen Schwangeren. Geburtsh u Frauheilk 37: 708
9. Murnaghan GA, Mitchell RH, Ruff S (1980) Circadian variation of blood-pressure in pregnancy. In: Bonnar J, MacGillivray I, Symonds EM (eds) MTP. Lancaster, pp 107—112
10. Sawyer MM, Lipshitz J, Anderson GD, Dilts PV, Halperin L (1981) Diurnal and short-term variation of blood pressure: Comparison of preeclamptic, chronic hypertensive, and normotensive patients. Obstet Gynaecol 58: 291
11. Schwarz R (1964) Das Verhalten des Kreislaufs in der normalen Schwangerschaft. I. Mitteilung: Der arterielle Blutdruck. Arch Gynaecol 199: 549

12. Page EW, Christianson R (1976) The impact of mean arterial blood pressure in the middle trimester upon the outcome of pregnancy. Am J Obstet Gynaecol 125: 740
13. Redman CWG, Beilin LJ, Bonnar J, Qunsted MK (1976) Fetal outcome in trial of antihypertensive treatment in pregnancy. Lancet II: 753
14. Rubin PC, Butters L, Clark DM, Reynolds B, Sumner DJ, Steedman D, Low RA, Reid JL (1983) Placebo-controlled trial of atenolol treatment of pregnancy-associated hypertension. Lancet I:431
15. Holzgreve H (1981) Forum hypertonicum. MMW Medizin, München
16. Chesley LC, Talledo OE, Bohler CS, Zuspan FP (1965) Vascular reactivity to angiotensin II and norepinephrine in pregnant and nonpregnant women. Am J Obstet Gynaecol 91: 837
17. Gant NF, Daley GL, Chand S, Whalley PJ, MacDonald PC (1973) A study of angiotensin II pressor response throughout primigravid pregnancy. J Clin Invest 52: 2682
18. Talledo OE (1966) Renin-angiotensin system in normal and toxemic pregnancies. I. Angiotensin infusion test. Am J Obstet Gynaecol 96: 141
19. Stumpe KO, Kolloch R, Higuchi M, Krück F, Vetter H (1977) Hyperprolactinaemia and antihypertensive effect of bromocriptine in essential hypertension. Lancet II: 211
20. Lehtovirta P, Ranta T, Seppalä M (1981) Elevated prolactin levels in oral contraceptive pill-related hypertension. Fertil Steril 35: 403
21. Kaulhausen H, Öney T, Feldmann R, Leyendecker G (1981) Decrease of vascular angiotensin sensitivity by l-dopa during human pregnancy. Am J Obstet Gynaecol 140:671

Blood pressure variability during athletics

P. Palatini, L. Mos, P. Mormino, A. Di Marco, L. Munari, M. Del Torre, F. Valle, A. C. Pessina and C. Dal Palù

1st Medical Clinic, University of Padova, Italy

Introduction

Blood pressure variability has long been a subject of intense interest [1, 2] even though its clinical significance has not been completely established [3, 4]. Physical activity has been shown to represent one of the predominant determinants of blood pressure variability [5] and the blood pressure changes determined by both isotonic and isometric exercise have been studied extensively by means of laboratory tests. Everyday physical activities, as well as sports activities, differ in many respects from stress testing, however, so that a direct comparison cannot be made [6]. In fact, during such activities the dynamic and the static components of the exercise are not as clearly separated as in laboratory tests, but there is a parallel, though different, contribution of each one of them.

In spite of these considerations the present knowledge on blood pressure variability during athletics is virtually based only on the results of stress testing, owing to the inability to measure blood pressure during sports activities.

The Oxford method [7] has provided us with a useful tool to continuously record blood pressure in freely ambulatory subjects, so it seemed to us the ideal system to be used in these circumstances.

In this paper the results are described of intraarterial blood pressure monitoring performed in three groups of athletes trained in different sports activities. A comparative evaluation of the hemodynamic effects of an overground training session and of a traditional laboratory test is made.

Subjects and Methods

Six normotensive (mean age 21.5 ± 6.3 years) and 14 hypertensive (mean age 24.1 ± 8 years) runners, three hypertensive cyclists (mean age 35.6 ± 2 years), one normotensive (25 years old) and one hypertensive (20 years old) weight-lifter participated in the study. They were trained to an amateur level. The normotensive subjects were all voluntees. In the hypertensives, the diagnosis of hypertension was made with the indirect auscultatory method, taking into account the mean of the measurements made on 3 separate days (mean casual blood pressure = 151 ± 7/96 ± 7 mm Hg). In all subjects, physical examination, routine blood tests, 12-lead ECG, stress test, M-mode and 2-D echocardiogram and fundoscopic examination were performed. In the hypertensives, creatinine clearance, plasma-renin activity and urinary aldosterone determination were also acquired to rule out the existence of secondary hypertension. All subjects underwent intraarterial blood pressure monitoring lasting for at least 12 h. The radial artery was cannulated and connected to an Oxford pressure transducer, held by the athlete at heart level [2]. To avoid

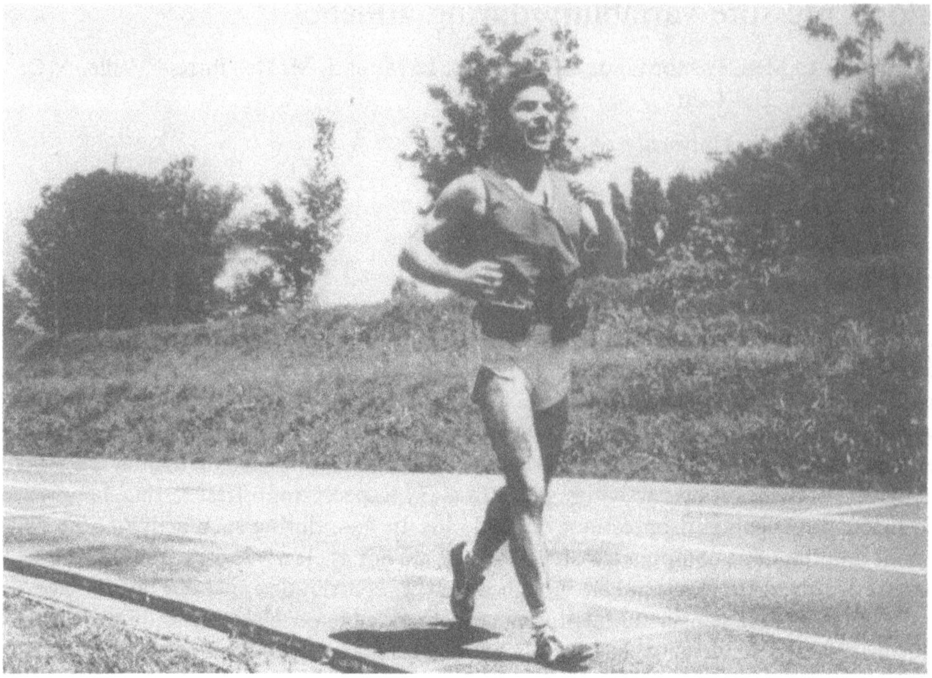

Fig. 1. Athlete wearing the Oxford system during track running.

the occurrence of artifacts on pressure tracings during running, the devices were accurately positioned and fastened to the subject's body with rubber bands and tapes (Fig. 1).

To evaluate whether the arm oscillations during running might have any effect on blood pressure behavior, the athletes were asked to keep the catheterized arm still alongside the body for at least 1 min while running. In three subjects the run was repeated after both the transducer and the recorder had been fixed on the outside of a car going beside them, to rule out the possibility of artifacts generated by the counterblow received by the devices during each foot-strike.

Blood pressure tracings were analyzed by means of a DG 10 computer as described elsewhere (8).

Tests protocol

After cannulation, all runners underwent a bicycle ergometric test and a track run in a random order to avoid the effect of fatigue. The three cyclists performed, besides bicycle ergometry, an outdoor cycling session and the lifters, a weight-lifting session.

Bicycle ergometry was preceded by a 10-min warm-up period, after which subjects pedalled at a 50 W workload, which was increased by 20 W every 2 min until exhaustion.

An average workload of 208 W was attained at peak exercise.

Track running was performed according to individual habits. In every case it began with a warm-up session lasting 10 to 15 min. Thereafter, athletes started running at submaximal speed as they used to do during their training sessions. Before the completion of exercise they were asked to run at maximal speed until exhaustion. The total running time ranged from 30 to 50 min.

The three cyclists performed an outdoor cycling session, which always included an upgrade and lasted on average 70 min.

The two weight-lifters performed a typical weight-training session, which included single-arm curls and over head presses with the non-catheterized arm, double-leg presses and squatting. In each exercise, repetitions were performed to the point of failure in successive sets with 50% — 80% — 90% — 100% of the maximum single lift. These athletes also performed a hand grip test at 30% maximal voluntary contraction for 5 min.

Statistics

Results are expressed as mean ± standard deviation; t-test for impaired data, one-way analysis of variance and the Bravet-Pearson test were used where indicated. The results were considered statistically significant for $p < 0.05$ or less.

Results

Runners

In 19 subjects, blood pressure proved lower than casual blood pressure, while in one normotensive it was higher. A weak correlation between ambulatory blood pressure and casual blood pressure was found only for systolic blood pressure ($r = 0.45$; $p < 0.05$). Considering a mean blood pressure level of 95 mm Hg as the threshold value between hypertension and normotension, nine athletes turned out to be hypertensive at continuous monitoring while the other 11 proved normotensive. Among the former, four individuals showed a I to II retinopathy stage, while in none of the latter subjects was any retinopathy detected. Left ventricular mass index was similar in the two groups.

Blood pressure response to bicycle ergometry was as follows: in all subjects systolic blood pressure progressively increased during the test, reaching maximal values a few seconds before exhaustion (Table 1). Diastolic blood pressure showed only minor changes throughout the test. Maximal blood pressure attained during exercise highly correlated with preexercise resting blood pressure (Fig. 2). Beat-by-beat analysis of the tracings showed a wide blood pressure variability during the test with continuous oscillations of the phasic waves.

Blood pressure response to track running (Table 1) was as follows: systolic blood pressure suddenly increased soon after the start, even though subjects were running at low speed. Thereafter, systolic blood pressure tended to decrease throughout the run, reaching minimal values at the end of the submaximal speed phase. During sprinting it rose again to values comparable to those reached during warm-up. Diastolic blood

Table 1. Blood pressure and heart rate changes in the 20 runners during bicycle ergometry and track running.

Bicycle ergometry						
	Resting	70 W	130 W	Peak	Rec. 1	Rec. 5
Systolic BP (mm Hg)	134±22	146±19	150±23	116±23	116±24	
Diastolic BP (mm Hg)	80±15	79±17	76±18	81±19	65±20	66±23
Heart rate (beats/min)	77± 9	123±18	150±20	179±13	144±12	116±15

Track running										
	Resting	1	2	4	8	S1	S2	Sprint	Rec. 1	Rec. 5
Systolic BP (mm Hg)	147±25	167±22	170±23	165±21	156±23	160±20	147±19	175±23	124±29	121±28
Diastolic BP (mm Hg)	85±15	71±17	75±14	69±16	63±13	67±13	66±12	69±14	71±20	70±17
Heart rate (beats/min)	82±11	144±12	153±14	157±13	164±14	174±13	178±14	191± 8	157±14	123± 9

BP = blood pressure. Rec. 1 and Rec. 5 = 1st and 5th minute of recovery.
S1 and S2 = First and last minute of running at submaximal speed.

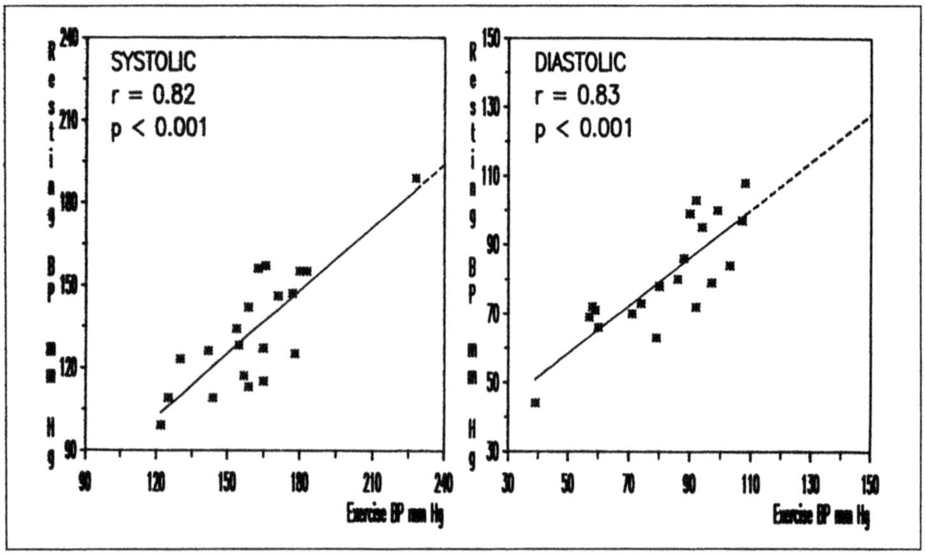

Fig. 2. Correlation between maximal blood pressure recorded during bicycle ergometry and preexercise resting levels in the 20 runners.

pressure showed a sharp fall at the beginning of the warm-up, then it remained virtually stable throughout the run and slightly increased on the final sprint. In ten subjects maximal blood pressure values were attained during warm-up, in the others during sprinting.

On average, systolic blood pressure reached higher values during running than during cycling, while diastolic blood pressure showed the opposite trend (Table 1). As a result, mean blood pressure levels did not substantially differ during the two tests.

A weak correlation, which reached the level of statistical significance only for systolic blood pressure, was found between resting blood pressure and the blood pressure recorded at peak exercise (Fig. 3).

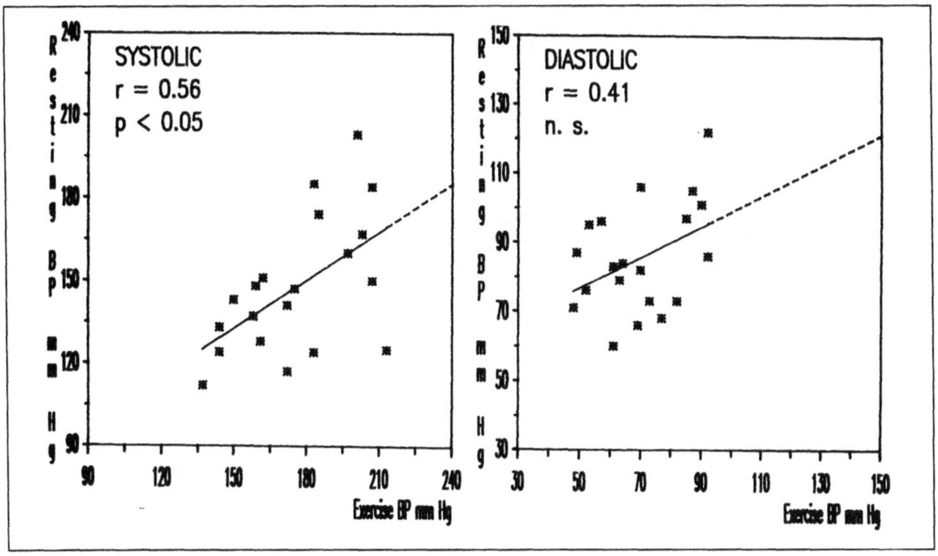

Fig. 3. Correlation between peak exercise blood pressure recorded during track running at submaximal speed and preexercise resting levels in the 20 runners.

Beat-by-beat analysis showed a peculiar behavior of the phasic waves during running. Rhythmic oscillations of pulse pressure were often observed during this exercise, chiefly when subjects were running at submaximal speed (Fig. 4). The frequency of the pressure cycles varied from 6—7 to 24—27/min and tended to increase with increasing heart rate and running velocity. Due to these wide oscillations, diastolic blood pressure approached, in some cases, zero levels; in three normotensive subjects even negative values up to -17 mm Hg were recorded at the end of the submaximal speed run. The shape of the cyclic pulse pressure variations did not change when, during running, the athletes kept the arm still alongside the body, nor did it vary when both the blood pressure transducer and the recorder were fixed on a car going alongside the runners. Breathing and stride rate during exercise always exceeded the frequency of pressure oscillations. No substantial changes in the blood pressure pattern were observed during breath-holding.

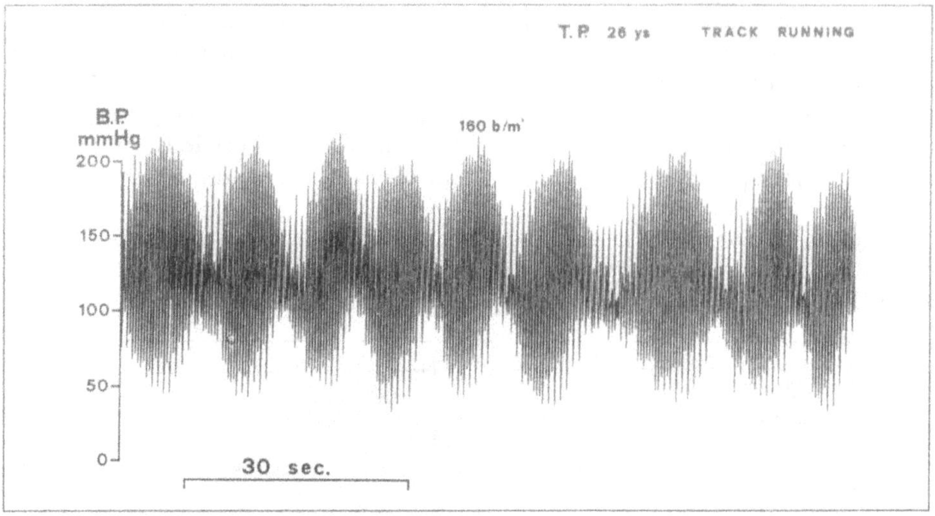

Fig. 4. Phasic waveforms of radial blood pressure recorded during track running at submaximal speed. Notwithstanding the high systolic and diastolic blood pressure variability, mean blood pressure remained substantially stable throughout the test, similarly to what was observed during ergometry.

Cyclists

Two cyclists considered as mildly hypertensive on the basic of their indirect blood pressure readings proved normotensive at intraarterial recording. In the third subject, who had exhibited a stage II retinopathy, the diagnosis of hypertension was confirmed by blood pressure monitoring.

Blood pressure response to outdoor cycling was as follows: in the three cyclists, blood pressure reached much higher values during cycling in outdoor conditions than during the ergometric test. Blood pressure showed a remarkable increase, especially when cycling uphill or when the athletes pedalled at maximal speed on the flat. Pressure phasic waves showed a behavior similar to that observed during ergometry. During track running, blood pressure reached levels comparable to those attained by the runners and on average lower than those observed during road cycling (Figs. 5—7).

Weight-lifters

The diagnosis made with the auscultatory method was confirmed by the intraarterial recording. The subject with hypertension showed a stage I retinopathy.

Blood pressure response to weight-lifting was as follows: extremely high blood pressure elevations were observed during this activity, which greatly exceeded the levels recorded in the other subjects during both running or cycling. Both systolic and diastolic levels sharply rose during the concentric contraction phase of the lift and then rapidly declined with the eccentric contraction. The pressure increase was proportional to the muscle mass employed and greatly exceeded the values observed during hand grip test. The highest blood pressure elevations, as high as 290/225 mm Hg were observed in the hypertensive athlete during squatting (Fig. 8).

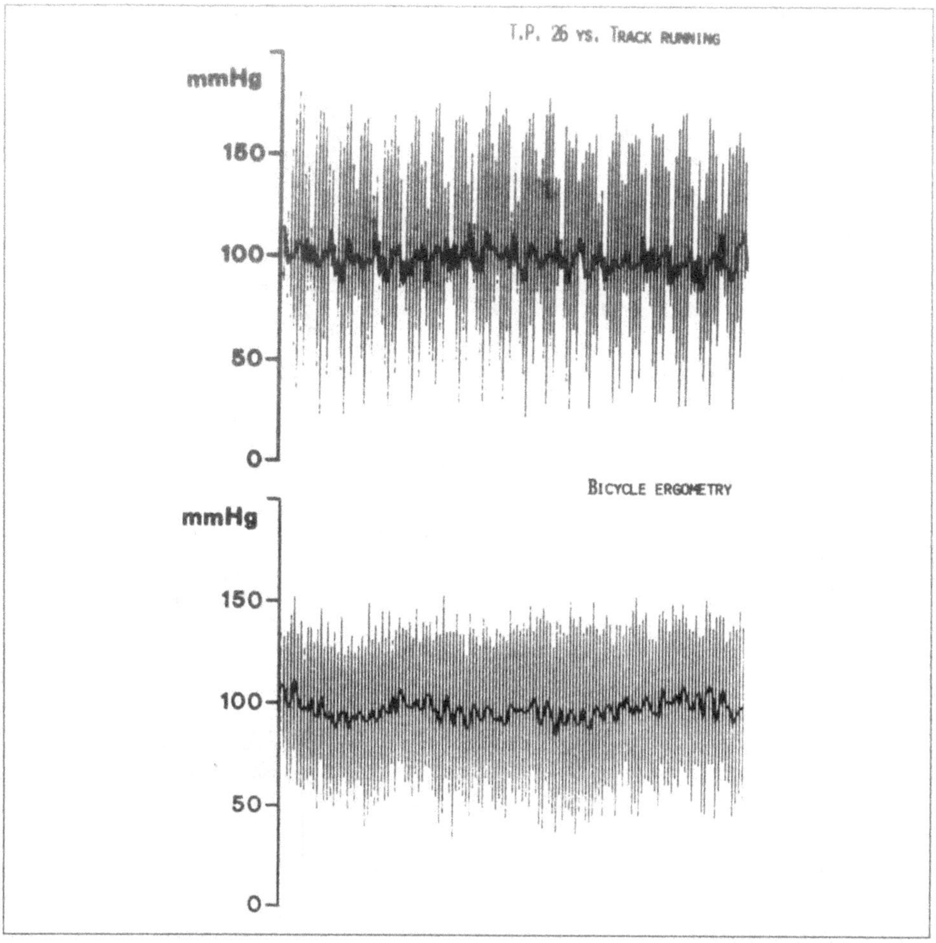

Fig. 5. Phasic waveforms and beat-by-beat mean blood pressure (represented by the line on the center of the tracings) during track running (top panel) and bicycle ergometry (bottom panel).

Discussion

Several studies have demonstrated that exercise is one of the most important determinants of blood pressure variability [5]. Although exercise-induced blood pressure elevations have been extensively studied by means of either static or dynamic stress testing, changes in blood pressure during athletics have never been investigated.

Our results, obtained by beat-by-beat direct recording of blood pressure, indicate that each sports activity brings about a peculiar blood pressure pattern and that laboratory tests are not accurate predictors of the blood pressure changes which actually occur during athletics.

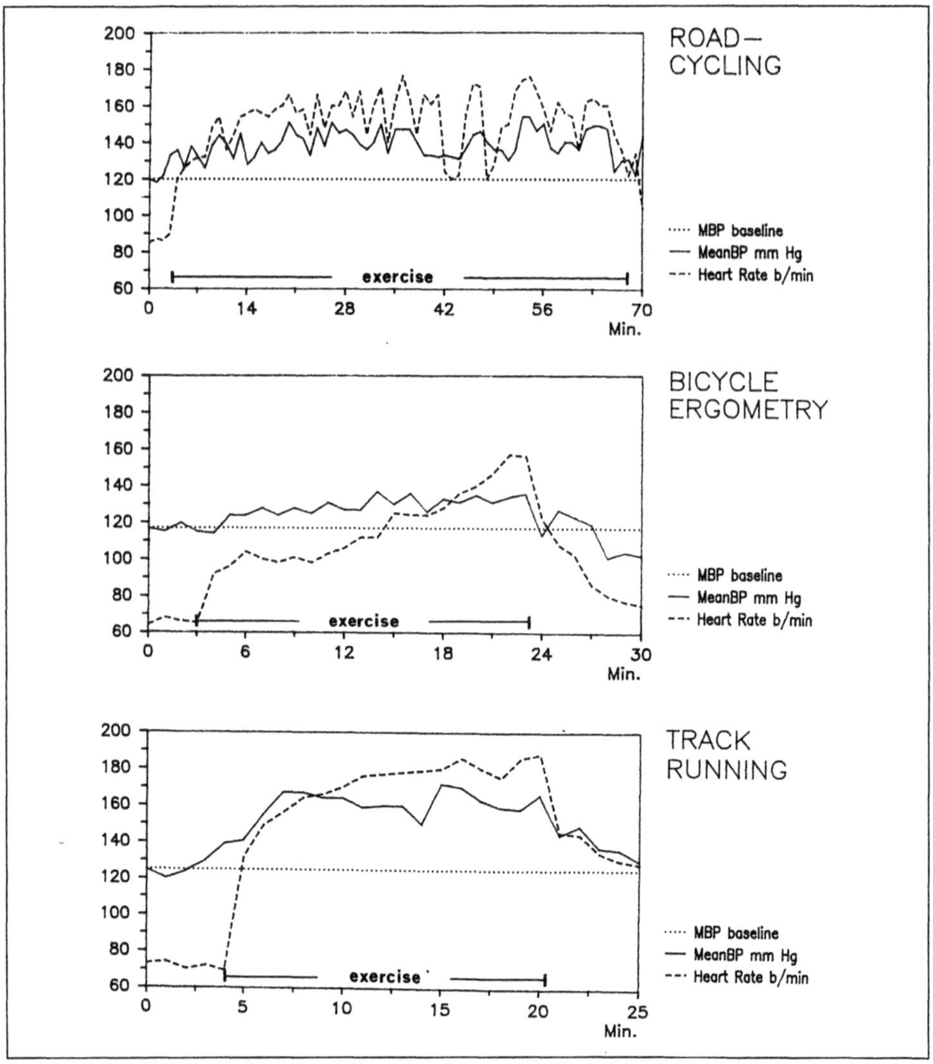

Fig. 6. Mean blood pressure and heart rate changes in a hypertensive cyclist during different types of exercise. Blood pressure levels during road cycling and track running exceed the values recorded during bicycle ergometry.

Track running

Contrary to what is currently observed by ergometry during a typical outdoor running session, blood pressure does not progressively increase throughout the effort, as the maximal blood pressure values are already attained after 2 min of warm-up. This is likely due to the heterostatic reflexes which come into action soon after starting exercising [9], when total peripheral resistance is still high. Subsequently, the vasodilation determines

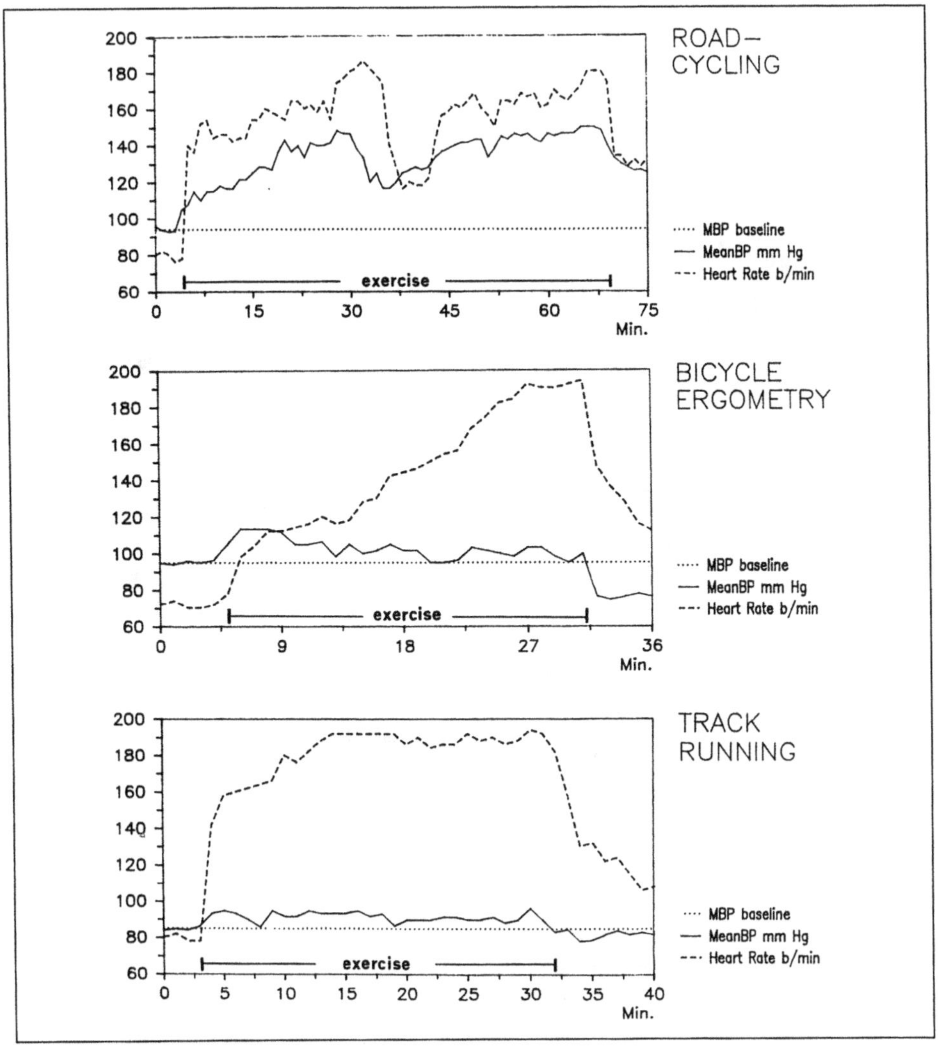

Fig. 7. Mean blood pressure and heart rate changes in a normotensive cyclist. Blood pressure levels during road-cycling exceed the values recorded during both bicycle ergometry and track running.

a progressive decline in blood pressure in spite of continuous increase in heart rate. During the final sprinting blood pressure just approaches the values observed during the warm-up period. The correlation tests demonstrate that the maximal ergometric pressure is strictly related to baseline preexercise values, while the blood pressure elevation determined by the "field test" is less predictable from the resting blood pressure levels. The reason for this discrepancy seems to be due to the fact that the ergometric test is strictly scheduled and implies a progressive increase in the work-load; during an overground race, by contrast, the athlete is free to run according to his individual habits.

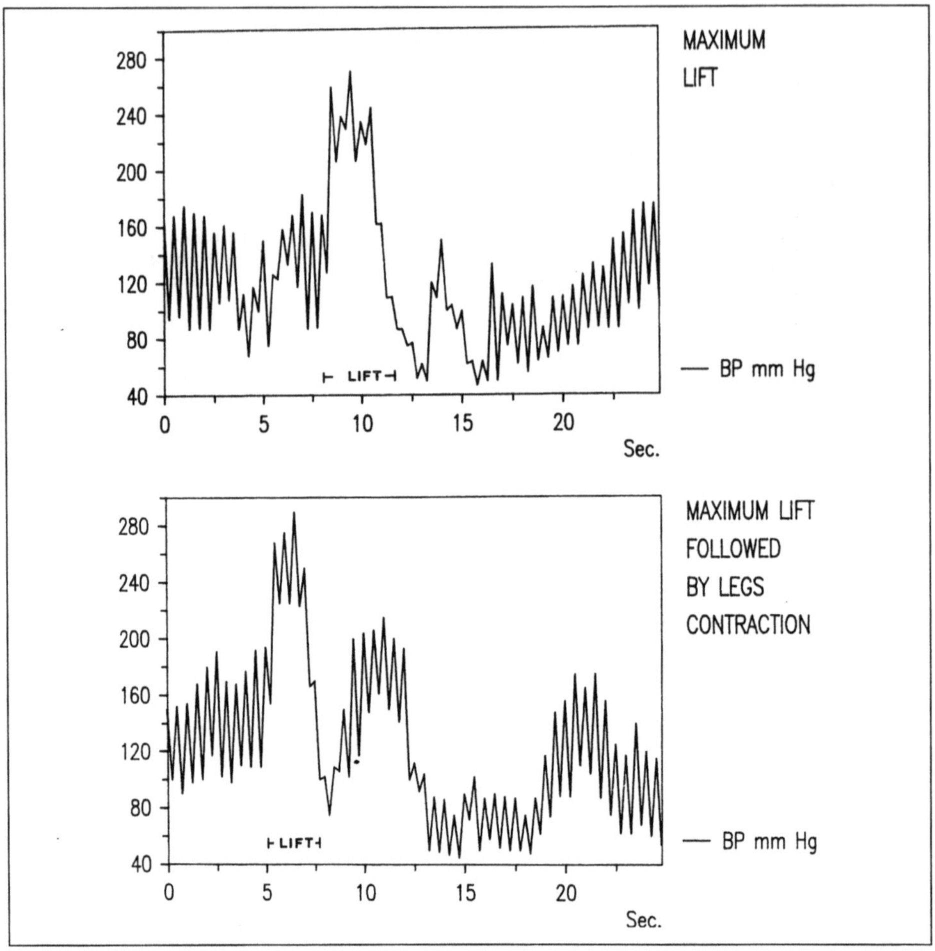

Fig. 8. Beat-by-beat pressure tracing during "maximal" sqatting in a mildly hypertensive weight-lifter. Blood pressure recording has been analysed by means of a computer and rebuilt by a plotter. In the bottom panel the single lift is followed by a short period of static contraction of legs.

Beat-by-beat analysis of the blood pressure tracings showed a completely different pattern during ergometry and running; while during cycling there are consensual oscillations of systolic and diastolic blood pressure, during running the variations of systolic blood pressure are not paralleled by those of diastolic blood pressure, so that a continuous widening and narrowing of pulse pressure is present. These oscillations were present throughout the various stages of the exercise and reached maximal frequency at the end of the submaximal running speed phase, when they also appeared sharper and more regular. These cyclic oscillations were unrelated to respiration, as measurements of respiratory activity during effort showed that breathing frequency was higher than the pressure variations. Furthermore, on breath-holding this pressure pattern remained unchanged. Pulse pressure periodic fluctuations were, by contrast, never observed during bicycle ergometry.

The peculiar blood pressure behavior recorded in our athletes while running cannot be ascribed to artifacts produced by arm oscillations or counterblows received by the recording devices at each impact of foot strike, as the behavior was still detectable when the catheterized arm or the devices were kept still. A source of error in the measurement of direct blood pressure is inadequate frequency response of the recording system. However, had the frequency response of the Oxford system been too low, we would have obtained exaggerately high blood pressure values during effort [10], but this was not the case with our recordings. Moreover, the Oxford system, which has successfully been used during effort by other investigators [11, 12], was validated in our laboratory against a Statham transducer with a frequency response flat to 16 Hz. Furthermore, during bicycle ergometry, where heart rates similar to those recorded during running were attained, no pulse pressure oscillations were recorded. Thus we are confident that the blood pressure pattern recorded during track running in our subjects is not due to measurement artifacts. A similar, though less striking pattern was found, on the other hand, by two groups of investigators [13, 14] during treadmill locomotion, but the mechanism of these cyclic pressure variations was not understood. In four subjects running on a treadmill, Rowell and Coll [13] recorded pulse pressure oscillations varying in frequency from 2 to 13 cycles/min both in the aorta and radial artery. Their amplitude varied from 42 to 100 mm Hg in the radial artery. Blood pressure oscillations of similar magnitude were observed by Rost [14], also during treadmill running. Rowell and Coll [13], in an attempt to speculate on the mechanisms responsible for this phenomenon, attributed it to "rhythmic peripheral vasomotor changes involved in thermal regulation". Rost, on the other hand, considered it to be the mere consequence of artifacts generated by the jarring running movements [14]. The particular shape of these cyclic pulse pressure changes prompted us to investigate whether they could be due to "beats". Beats are generated when two sine waves of nearly equal frequency propagate through a fluid: the combined effect of the two waves gives rise to a harmonic where the elongations of the two component waves periodically sum up and subtract (Fig. 9). Beat frequency is determined by the difference in frequency of the two component waves; when the frequencies of the two waves become equal, beats disappear. By summing up an artificial sine wave with a 150/min frequency and an intraarterial blood pressure tracing recorded during bicycle ergometry, we obtained a tracing with the same characteristics as that recorded in our athletes during running (Fig. 10). This frequency was chosen because the retrospective analysis of the blood pressure tracings had revealed that the frequency of the hypothetical accessory wave had to be around 150/min. This may easily be deduced from the tracing of Fig. 11; beats are discernible from the onset of the run, when heart rate is 120 beats/min. As heart rate increases, beat frequency progressively declines to temporarily disappear when heart rate reaches 152 beats/min. When it exceeds 152 beats/min, the beat phenomenon reappears and subsequently beat frequency gradually increases with a progressive rise in heart rate. This is why we have put forward the hypothesis that the wave frequency was around 150/min. During sprinting, which is accompanied by a sudden temporary increase in stride frequency, beat frequency sharply decreases. As the frequency of the accessory wave seemed to correspond to that of the athlete's strides, we presumed that the source of this stride-dependent wave would be identified with the shakes received by the aorta and the great vessels during the run. As a matter of fact, pressure variations up to 125 mm Hg were recorded during the run in the container fixed on the athletes chest. The characteristics of these pressure waves

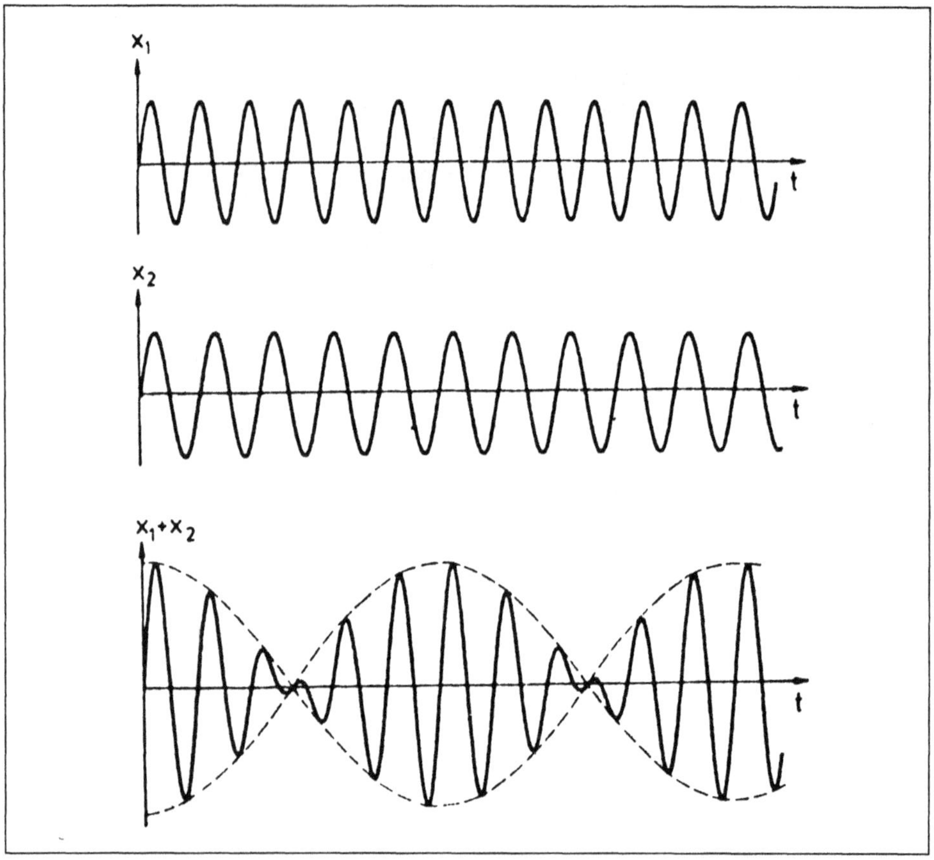

Fig. 9. The "beat" phenomenon. For an explanation, see text.

varied according to the style of the runners, their magnitude being dependent on the shock at each heel-strike impact and the power of the subsequent leg push-off. The lowest pressure variations were recorded in the subjects running with a shock-absorbing technique. Intermittent large and small waves were often recorded, reflecting the different forward-thrust developed by the two legs, an effect which was clearly discernible on the intraarterial tracings. A striking feature of the present results is represented by the unusual detection of negative blood pressure values up to -17 mm Hg. The negative values were observed in the three normotensive runners exhibiting the highest pressure variations of the saline-filled container. This finding may appear less surprising if one considers the mechanism behind the phenomenon. At the end of a prolonged strenuous effort, it is not unusual to detect, especially in the upright posture, diastolic pressures as low as 40 mm Hg [15, 16]. If a negative pressure of 55—60 mm Hg (such as that reeorded in the container of some of our athletes) is periodically added to this pressure, levels of -15 to -20 mm Hg will be intermittently obtained. On the other hand, during bicycle ergometry, where heart rates comparable to those recorded during running were achieved, in no subject was a diastolic blood pressure lower than 40 mm Hg recorded.

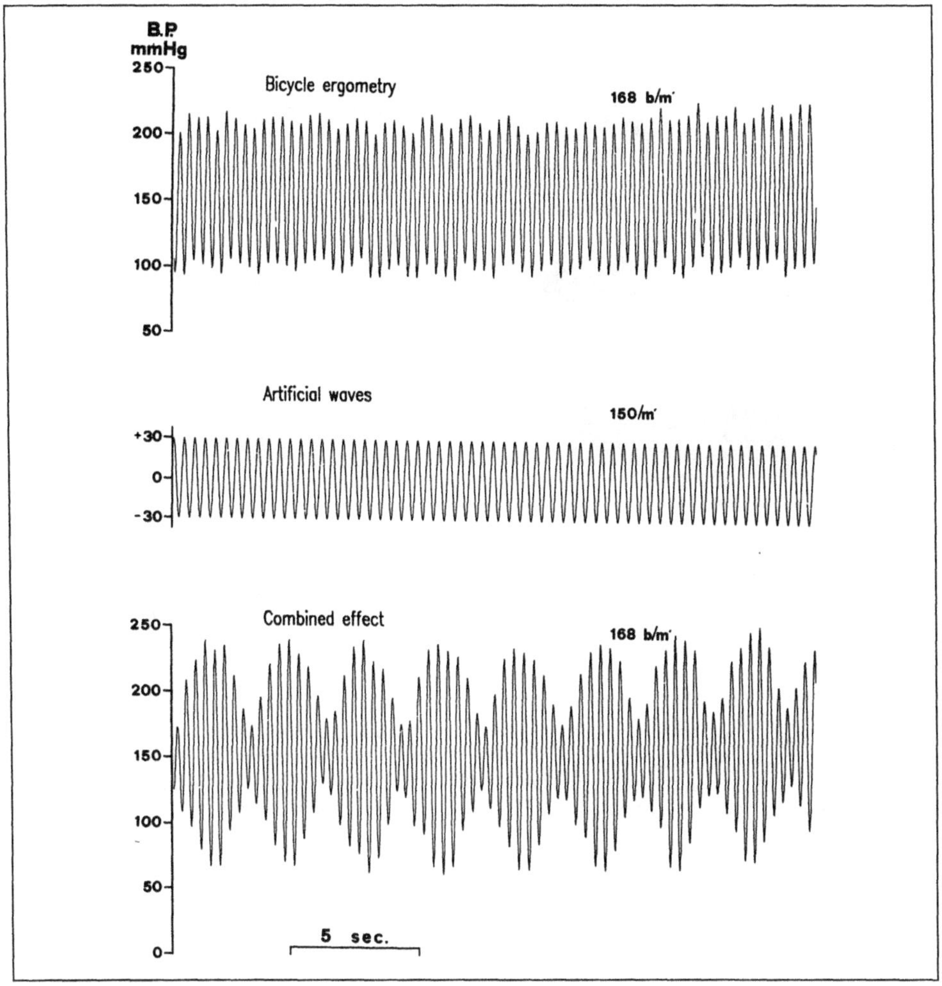

Fig. 10. A blood pressure tracing recorded during bicycle ergometry (top) is summed up to an artificial sine wave (middle) by means of a computer. The resultant harmonic (bottom) shows the "beat" phenomenon.

Road cycling

Outdoor cycling caused a far higher increase in blood pressure than bicycle ergometry, confirming that the blood pressure response to the laboratory test is not a good predictor of the blood pressure changes which actually occur in overground activities. The greatest blood pressure elevations were detected when the cyclists pedalled uphill or at maximal speed on the flat, probably as a consequence of the higher isometric component developed by the subjects during these phases of the exercise. The blood pressure values attained during road-cycling on average also exceeded the levels reached by the same subjects during track running. This indicates that cycling determines a greater increase in

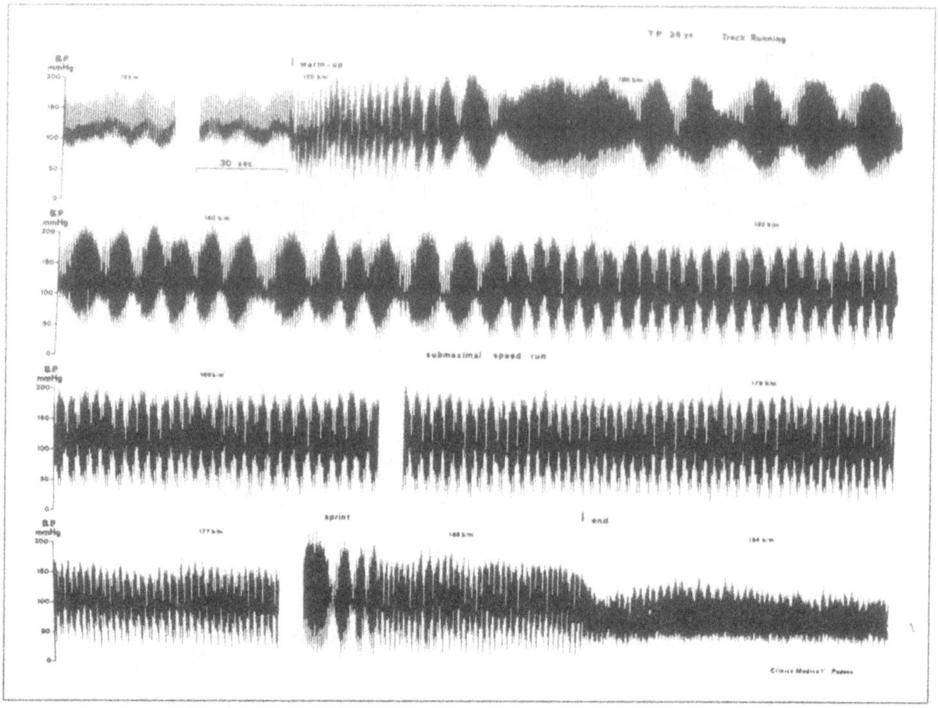

Fig. 11. Intraarterial blood pressure tracing recorded during running in an athlete. Beats, which in this example are particularly striking, are present throughout the various stages of the effort and temporarily disappear when heart rate equals stride frequency. The square waves correspond to the event markers. Figures indicate heart rate (beats/min). For a more detailed explanation, see text.

blood pressure than running, thereby justifying the higher degree of left ventricular hypertrophy found by some authors in cyclists [17].

Weight-lifting

To our knowledge there is only one report in the literature by MacDougall and Coll [18] dealing with this matter. In keeping with their results, our data demonstrate that weight-lifting brings about extremely high elevations of blood pressure. During each set of lifting repetitions, a progressive increase in blood pressure was observed with each lifting, probably due to an increasingly high recruitment of active muscles during each bout of exercise [18]. The magnitude of blood pressure elevations was proportional to the muscle mass involved and was therefore higher during legs than arm exercises. In the two weight-lifters both dynamic and static stress testing determined a much lower increase of blood pressure.

Conclusions

The present results clearly demonstrate that the blood pressure variations recorded during athletics are not well reproduced by the laboratory tests. Extensive use has been made of either treadmill or bicycle ergometry in evaluating exercise-induced blood pressure increase in both normotensive and hypertensive subjects. In the light of the present results it would appear that many of the reported data are under-estimates of the blood pressure changes as they exist in real-race situations. Several factors can explain the discrepancies between overground activities and stress tests reported in our study. First of all, each sports activity implies a different contribution of the dynamic and static components of muscle contraction, which are not so clearly separated as in laboratory tests. Secondly, psychologic factors can limit the workload one tolerates while exercising on an ergometer, as the threshold of fatigue is felt earlier. The air-induced coll- cooling of the skin during outdoor activities determines an increase of total peripheral resistance in the skin vascular bed, which produces a considerable increase in blood pressure [19]. Air resistance, which is particularly high during cycling, increases the energy demands of the effort, thereby making overground activities much more costly than working on an ergometer [20]. Obviously, any environmental factors outside the ideal conditions encountered with laboratory tests add even more to the demands of actual race situations.

References

1. Watson RDS, Stallard TJ, Flinn RM, Littler WA (1980) Factors determining direct arterial pressure and its variability in hypertensive man. Hypertension 2: 333—341
2. Pessina AC, Mormino P, Semplicini A, Palatini P, Casiglia E, Hlede M, Dal Palù C (1980) The blood pressure in labile and established hypertension: computer analysis of the continuous blood pressure recording. Stott FH (ed) Proceedings of 3rd ISAM, London 1979. Academic Press, London p 273
3. Palatini P, Mormino P, Di Marco A, Libardoni M, Mos L, Munari L, Pessina AC, Dal Palù C (1985) Ambulatory blood pressure versus casual pressure for the evaluation of target organ damage in hypertension: complications of hypertension. J Hypertension 3 (suppl 3): S425—S427
4. Skolow M, Werdegar D, Kain HK, Hinman AT (1966) Relationship between level of blood pressure measured casually and by portable recorders and severity of complications in essential hypertension. Circulation 34: 279—287
5. Mancia G, Ferrari A, Gregorini L, Parati G, Pomidossi G, Bertinieri G, Grassi G, Di Rienzo M, Pedotti A, Zanchetti A (1983) Blood pressure and heart rate variabilities in normotensive and hypertensive human being. Circ Res 53: 96—104
6. Strong WB (1979) Hypertension and sport. Pediatrics 64: 693—695
7. Bevan AT, Honour AJ, Stott FH (1969) Direct arterial pressure recording in unrestricted man. Clin Sci 361: 329—344
8. Mormino P, Palatini P, Di Marco A, Sperti G, Cordone L, Casiglia E, Pessina AC, Dal Palù C (1985) Computer analysis of continuous direct blood pressure recording. Clin Exper A7: 455—461
9. Ludbrook J (1983) Reflex control of blood pressure during exercise. Ann Rev Physiol 45: 155—168
10. Rasmussen PH, Staats BA, Driscoll DJ, Beck KC, Bonekat W, Wilcox WD (1985) Direct and indirect blood pressure during exercise. Chest 87: 743—748
11. Gould AB, Hornung R, Altman D, Cashman PMM, Raftery EB (1985) Indirect measurement of blood pressure during exercise testing can be misleading. Med J 53: 611—615
12. Kieso HA, Gould BA, Mann S, Hornung RS, Altman DG, Raftery EB (1983) Effect on intraarterial blood pressure of slow release metoprolol combined with placebo or chlortalidone. Br Med J 287: 717—720
13. Rowell LB, Brengelmann GL, Blackmon JR, Bruce RA, Murrey JA (1968) Disparities between aortic

and peripheral pulse pressures induced by upright exercise and vasomotor changes in man. Circulation 37: 954—964
14. Rost R (1983) Sportliche Aktivität des Hypertonikers. Munch Med Wschr 125: 1025—1033
15. Pugh LGCE (1969) Thermal, metabolic, blood, and circulatory adjustments in prolonged outdoor exercise. Br Med J 2: 657—662
16. Fleg JL, Lakatta EG (1986) Prevalence and significance of postexercise hypotension in apparently healthy subjects. Am J Cardiol 57: 1380—1384
17. Fagard R, Aubert A, Staessen J, Vandeneynde E, Vanhees L, Amery A (1984) Cardiac structure and function in cyclists and runners. Comparative echocariographic study. Br Heart J 52: 124—129
18. MacDougall JD (1985) Arterial blood pressure response to heavy resistance exercise. J Appl Physiol (3): 785—790
19. Rowell LB (1974) Human cardiovascular adjustment to exercise and thermal stress. Physiol Rev 54: 75—159
20. Daniels JT (1985) A physiologist's view of running economy. Med Sci Sports 17: 332—337

Blood pressure variability and reactivity in the natural environment

G.A. Harshfield[1], T.G. Pickering[2], G.D. James[2] and S.G. Blank[2].

[1] The Hypertension Center, Department of Medicine, The Charles R. Drew Postgraduate Medical School, Los Angeles, California,
[2] The Hypertension Center, The New York Hospital-Cornell Medical Center, New York, New York, USA

Introduction

Laboratory studies have found that individuals with mild hypertension differ from normotensives in their degree of blood pressure variability and reactivity, defined as the change in blood pressure to specific stimuli. Based on the assumption that mild hypertension represents an intermediate stage in the development of established hypertension, these studies have led to the speculation that exaggerated blood pressure variability and/or reactivity plays an etiological role in the development of established hypertension [1—3]. These findings, however, have not been extended to blood pressure functioning under natural, day-to-day conditions. In the present study we examined blood pressure variability and reactivity over a 24-h period in three groups of individuals: a) normotensive control subjects, defined as a clinic blood pressure ≧ 120/80 mm Hg, b) mild hypertensive subjects, defined as a clinic blood pressure > 120/80 mm Hg < 160/104 mm Hg; and c) established hypertensive subjects, defined as a clinic blood pressure > 160/104 mm Hg. There are no generally accepted ways of measuring blood pressure variability and reactivity in the natural environment [4]; therefore, in this study we have chosen to define variability in three different ways: a) the blood pressure pattern based upon the location/activity in which the measurement was obtained; b) the overall variability of blood pressure; and c) the range in blood pressure. Reactivity was defined as a) blood pressure responses obtained during the performance of activities with either physical or b) psychological demands relative to blood pressure during relaxation, as well as c) the percentage of readings less than the individual's own clinic reading.

Methods

The subjects were 644 hypertensive patients and 58 normotensive controls from the Hypertension Center of The New York Hospital-Cornell Medical Center. The subjects were divided into two groups based on the level of their clinic blood pressure: 1) 578 patients with "mild" hypertension, defined as a clinic systolic blood pressure (SBP) ≧ 120 mm Hg but ≦ 160 mm Hg and a clinic diastolic blood pressure (DBP) > 80 mm Hg but < 105 mm Hg; and 2) 66 patients with "established" hypertension, defined as a clinic SBP > 160 mmHg and a clinic DBP > 105 mmHg. The hypertensive patients were off all forms of hypertensive medication for at least 3 weeks prior to testing. The demographics for the three groups are shown in Table 1. The three groups showed comparable male/female ratios, but the established group was significantly older than the normal group ($p < .05$). The ambulatory blood pressure recorders (Del Mar Avionics Pressurometer II, III, ICR 5200) and procedures used in this study have been previously described in detail [5, 6]. The subject arrived at the Hypertension Center on the morning of the day of testing and was fitted with the recording device. Five calibration readings were obtained in the seated position to insure the readings obtained by the recorder agreed with those obtained by a trained observer using a mercury column and stethoscope. If an adequate calibration was not obtained the procedure was abandonned. The automatic timer was then set to obtain a reading every 15 min during the day and every 30 min at night. Each time the recorder took a reading the subject was instructed to keep their arm as motionless as possible to prevent artifactual readings and to record in a diary their location (work, home, miscellaneous), position (sitting, standing, reclining) and specific activity (e.g., watching television, in a business meeting, etc.).

Table 1. Demographic characteristics of subjects

	Normal	Mild	Established
N	58	578	66
Age	38 ± 12	46 ± 12	51 ± 11*
Sex	39 M	389 M	20 M
	19 F[2]	128 F	44 F

*Significantly different from normal group ($p<.05$).
M = males, F = females

The data reduction techniques for the ambulatory recordings have also been described in detail [7]. Each data point was scanned by a trained observer for the elimination of artifactual readings and the readings were coded for location, position and specific activity. Average values were then calculated for each individual for each variable of interest.

Results

Data were analyzed by analysis of variance and t-tests where appropriate. Data are expressed as means ± standard deviation.

Blood pressure patterns

The average level of both SBP and DBP during each of the situations for each of the three groups of subjects are displayed in Fig. 1. The highest SBP for the established group was in the clinic (177 ± 15) with a 10 mmHg difference between the clinic and work ($p < 0.001$), an 11 mmHg difference between work and home ($p < 0.001$) and a 17 mmHg difference between home and sleep ($p < 0.001$). The highest level of DBP for the established group was also in the clinic (115 ± 15), with an 8 mmHg difference between the clinic and work ($p < 0.001$), a 7 mmHg difference between work and home ($p < 0.05$) and a 13 mmHg difference between home and sleep ($p < 0.001$). The mild group showed a similar pattern. The highest SBP for the mild group was at work (144 ± 12) with a 3 mmHg difference between the clinic and work ($p < 0.001$), an 8 mmHg difference between work and home ($p < 0.001$) and a 14 mmHg difference between home and sleep ($p < 0.001$). The highest DBP was also at work (94 ± 8), with 1 mmHg difference between the clinic and work (ns), a 6 mmHg difference between work and home ($p < 0.001$) and a 12 mmHg difference between home and sleep ($p < 0.001$). The normal group also showed the highest level of SBP at work (116 ± 9) with a 3 mmHg difference between work and home ($p < 0.06$), a 5 mmHg difference between home and the clinic ($p < 0.05$) and a 12 mmHg difference between home and sleep ($p < 0.001$). DBP for the normal group showed the same pattern with the highest level at work (79 ± 6), a 2 mmHg difference between work and home ($p < 0.05$), a 4 mmHg difference between home and the clinic ($p < 0.05$) and a 10 mmHg difference between home and sleep ($p < 0.001$).

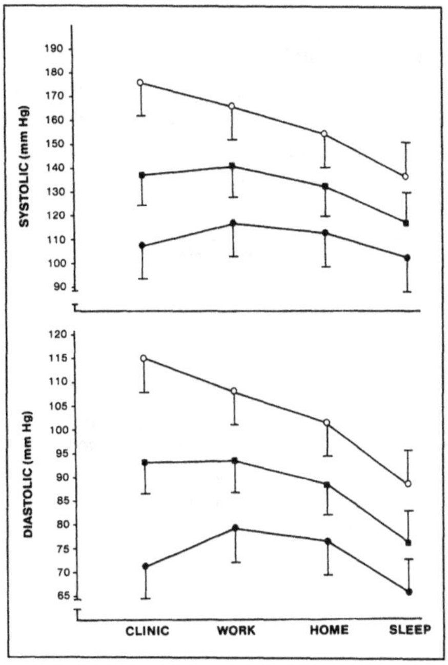

Fig. 1. Systolic (above) and diastolic (below) ambulatory blood pressure patterns for the three groups. The primary difference between the three groups is in the hypertensive's pressor response to the clinic.

A comparison of the level of the three groups showed the SBP and DBP of the established group was higher than the mild group in the clinic ($p < 0.001$ for both) at work ($p < 0.001$ for both), at home ($p < 0.001$ for both) and during sleep ($p < 0.001$ for both). The mild group, in turn, showed higher levels of SBP and DBP than the normal group in the clinic ($p < 0.001$ for both), at work ($p < 0.001$ for both) at home ($p < 0.001$ for both) and during sleep ($p < 0.001$ for both).

We compared the percent change in blood pressure between the different situations for the three groups. The established group showed a 6% decrease in SBP from the clinic to work, which was different from the 2% increase shown by the mild group ($p < 0.001$). The established group also showed a 7% decrease in DBP from the clinic to work, which was also different from the 0.05% decrease shown by the mild group ($p < 0.001$). The normal group showed a 7% increase in SBP from the clinic to work which was different from the mild group ($p < 0.001$) and a 8% increase in DBP which was also different from the mild group ($p < 0.001$). The established and mild groups showed no differences in percent change in either SBP or DBP from work to home. The 6% decrease in SBP for the mild group, however, differed from the 2% decrease of the normal group ($p < 0.001$) as did the 7% decrease in DBP by the mild group compared to the 4% decrease for the normal group ($p < 0.05$). The three groups did not differ in the percent drop in either SBP or DBP between home and sleep, with all three groups showing about a 13% drop in SBP and 16% drop in DBP.

Blood pressure variance

The values for blood pressure variance are presented in Table 2, with a frequency histogram for SBP presented in Fig. 2. The established group showed no significant differences between the three conditions of work, home and sleep for either SBP or DBP variance. The mild group showed no difference in SBP variance between work and home, but did show greater DBP variance at work ($p < 0.001$). The mild group also showed a greater variance at home than during sleep for both SBP ($p < 0.001$) and DBP ($p < 0.01$). The normal group showed no differences between conditions for either SBP or DBP.

Table 2. Average systolic and diastolic (± S. D.) blood pressure variance*

Location	Normal	Mild	Established
Work	92/55 ± 66/36	134/69 ± 106/53	200/85 ± 127/60
Home	104/83 ± 70/56	139/91 ± 92/55	207/101 ± 142/80
Sleep	106/66 ± 118/62	113/77 ± 100/66	154/87 ± 167/90
Awake	130/87 ± 100/53	145/99 ± 105/64	244/119 ± 188/86
24 hour	157/105 ± 128/72	223/99 ± 65/64	309/153 ± 231/105

*See text for significant differences

We next compared the variances of the three groups for each of the conditions. The established group showed a greater SBP variance at work than the mild group ($p < 0.001$), which in turn showed a greater SBP variance at work than the normal group ($p < 0.001$). There were no differences between the groups in DBP variance at work. The established group showed a greater SBP variance at home than the mild group ($p < 0.001$), which in turn showed greater SBP variance at home than the normal group ($p < 0.001$). There were again no differences between the three groups in DBP at home. The established group showed a greater SBP variance than the mild group during sleep ($p < 0.05$). There was no difference between the mild and normal groups for sleep SBP or DBP. Finally, the established group showed a greater awake variance than the mild group for both SBP ($p < 0.001$) and DBP ($p < 0.01$). The mild group and the normal group did not differ.

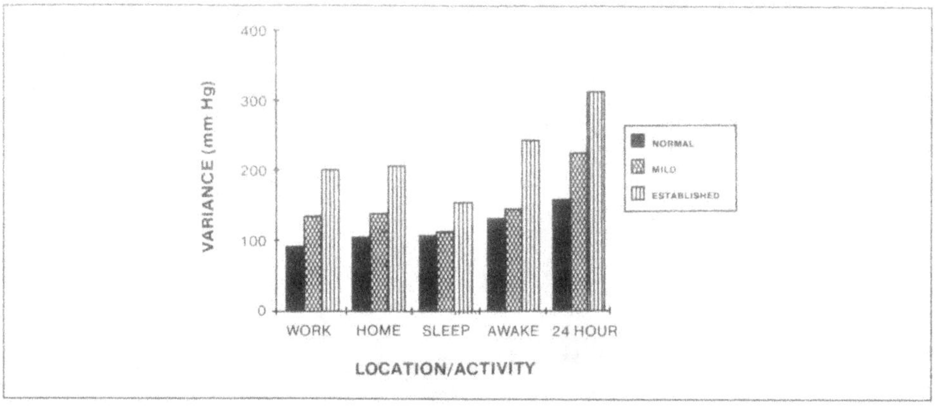

Fig. 2. A frequency histogram of systolic blood pressure variance by recording location/activity for the three groups. The established group showed the greatest variance followed by the mild group and the normal group. Variance did not, in general, differ by the recording locations of work, home and sleep.

Blood pressure range

The range of SBP and DBP for each condition was defined as the highest 5% of readings minus the lowest 5%. This definition was chosen to protect against spurious artifactual readings which may affect the range. These values are presented in Table 3 and displayed for SBP in Fig. 3. The established group showed no differences in range between work and home for either SBP or DBP. They did, however, show significantly greater range at home than during sleep for both SBP ($p < 0.001$) and DBP ($p < 0.01$). The mild group showed a difference in range between work and home for both SBP and DBP ($p < 0.01$ for both) as well as between home and sleep for both SBP and DBP ($p < 0.01$ for both). The normal group also showed no differences in range between work and home for SBP but did for DBP ($p < 0.001$). The normal group also showed a difference in the range between home and sleep for both SBP ($p < 0.05$) and DBP ($p < 0.01$).

Table 3. Average systolic diastolic blood pressure range (± S. D.)*

Location	Normal	Mild	Established
Work	31/25 ± 13/9	41/29 ± 19/21	47/30 ± 14/13
Home	37/33 ± 18/12	44/34 ± 17/12	51/34 ± 18/12
Sleep	29/24 ± 17/14	47/35 ± 19/12	35/27 ± 19/13
Awake	37/33 ± 15/11	44/34 ± 15/11	51/34 ± 19/12

*See text for significant differences.

A comparison of the established and mild groups showed no differences in the range for either SBP or DBP at work. The mild group did differ from the normal group for range in SBP at work ($p < 0.05$). The established group showed a greater range than the mild group at home for SBP ($p < 0.001$) but not for DBP. The mild group, in turn, showed a greater range than the normal group for SBP at home ($p < 0.001$), but not for DBP. The established group also showed a greater range in SBP than the mild group during sleep for SBP ($p < 0.01$) and DBP ($p < 0.001$). The mild group, in turn, showed a greater range during sleep than the normal group for both SBP and DBP ($p < 0.001$ for both). Finally, the established group showed a greater range in awake SBP than the mild group ($p < 0.001$) and the mild group showed a greater awake SBP range than the normal group ($p < 0.001$). There were no group differences in DBP.

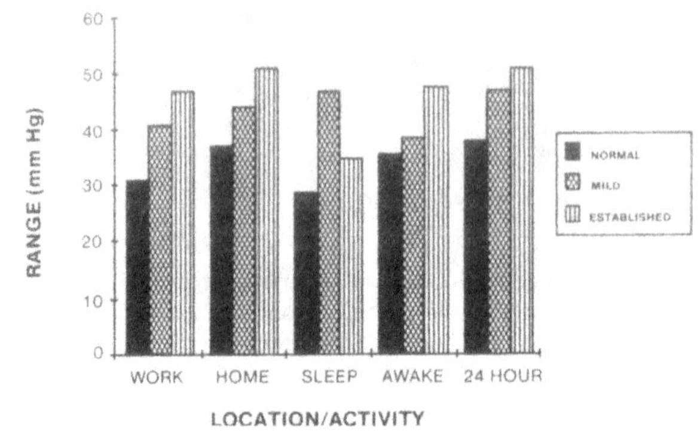

Fig. 3. A frequency histogram of systolic blood pressure range by recording location/activity for the three groups. The established group showed the greatest variance followed by the mild group and the normal group. Variance did not, in general, differ between work, home and sleep.

Blood pressure responses during specific activities

We calculated the average SBP and DBP during the performance of the 11 most frequently reported activities, as well as for relaxation. We divided the activities into those with primarily physical and those with primarily psychological demands. Activities with primarily physical demands included walking, shopping, eating, drinking and house cleaning. Activities with primarily psychological demands included talking, talking on the telephone, working, business-related activities at home, reading and watching television. The absolute values can be found in Table 4. We calculated blood pressure reactivity by determining the percent change from relaxation for each activity.

The established group showed a significant response to the physical activities for both SBP ($p < 0.001$) and DBP ($p < 0.001$). They also showed a significant response to the psychological activities for both SBP and DBP ($p < 0.001$ for both). A comparison of the responses for the two types of activities showed no differences in SBP but the physical activities were associated with a greater DBP response ($p < 0.01$). The mild group showed a similar pattern, showing a significant increase in SBP and DBP ($p < 0.001$ for both) during the physical activities as well as an increase in SBP and DBP ($p < 0.001$ for both) during the psychological activities. They also showed a difference between activities for SBP ($p < 0.01$) but not for DBP. The normal group showed an increase during the physical activities for SBP and DBP ($p < 0.001$ for both) but only showed a significant increase in DBP to the psychological activities ($p < 0.01$). The normal group also showed greater responses to the physical activities for both SBP ($p < 0.01$) and DBP ($p < 0.05$).

Table 4. Blood pressure during activities with either physical or psychological demands*

Activity	Normal	Mild	Established
Physical			
Walking	121/78	145/92	164/105
Shopping	119/78	142/93	150/108
Eating	119/78	139/94	166/110
Drinking	122/82	140/92	162/108
Housework	113/78	145/90	162/111
Psychological			
Telephone	118/78	139/94	162/106
Talking	115/78	139/93	158/101
Working (work)	112/78	139/93	159/103
Working (home)	112/76	136/91	155/106
Reading	107/71	131/87	155/104
Television	110/73	130/84	147/98
Relaxation	113/73	130/84	146/96

*See text for significant differences.

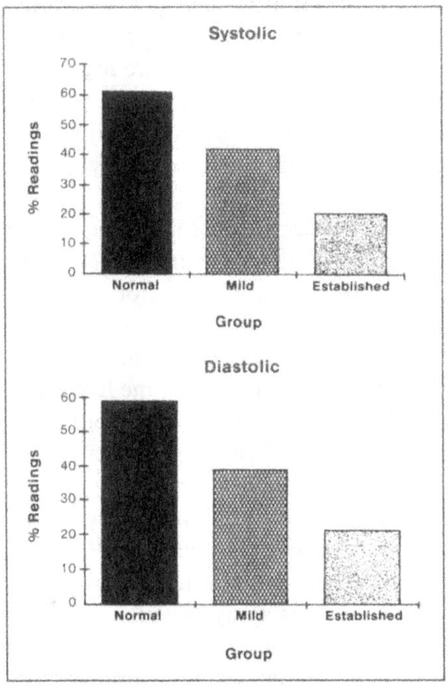

Fig. 4. The average percentage of systolic (above) and diastolic (below) readings by individual greater than their own clinic readings for each of the three groups.

A comparison of the established group to the mild group showed no differences in SBP responses for either type of activities. The established group did show a greater DBP response to the physical activities ($p < 0.05$). A comparison between the mild group and the normal group showed a greater response by the mild group for SBP during the physical activities ($p < 0.05$ and psychological activities ($p < 0.05$) but no differences for DBP.

Percentage of readings greater than the clinic reading

The average percentage of readings greater than the clinic reading for both SBP and DBP is displayed in Fig. 4. The normal group showed the greatest percentage of readings during the day greater than their own clinic reading, followed by the mild group, with the established group showing the least.

Discussion

The role blood pressure variability in the hypertensive process has been the focus of a considerable research effort over the past several years. One position is that exaggerated blood pressure variability leads to the development of essential hypertension. Two hypotheses have been developed to explain the mechanisms involved, one suggesting that exaggerated variations in pressure result in damage to the peripheral circulation which in turn results in autoregulatory changes leading to increases in peripheral resistance. The other hypothesis suggests that increased variability leads to target organ damage, particularly in the kidney and/or the heart which leads to increases in cardiac output and elevated blood pressure. A second position suggests that it is not the increased variability of blood pressure per se that leads to the development of hypertension, but rather exaggerated pressor responses to specific stimuli, i.e., exaggerated blood pressure reactivity. This position relies on similar hypotheses as above, suggesting the exaggerated pressor responses to a series of specific stimuli lead to either vascular or target organ damage. The third position is that exaggerated blood pressure variability and/or reactivity is a marker for the development of essential hypertension, i.e., is indicative of a genetic "abnormality" which predisposes the individual to the development of hypertension. A fourth and final possibility is that exaggerated blood pressure variability and/or reactivity is a consequence of the hypertensive process, rather than a cause (for extensive reviews see refs. [1, 2, 8, 9, 10]).

Support for the former three hypotheses comes primarily from laboratory studies which have a) compared the responses of individuals with mild, or borderline hypertension with those of normotensive individuals, with the assumption that borderline hypertension represents an intermediate stage in the development of established hypertension; or b) compared the responses of individuals with a positive family history of hypertension to those with a negative family history. These studies have, in general, yielded positive results, although the findings have not been totally convincing. Previous research by our group using 24-h ambulatory blood pressure monitoring, however, has questioned the validity of these findings. Firstly, in a previous study in which we compared the ambulatory blood pressure patterns of 25 normotensive, 25 borderline hypertensive and 25 established hypertensive subjects [11] we found that the primary difference between the normotensives and the hypertensives, other than the level of pressure per se, was in the hypertensives' pressor response to the clinic. Previous data collected on mild hypertensives under laboratory conditions, which has shown increased reactivity in this group relative to normals, is probably confounded by this pressor response exhibited by the hypertensives to the laboratory situation. Although this is undoubtedly true in normotensives as well, it seems to be a much stronger effect for the hypertensives. Thus, earlier data which has shown differences between the two groups must be interpreted with this in mind. Furthermore, most of these studies have not included a comparison group of individuals with consistently elevated blood pressures to compare with the borderline group. Secondly, we have found that the level of blood pressure measured in the clinic does not generalize to blood pressure measured under natural conditions outside of the laboratory [12].

The ambulatory blood pressure patterns of the mild and established hypertensive subjects in this study are similar to the patterns we have previously found in a much smaller sample [13], with differences in blood pressure based on the condition in which the measurement was obtained. In general, blood pressure was elevated in the clinic and at work, decreased at home, and decreased still further during sleep. The normotensive group also showed a pattern similar to the pattern previously reported, with the highest pressure at work, followed by home, the clinic and sleep [11].

A comparison of the patterns of the mild and established groups shows the primary difference between the groups is their level of pressure, with both groups showing similar blood pressure patterns and comparable changes between the different conditions. A comparison of the pattern of the hypertensive groups with the normotensive group, however, demonstrated two important differences. Firstly, both hypertensive groups maintained a higher level of blood pressure than the normotensive group throughout the day. This was not only true for the clinic pressure (which is true by definition) but also for pressure at work at home, and during sleep. Furthermore, the differences between the groups remained relatively constant at work, at home and during sleep with the established group averaging 22/13 mmHg higher pressures than the mild group which in turn averaged 20/12 mmHg higher pressures than the normal group. (These values were calculated by averaging the values of systolic/diastolic pressure for work, home, and sleep are plotted in Fig. 1). Second, the hypertensive groups showed a pressor response to the clinic situation which the normal group did not. This can be demonstrated by calculating the differences in the level of blood pressure between the groups for the clinic and comparing this difference to the above differences calculated while at work, home and sleep. The difference between the mild and established groups in the clinic was 39/22 mmHg, 19/10 mmHg higher than the average difference between the two groups during the other conditions (see above), while the difference between the mild and normal groups was 30/21 mmHg, 8/8 mmHg greater than the average difference between these two groups during the other conditions.

Values of blood pressure range and variance during work, while at home and during sleep for groups similar to the three groups in this study have not been previously reported. An examination of these values, which were presented in Tables 2 and 3, reveals the following. Firstly, there is considerable variability in blood pressure during the day. This can readily be seen in the average awake variance of 173/102 mmHg and average awake range of 45/34 mmHg displayed by the three groups. (These values were obtained by averaging the awake values for the three groups). Secondly, the majority of the significant differences between conditions are, as one would expect, between work or home, periods associated with activity, and sleep, a period associated with inactivity. Perhaps surprisingly, however, is the comparison of ranges and variances between work and home. Contrary to what one might expect, the average variance across groups is 8/26 mmHg greater at home than at work and the average range is 5/12 mmHg greater at home than at work. (These values were calculating by averaging of the three groups for work and home). Thirdly, there are large standard deviations which reflect a considerable degree of individual differences.

The results for blood pressure responses to the specific activities were similar to those we previously reported [14]. Both the physical and psychological activities resulted in significant elevations in blood pressure relative to periods of relaxation. Furthermore, the physical activities produced an average of 6/4 mmHg greater elevations than the psychological activities (These values were derived by averaging the values for the activities across groups which are found in Table 4). A comparison of the three groups once again yielded similar results to those found for blood pressure patterns and blood pressure variability. Once the initial level of pressure was taken into account, the groups did not differ in reactivity. This was true for both tasks with pyhsical and psychological demands.

Conclusions

A recent editorial by Weder and Julius [9] questioned the validity of theories of essential hypertension which are based upon exaggerated blood pressure variability and reactivity. They point out that research to date has yet to demonstrate a) that blood pressure changes obtained under laboratory conditions predict blood pressure changes occurring in response to natural behaviors, and b) that mild hypertensives show greater blood pressure reactivity than normotensives during natural behaviors. The results of this study address both of these criticisms. Firstly, the only differences in blood pressure patterns between the normotensive and hypertensive groups was in the pressor response exhibited by the hypertensive groups to the clinic situation. Furthermore, the established group showed a greater pressor response than the mild group. This suggests that previous differences found between normotensives and hypertensives to laboratory stressors is probably somewhat confounded by the pressor response exhibited by the hypertensives to the laboratory situation which could act to potentiate the response. Although this is undoubtedly true in normals as well, it seems to be much more so for hypertensives for whom "blood pressure" has much greater saliency.

Secondly, the finding that the established group showed even greater pressor responses to the clinic than the mild group suggests that the level of the response is dictated by the level of pressure per se. Few previous laboratory studies have included a comparison group with blood pressures at this level and therefore would not have been able to observe this finding. (It is part of our standard practice to perform a hypertensive evaluation on everyone while they are off medication to get an accurate biochemical profiling, affording us the opportunity to collect 24-h recordings on these individuals which were also used as part of their evaluation. We have observed that 5% of individuals with pressures even in this range show "normal" pressures outside of the clinic [15]). This is further supported by the differences in variability and reactivity found outside of the laboratory. These data show increases in variability and reactivity as blood pressure increases. If exaggerated variability and reactivity were a "cause" of hypertension we would expect to see the greatest variability and reactivity in the mild group, which may represent the developmental stage of hypertension, not in the established group. It is possible, however, that the variability of the mild group represents hypertension in the "developmental stage" while the even greater variability of the established group represents the response to already existing target organ damage. This, however, seems unlikely.

References

1. Obrist PA (1981) Cardiovascular Psychophysiology. New York, Plenum Press
2. Krantz DS, Manuck SB (1984) Acute psychophysiologic reactivity and risk of cardiovascular disease: A review and methodologic review. *Psychol Bull* 96: 435—464
3. Steptoe A, Melville D, Ross A (1984) Behavioral response demands, cardiovascular reactivity, and essential hypertension. *Psychosom Med* 46: 33—47
4. Pickering TG, Harshfield GA, Devereux RB, Laragh JH (1985) What is the role of ambulatory blood pressure monitoring in the management of hypertensive patients? *Hypertension* 7: 171—177
5. Harshfield GA, Pickering TG, Laragh JH (1979) A validation study of the Del Mar Avionics Ambulatory Blood Pressure System. *Ambulatory Electrocardio* 1: 7—12
6. Harshfield GA, Pickering TG, Blank S, Lindahl C, Stroud L, Laragh JH (1984) Ambulatory Blood Pressure Monitoring: Records, applications, and analysis. *In*: Weber MA, Drayer JIM, (eds) Ambulatory Blood Pressure Monitoring. Dannstadt, Steinkopff Verlag, pp 1—7
7. Harshfield GA, Hwang C, Blank SG, Pickering TG. Research techniques for ambulatory blood pressure monitoring. In: Schneiderman N, Kaufman P, Weis SM, (eds) New York, Plenum (in press)
8. Folkow B (1982) Physiological aspects of primary hypertension. *Physiolog Rev* 62: 347—504
9. Weder AB, Julius S (1985) Behavior, blood pressure variability, and hypertension. *Psychosom Med* 47: 406—414
10. Julius S, Johnson E (1985) Stress, autonomic hyperactivity and essential hypertension: An enigma. *J Hyperten* 3: S 11—S 17
11. Pickering TG, Harshfield GA, Kleinert HD, Blank SG, Laragh JH (1982) Comparisons of blood pressure during normal daily activities, sleep, and exercise in normal and hypertensive subjects. *J Am Med Ass* 247: 992—996
12. Harshfield GA, James GD, Schlussel Y, Yee L, Blank SG, Pickering TG. Do laboratory tests of blood pressure reactivity predict blood pressure variability in real life? (in press)
13. Harshfield GA, Pickering TG, Kleinert HD, Blank SG, Laragh JH (1982) Situational variations of blood pressure in ambulatory hypertensive patients. *Psychosom Med* 44: 237—245
14. Clark LA, Denby L, Pregibon D, Harshfield GA, Pickering TG, Blank SG, Laragh JH. The effects of activity and time of day on the diurnal variations of blood pressure. *J Chron Dis* (in press)

Diurnal blood pressure rhythm: dependence on internal and external time triggers

P. Baumgart

Medizinische Poliklinik, Universität Münster, FRG

Introduction

Biphasic fluctuations with lower levels during the night and higher levels during the day usually characterize the 24-h blood pressure curve.
The diurnal rhythms of some biological parameters are dependent on internal time triggers and thus resistant to shifts of activity and sleeping periods, others are exclusively determined by the diurnal activities. Rotated shift work is a suitable model for investigation of influences of external and internal time triggers on bioparameters. The 24-h body temperature curves are not yet reversed within one week after shift rotation [14]. Some hormones retain their 24-h rhythm for a few days [8], others immediately follow the new sleeping and activity phases [4, 8].
There are only sporadic reports about the effect of rotated working and sleeping phases on the blood pressure, based on casual blood pressure measurements (3, 6). Ambulatory blood pressure monitoring has meanwhile become suitable for recording representative 24-h blood pressure profiles at physical work without significant impairment of the working performance.
In this study, the dependence of the 24-h blood pressure on internal and external time triggers was investigated in shift workers by repeated ambulatory blood pressure monitoring.
Between the two shifts, the mean blood pressure values in 24-h and in various time and activity phases, and the amplitudes of diurnal fluctations of the 24-h blood pressure curves were compared.

Patients and methods

Fifteen shift workers (men aged 34—53 years) underwent repeated ambulatory 24-h blood pressure monitoring. They were employed at a chemical factory and performed manual labor on a weekly rotated three-shift system (weekends free).
At routine blood pressure readings after five min rest in a sitting position (average of three subsequent readings) all were normotensive ($<$140/90 mmHg). At physical examination they were also otherwise healthy. None had been taking drugs.
Indirect pressure recordings of the 24-h blood pressure were performed on the last day (Friday) of morning and night shift weeks.
Work lasted from 0600 hours—1100 hours in the morning shift and from 2200—0600 hours in the night shift.
Five of the 15 workers underwent 24-h blood pressure monitoring a third time on the first day (Monday) of a night-shift period.

The readings of the blood pressure and heart rate were taken intermittently at intervals of 30 min throughout the 24-h. Portable automatic recorders (SL 90202, SpaceLabs) were used to read the blood pressure. These are lighter (660 g including batteries), smaller, and more accurate than previous recorders [1]. This oscillometric recorder does not use patient electrodes which were usually applied for ECG triggered microphone-gating in sphygmomanometric recorders. Thus the working performance was not impaired subtantially and the devices seemed particularly suited for measurements during physical work. The workers recorded their sleeping and working phases during the measurements on standard protocol sheets. They additionally rated the impairment at work and during sleep, respectively, on a scale of four degrees (0—3) in standard questionnaires.
The averages of blood pressures and heart rates of the entire group were calculated for every single hour, for the day (0800—2000 hours), night (2000—0800 hours) and for the total 24-h-periods from the individual hourly mean values. Likewise the mean blood pressures and heart rates during sleep and at work were calculated from the individual mean blood pressures during the respective phases.
The 24-h blood pressure (and heart rate) courses of two shifts were compared by the cross correlation procedure for time series. The hourly mean blood pressure (and heart rate) values in the two shifts were used as data vectors for calculation of correlation coefficients at hourly increasing phase shifts (from —12 h to +12 h) between the two 24-h-cycles.

Results

The average blood pressure and heart rate values in the various time periods and activity phases are presented in Table 1.

Table 1: Mean + SEM of the systolic/diastolic blood pressure [mmHg] and heart rate [puls/min] in 24-h, during sleep and at work of 15 shift workers in their morning and night shifts.

	Morning shift	**Night shift**
	Blood Pressure	
24-h	126.7+2.0/77.6+1.6	126.6+1.4/77.3+1.3
during sleep	112.8+2.0/64.5+1.9	113.5+1.6/65.4+1.5
at work	131.4+2.2/83.1+1.8	132.8+1.8/83.7+1.7
	Heart Rate	
24-h	80.4+2.2	77.3+2.1
during sleep	66.8+2.4	65.0+2.4
at work	87.7+2.3	85.1+2.5

The mean 24-h blood pressures were identical in the morning shift and in the night shift. The nocturnal blood pressure during the morning shift corresponded to the daytime blood pressure during the night shift; the daytime blood pressure during the morning shift did not differ from the nighttime blood pressure during the night shift.
There were also no blood pressure differences between the sleeping phases or between the working phases of the two shifts.

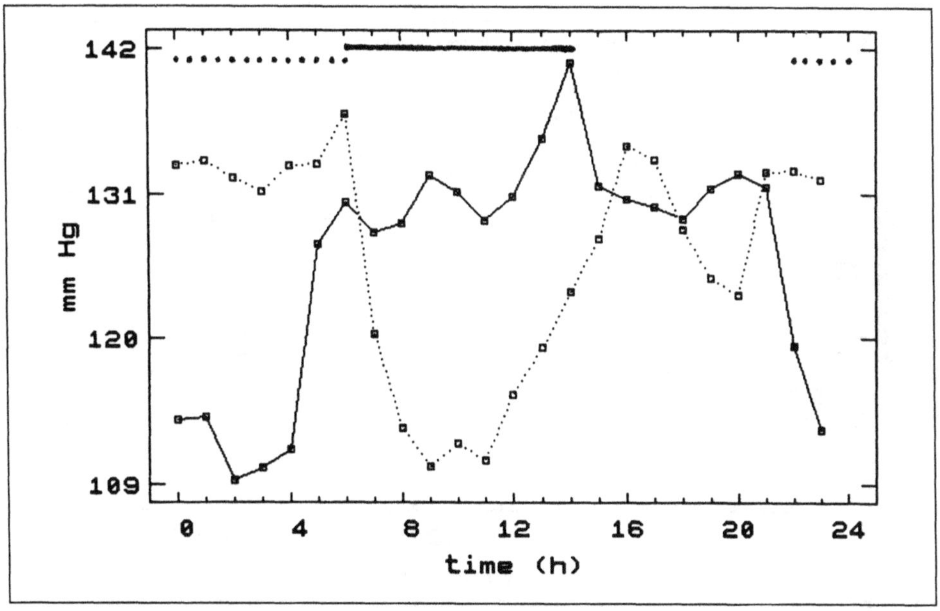

Fig. 1. Systolic and diastolic blood pressure (hourly group averages) of shift workers during morning (—) and night (. . .) shifts (N = 15). Continuous and pointed straight lines indicate working times.

The mean hourly blood pressure values during the morning and night shifts are plotted in Fig. 1.

The minimal and maximal hourly values occuring in 24-h were comparable in the two cycles. Hence the amplitudes of diurnal blood pressure fluctuations were in the same range. The mean duration of high (and low) blood pressure periods in 24-h were roughly equal.

Figure 2 shows the corresponding mean values of the heart rate during the two shifts. The heart rate curve is similarly reversed by shift rotation as is the blood pressure profile. The cross correlation coefficients between the hourly mean systolic blood pressure values in the morning and night shifts at increasing phase shifts (lags) between the two 24-h curves are presented in Fig 3. There was a periodic increase and decrease of the correlation, the maximum occuring at a lag of 8 h. This corresponded to the lag between the working periods. Shifting the curve of the night shift along the curve of the morning shift by 8 h, a high correlation coefficient ($r = 0.68$) was achieved. The mean hourly heart rates in the two shifts showed minor maximal correlation coefficients ($r = 0.59$), however this maximum also occurred after a shift of 8 h (not shown). The cross-correlation procedures indicates, that the shape of the 24-h blood pressure curve is highly consistent after shift rotation. The shape alterations of the heart rate profiles even exceed those of the systolic blood pressure profiles.

Figure 4 shows the average systolic blood pressures curve of five subjects during the first and last day of a five-day night shift week.

The courses of the two curves are similar. The correlation of the mean hourly blood pressures between the two days was very close ($r = 0.86$). The respective correlation of

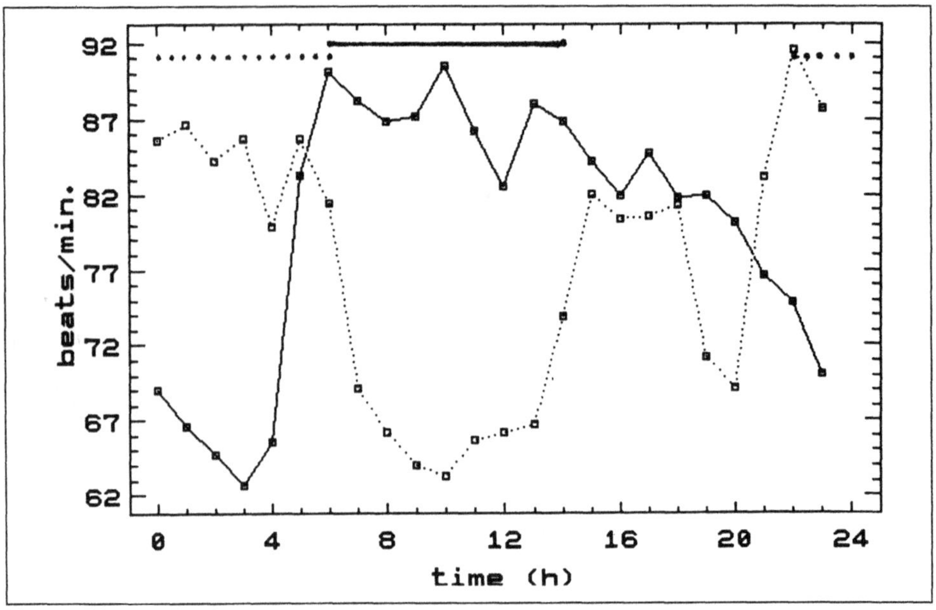

Fig. 2. Hourly group averages of the heart rate of shift workers during morning (—) and night (. . .) shifts (N = 15). Continuous and pointed straight lines indicate working times.

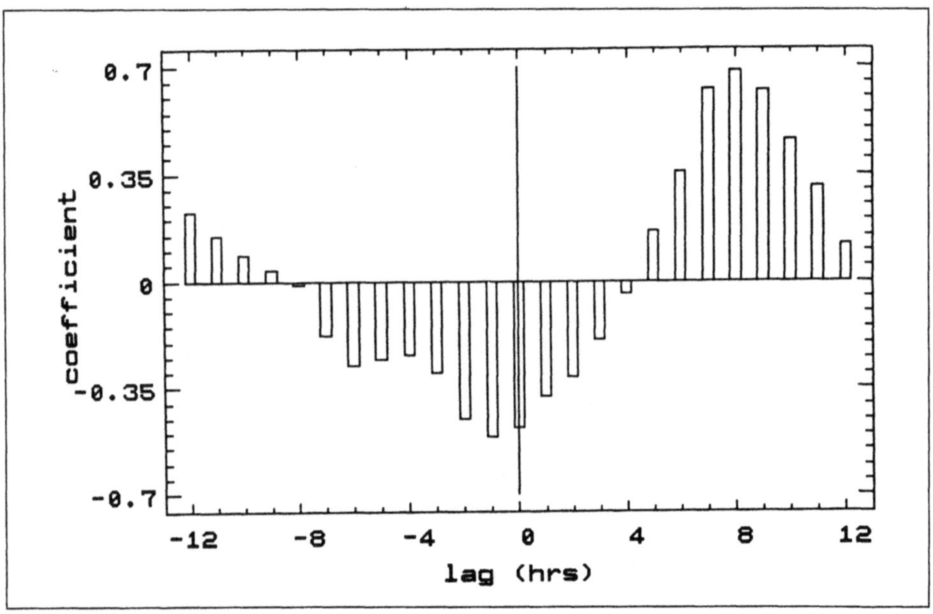

Fig. 3. Cross correlations between the hourly mean systolic blood pressures in the morning and night shift at hourly increasing phase shifts.

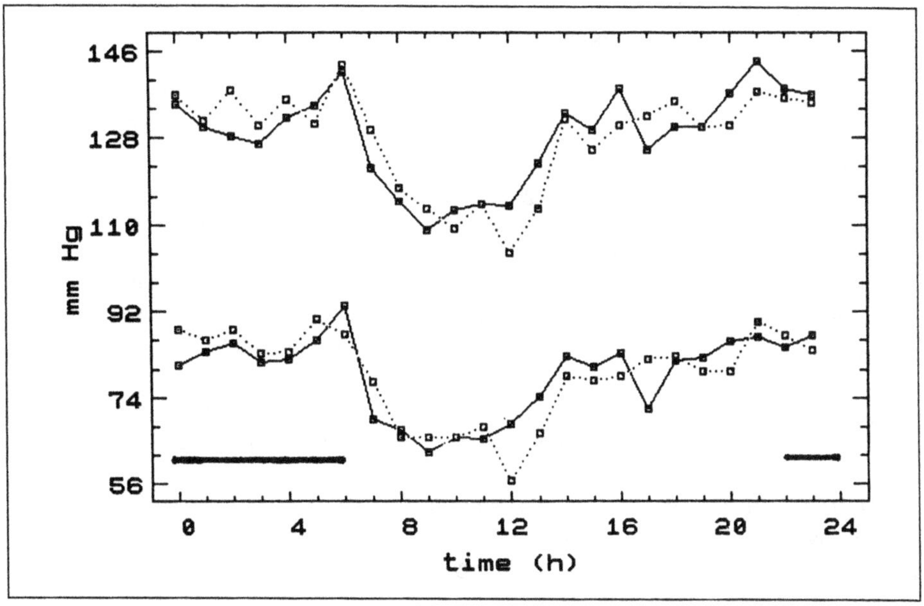

Fig. 4. Systolic and diastolic blood pressures (hourly group averages) of shift workers in the first (. . .) and last (—) day of a night shift week (N = 5).
Straight line indicates working time.

the heart rates was comparably close (r = 0.82). Hence the adaptation of the 24-h blood pressure and heart rate profiles after rotation to the night shift were immediately developed by full extent.

None of the 15 subjects had noted substantial impairments of work by the blood pressure recorders. Four noted slight impairment of sleep (grade 1 on a scale of 0—3), however the durations of the sleeping periods were judged "as usual" by every worker. According to the questionnaire, the quality of sleep between the two shifts did not differ, the sleeping periods lastet 78 h 30 min + 75 min (mean+sd) in the morning shift and 7 h + 75 min in the night shift.

Conclusion

The results indicate that the 24-h blood pressure profile is largely independent of internal time triggers and is mainly determined by external time triggers.

Contrasting to other bioparameters such as body temperature [14], secretion of growth hormone [8] and urinary electrolyte excretion [21, 25], the blood pressure and heart rate are immediately adapted after reversed sleeping and working phases by shift rotation.

In various pathologic conditions like preeclampsia [23], autonomic failure [18], and Cushing's syndrome [13], the nocturnal blood pressure reductions were found to be attenuated or abolished. This suggested that activities and sleep do not necessarily induce a day and night rhythm of the blood pressure.

There are reports on a regular blood pressure increase during the early morning before arousal [20, 24] indicating that blood pressure variations are independent of activities. In contrast, other investigators assumed that the diurnal variations of the blood pressure in essential hypertension and in healthy normotensive subjects were mainly due to activities and sleep [2, 9, 16]. Mancia et al. concluded against an internal rhythm shaping the 24-h blood pressure curve, since they found no blood pressure increase before arousal [17]. The variability of the blood pressure at various activities were investigated in regular sleeping and waking schedules sleeping in the night) [5]; the blood pressure fluctuated parallel to the activities during the waking phases. This led to the conclusion that there is no substantial internal rhythm of the blood pressure. Our direct comparisons of shifted sleep and activity phases have now clearly indicated that this assumption is correct.

The mean 24-h blood pressures and the ranges of the diurnal variations were equal in the morning and night shifts. The only major alteration of the 24-h blood pressure curve was a phase shift. This phase difference exactly reflects the lag between the periods of work (8 h). Contrasting reports on attenuation of the diurnal blood pressure variability after shift rotation were based on single blood pressure measurements in long intervals [6].

The effects of shift rotation on the 24-h blood pressure curve are fully developed within the first day and there is no important blood pressure rhythm with a longer period (> 24-h). This can be concluded from the equality of the 24-h blood pressure profiles during the first and last day of the night-shift week.

The alteration of the 24-h heart rate profile occurred as rapidly as those of the blood pressure. Thus, there is no substantial interference with an internal rhythm of the heart rate at a period exceeding 24-h.

The diurnal blood pressure fluctuation in patients dependent on cardiac pacemakers with fixed heart rate are blunted, but preserved [7]. Hence heart rate fluctuations cannot be the only determinants of the blood pressure variations. It can be concluded that in the present study the heart rate curve was shaped by external time triggers parallel to the blood pressure curve.

It is controversely discussed, whether shift work with rotated day and night shifts causes elevated prevalence of hypertension or other arteriosclerotic risk factors [10—12, 15, 19, 22]. Up to now, there are no longitudinal studies on hypertension development in slowly rotated shift systems. In the day and night shifts the mean 24-h blood pressures as the 24-h peak pressures were equal in this study. Thus there is no short-term blood pressure elevation by shift rotation.

References

1. Baumgart P, Dorst K, Walger P, Vetter H (1987) Ambulantes Langzeit-Blutdruckmonitoring: Vergleich des neuen SL 90202 mit bisherigen Meßsystemen. Hochdruck 7: 53—54
2. Bevan AT, Honour AJ, Stott FH (1969) Direct arterial pressure recording in unrestricted man. Clin Sci 36: 329—344
3. Bicakova-Rocher A, Gorceix A, Reinberg A (1981) Possible circadian rhythm alterations in certain healthy human adults (effects of placebo). In: Reinberg A, Vieux N, Andlauer P (eds) Night and shift work — biological and social aspects Pergamon press Oxford New York Toronto Sydney Paris Frankfurt pp 297—310
4. Bolm-Audorff U, Schreml N, Ehlenz K, Knecht U, Hahne H, Woitowitz HJ (1985) Belastung und Beanspruchung von Rettungssanitätern. Verh Dt Ges Arb Med 25: 395—400

5. Clark LA, Denby L, Pregibon D, Harshfield GA, Pickering TG, Blank S, Laragh JH (1987) A quantitative analysis of the effects of activity and time of day on the diurnal variations of blood pressure. J Chron Dis 40: 671—681
6. Costa G, Gaffuri E, Perfranceschi G, Tansella M (1979) Reentrainment of diurnal variation and psychological and physiological performance at the end of a slowly rotated shift system in hospital workers. Int Arch Occup Health 44: 165—175
7. Davies AB, Gould BA, Cashman PMM, Raftery EB (1984) Circadian rhythm of blood pressure in patients dependent on ventricular demand pacemakers. Br Heart J 52: 93—98
8. Desir D, Van Cauter E, Golstein J, Fevre M, Jadot C, Refetoff S, Copinschi G (1981) Adaption of the nyctohemeral variations of pituitary and related hormones after transmeridian transportation in normal man. In: Reinberg A, Vieux N, Andlauer P (eds) Night and shift work — biological and social aspects Pergamon Press Oxford New York Toronto Sydney Paris Frankfurt p 365
9. Floras JS, Jones JV, Johnston JA, Brooks DE, Hassan MO, Sleight P (1978) Arousal and the circadian rhythm of blood pressure. Clin Sci Mol Med 55: 395 s—397 s
10. Fouriaud C, Jaquinet-Salord MC, Degoulet P, Aime F, Lang T, Laprugne J, Main J, Oeconomos J, Phalente J, Prades A (1984) Influence of socioprofessional conditions on blood pressure levels and hypertension control. Am J Epidemiol 120: 72—86
11. Harrington JM (1978) Shift work and health. A critical review or the literature. Her Majesty's Stationary Office, London
12. Helmert U, Groetschel R, Herman B, Klesse R, Greiser E (1986) Risikofaktoren für koronare Herzkrankheiten bei männlichen Betriebsangehörigen — Ergebnisse von Screening-Untersuchungen in zwei norddeutschen Großbetrieben. Öff. Gesundh-Wes 48: 249—254
13. Imai Y, Abe K, Sasaki S, Minami N, Nihei M, Munakata M, Murakami O, Matsue K, Sekino H, Miura Y, Yoshinaga K (1988) Altered circadian blood pressure rhythm in patients with Cushing's syndrome. Hypertension 12: 11—19
14. Knauth P, Emde E, Ruthenfranz J, Kiesswetter E, Smith P (1981) Re-entrainment of body temperature in field studies of shiftwork. Int Arch Occup Environ Health 49: 137—149
15. Kornhuber HH, Lisson G (1981) Bluthochdruck — sind Industrie-Stressoren, Lärm oder Akkordarbeit wichtige Ursachen? Dtsch Med Wschr 106: 1733—1736
16. Littler WA (1979) Sleep and blood pressure: Further observations. Am Heart J 97: 35—38
17. Mancia G, Ferrari A, Gregorini L, Parati G, Pomidossi G, Bertinieri G, Grassi G, di Rienzo M, Pedotti A, Zanchetti A (1983) Blood pressure and heart rate variabilities in normotensive and hypertensive human beings. Circ Res 53: 96—104
18. Mann S, Altman DG, Raftery EB, Bannister R (1983) Circadian variation of blood pressure in autonomic failure. Circulation 68: 477—483
19. Michel-Briand C, Chopard J L, Guiot A, Paulmier M, Studer G (1981) The pathological consequences of shift work in retired workers. In: Reinberg A, Vieux N, Andlauer P (eds) Night and shift work — biological and social aspects Pergamon Press Oxford New York Toronto Sydney Paris Frankfurt pp 399—407
20. Millar-Craig MW, Bishop CN, Raftery EB (1978) Circadian variations in blood pressure. Lancet 1: 795—797
21. Minors DS, Waterhouse JM (1981) Endogenous rhythms during anchor sleep experiments. In: Reinberg A, Vieux N, Andlauer P (eds) Night and shift work — biological and social aspects Pergamon Press Oxford New York Toronto Sydney Paris Frankfurt pp 169—170
22. Piorkowski P, Günther KH, Harig H, Wandreg W, Braun H (1982) Risikofaktoren des Herzinfarktes und soziale Parameter — Studie Cottbus. Dt Gesundh-Wes 37: 1680—1682
23. Redman CWG, Beilin LJ, Bonnar J (1976) Reversed diurnal blood pressure rhythm in hypertensive pregnancies. Clin Sci Mol Med 51: 687 s—689 s
24. Rowlands DB, Stallard TJ, Watson RDS, Littler WA (1980) The influence of physical activity on arterial pressure during ambulatoriy recording in man. Clin Sci 58: 115—117
25. Vokac Z, Gundersen N, Magnus P, Jebens E, Bakka T (1981) Circadian rhythm of urinary excretion of mercury. In: Reinberg A, Vieux N, Andlauer P (eds) Night and shift work — biological and social aspects Pergamon Press Oxford New York Toronto Sydney Paris Frankfurt pp 425—431

Blood pressure in normal subjects

M. A. Weber and J. I. M. Drayer.

Hypertension Center, Veterans Administration Medical Center, Long Beach, California and the University of California, Irvine, California, USA

Introduction

There is no clear separation between normal blood pressure and hypertension. Actuarial data have shown a continuous relationship between blood pressure and the probability of major cardiovascular events, but there is no agreement concerning the level of blood pressure at which a diagnosis of hypertension should be made. It is possible to suggest a functional definition of hypertension as being the lowest level of blood pressure at which therapeutic intervention could be predicted to lessen the likelihood of cardiovascular complications. In the United States, the Joint National Committee on the Detection, Evaluation and Treatment of High Blood Pressure [1] has recommended that conventionally-measured office or clinic diastolic blood pressures of 84 mmHg or less be considered normal; that 85—89 mmHg be considered high-normal; and that levels of 90 mmHg or above define a hypertensive range that may justify treatment.

Whole-day blood pressure monitoring and normalcy

Because the whole-day measurement of blood pressure using automated non-invasive portable equipment is still a new technique, it has not yet been possible to establish data linking this type of measurement to cardiovascular outcomes. Moreover, since whole-day monitoring procedures are obviously more inconvenient and expensive to perform than conventional blood pressure measurements, it is likely that we will never develop the same depth of epidemiologic experience with this newer technique as with the conventional methods. Only one study has attempted to link whole-day repetitive blood pressure measurements with cardiovascular prognosis [2], and even this study depended primarily on differences between the clinic and the long-term blood pressure values rather than on the actual blood pressure measurements.

Probably the simplest way of defining normal blood pressure during 24-hour monitoring is to extrapolate from the data already arbitrarily suggested for conventional blood pressure readings [1]. For example, it has been shown that the average of the whole-day blood pressure (mean of all readings obtained during a 24-hour period) typically is approximately 5 mmHg lower than the corresponding conventional office reading obtained during the same day [3]. Thus, based on the recommendations of the Joint National Committee described above [1], a whole-day diastolic blood pressure average of 79 mmHg or below would be considered normal; 80—84 mmHg would be high normal; and values of 85 mmHg or above would be regarded as hypertensive. From a practical point of view, this simple approach at present probably provides the best basis for the diagnostic use of whole-day blood pressure monitoring techniques. Admittedly, this method fails to take into account potentially important information that could be obtained from analysis of the patterns of blood pressure throughout the day, but as yet there are insufficient data to provide a basis for this type of approach.

Theoretically, the best definitions of normalcy and hypertension based on whole-day blood pressure monitoring would be to establish relationships between the blood pressure and the status of underlying target organs of hypertension such as the heart. It has already been shown that whole-day blood pressure monitoring correlates more strongly with echocardiographically measured left ventricular muscle mass than do conventional blood pressure readings [4, 5]. Moreover, we have previously shown that this relationship appears strongest in the normal to mildly hypertensive range of blood pressure [6], a finding that tends to emphasize the potential sensitivity of whole-day monitoring in discriminating evidence for left ventricular hypertrophy or other cardiac consequences of early hypertension.

Most of the information concerning normal blood pressure patterns with whole-day monitoring has come from studies of subjects designated as normal by conventional office blood pressure measurements. Because of the potential inaccuracies of this method of measuring blood pressure, it is possible that some of the data concerning normalcy during whole-day monitoring may be partly based on patients whose blood pressures may not have been truly "normal". However, these findings are sufficiently different from those found in hypertensive patients to justify their use as a basis for considering the characteristics of the normal whole-day blood pressure.

The circadian pattern

As shown in Figs. 1 and 2, blood pressure in normal individuals follows a clear circadian pattern; during the daytime hours, from approximately 0800 to 1800 hours, the blood pressure is mainly at a plateau although there are modest elevations at the beginning and end of this period. Thereafter, blood pressure falls steadily to a nadir at midnight or soon afterwards, and then prior to arousal from sleep it rises again in a fairly sharp fashion until it regains the higher daytime levels. A comparison between age-matched normotensive and hypertensive men is shown in Fig. 1 [7]. It is evident that the circadian pattern is similar for both the hypertensive and normotensive individuals; there is a slight tendency for the blood pressures amplitude (difference between the highest and lowest periods of the day) to be slightly greater in the normals than in the hypertensives, but this is not significant.

A key issue in evaluating whole-day blood pressure monitoring in normals is to determine its reproducibility. The data shown in Fig. 2 summarize values in 56 normal volunteers, each of whom was subjected to whole-day ambulatory blood pressure monitoring on two separate occasions, approximately 6 weeks apart, while following their normal routines at work and domestically [8]. It is clear that the blood pressure patterns (based on the averages during each of the 12 two-hours periods constituting the whole day) were similar during the two separate 24-h periods of monitoring. But if the patients were considered individually rather than as a group as a whole, it was found that the average systolic blood pressure for the full day was at least 10 mmHg different during the two days of monitoring in about 20% of subjects, and the diastolic blood pressure averages were at least 5 mmHg different in approximately 35% of subjects [9]. The

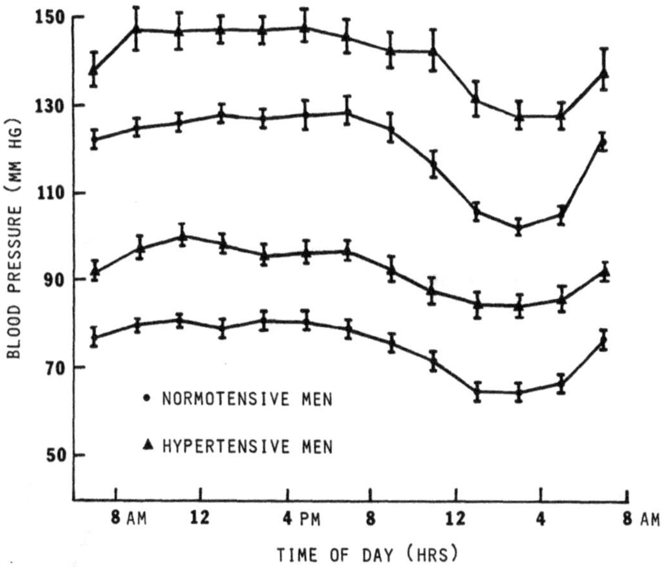

Fig. 1. Average systolic and diastolic blood pressure values of 29 age-matched normotensive-hypertensive pairs of men during whole-day ambulatory blood pressure monitoring. Points shown are the means (± SD) of the readings obtained during each of 12 2-h periods comprising the day.

reason for this inconsistent reproducibility in some individuals cannot readily be explained, and underscores a fundamental question in ambulatory blood pressure monitoring: Are differences in blood pressures between 2 separate monitoring days due to intrinsic variations in the blood pressures, or does it simply reflect the possibility that subjects were undertaking different types of activity during the 2 days? Unfortunately, there have been insufficient studies carried out in patients under controlled conditions and environments to allow this important question to be answered. It is evident, however, that whole-day blood pressure values within individual patients are more reproducible than conventional single measurements.

Beyond the question of the blood pressure averages, it is important to note that the circadian pattern itself is reproducible. Thus, if instead of using actual blood pressure values during each of the 12, 2-h periods of the day, we substitute their rank values (that is, we assign each of the 2-h periods during the day a value of from 1 to 12 based on its blood pressure value relative to the other periods) we find that the patterns for two separate days of monitoring in normal subjects are virtually identical (Fig. 3) [9]. Moreover, we have found that the amplitude (the difference between the blood pressure during the highest and lowest 2-h periods) of the blood pressure during the two separate days of monitoring in the normal subjects is closely reproducible [10]. Amplitude is a simple expression of the overall blood pressure variability during the day, and future studies may show it to be an important determinant of normal and hypertensive whole-day blood pressure characteristics. It is also possible that the blood pressure amplitude, independently of the actual levels of blood pressure, may be linked to cardiovascular prognosis. We have noted that the amplitude for the whole day correlates with the

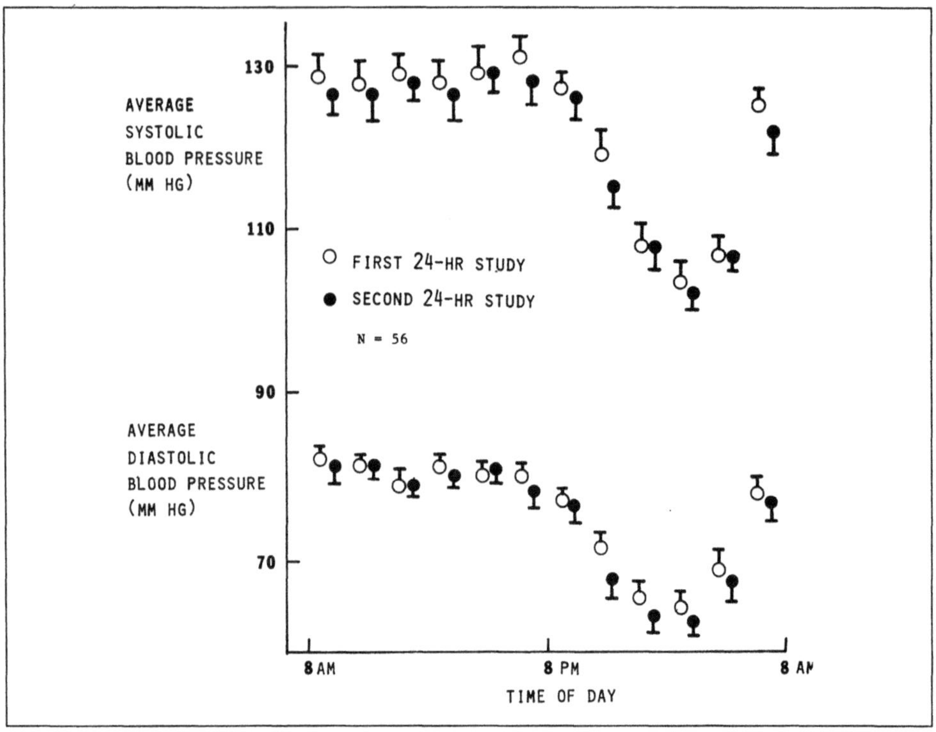

Fig. 2. Average systolic and diastolic blood pressure values of 56 normotensive subjects during 2 separate days (approximately 6 weeks apart) of whole-day ambulatory blood pressure monitoring. Points shown are the means (± SD) of the readings obtained during each of 12, 2-h periods comprising the day.

standard deviation (as an index of variability) of the mean of the blood pressure values obtained throughout the day by automated monitoring [10]. Additionally, we have noted that in normal subjects the amplitude of the systolic blood pressure appears to be dependent primarily on the height to which the systolic blood pressure rises during the daytime hours, whereas the amplitude of the diastolic blood pressure appears more dependent upon the nadir values of blood pressure observed during the night [10]. This suggests that differing factors may mediate the systolic and diastolic blood pressure patterns and may provide a future basis for characterizing blood pressure and hypertension.

Normal blood pressure and hypertension

One of the main arguments used to support ambulatory blood pressure monitoring is that conventional blood pressures measured in the office or clinic may be falsely high owing to a so-called "white coat effect" [11]. Thus, it has been assumed that blood pressures measured throughout the day would average less than the values obtained in the office. But this may not be true for all individuals [3, 12]. A comparison between office blood pressures and whole-day averages are shown in Fig. 4 for both hypertensive

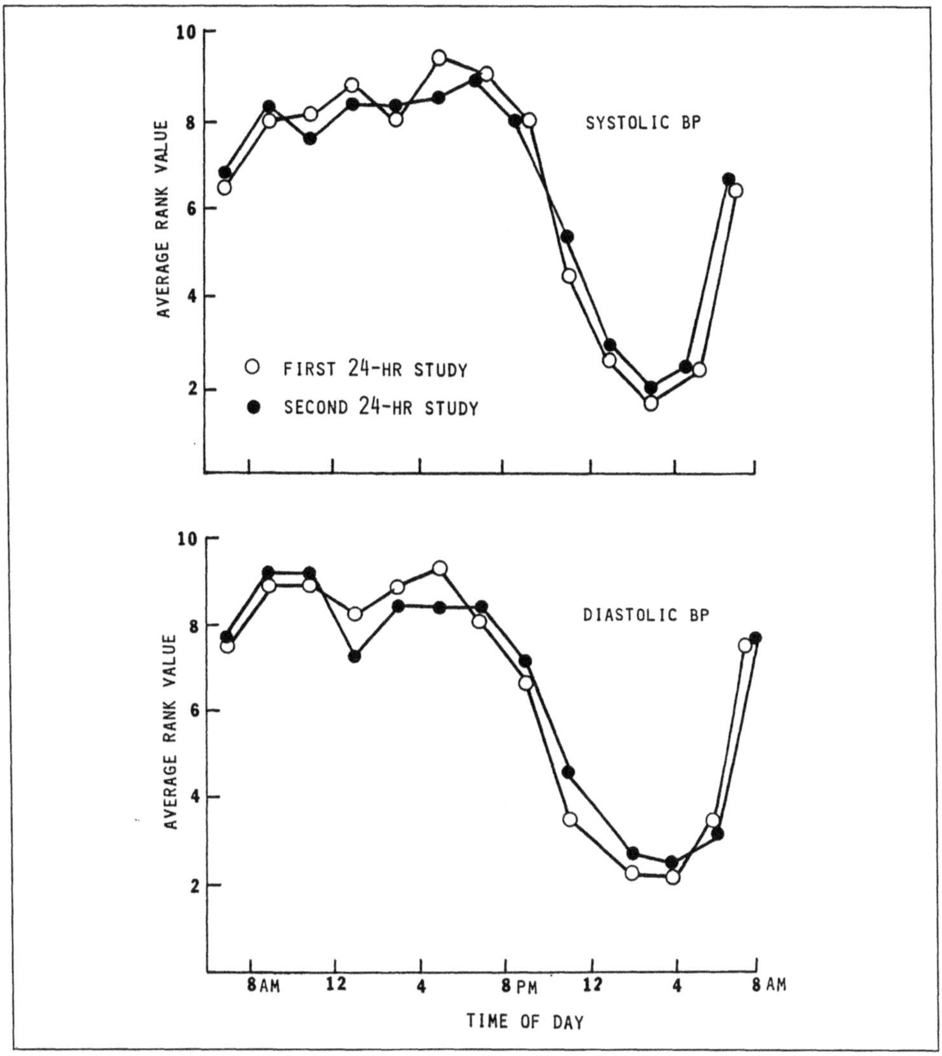

Fig. 3. Average rank values (as defined in the text) in 33 normal volunteers during 2 separate days of ambulatory blood pressure monitoring.

patients (diagnosed previously by conventional means) and normal subjects (confirmed by repeated conventional measurements). It is evident that for many individuals, either hypertensive or normal, their differences are beneath the "zero" line, indicating that their whole-day blood pressure averages actually are lower than their office measurements. But there are a number of exceptions, both among the hypertensives and the normals, suggesting that conventional blood pressure measurements may provide readings that are misleadingly low. This has already been shown to have prognostic importance for hypertensive patients, for it has been found that those individuals whose whole-day averages are actually higher than their clinic values are more likely to

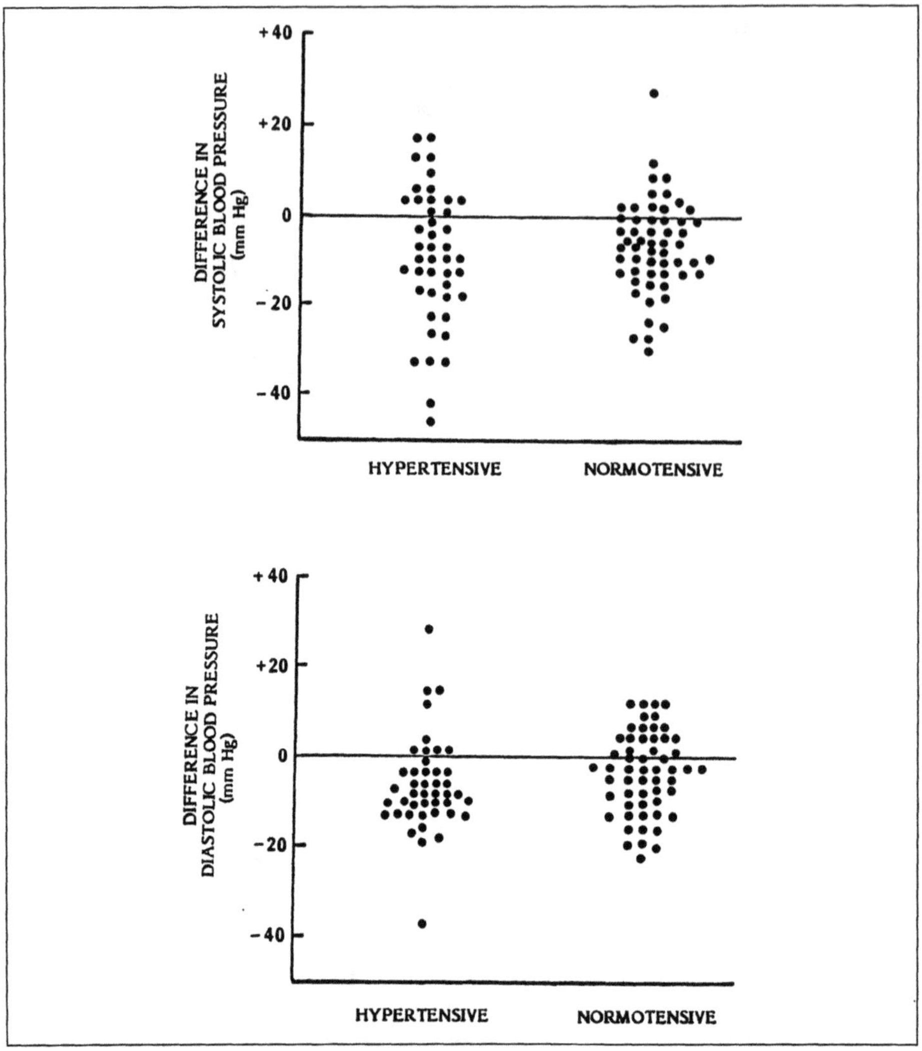

Fig. 4. Differences in hypertensive and normotensive patients between conventionally measured office blood pressures and whole-day blood pressure averages. Individuals shown above the zero line are those whose whole-day averages were higher than the office measurements.

experience serious cardiovascular complications than those whose blood pressure averages are lower than their clinic readings [2]. This finding may also have implications for those subjects who appear to have normal blood pressures when checked by standard methods in the office. As indicated by Fig. 4, almost 20% of such persons appear to have clearly higher diastolic blood pressures during the rest of the day and may even be hypertensive and vulnerable to a heightened cardiovascular risk. This raises the possibility that whole-day blood pressure monitoring may not only be a useful tool for determining which apparently hypertensive patients may really be normal, but also for deciding which patients who appear to be normal during office visits may actually be hypertensive and possibly in need of additional observation.

The influence of age

Cross-sectional studies of populations have shown that blood pressure tends to increase with age. This is especially so for systolic blood pressure, and results in a gradual widening of the pulse pressure as individuals become more elderly. There has been a growing interest in systolic hypertension of the elderly, especially as it is now recognized as a major risk factor for cardiovascular complications. In studies with whole-day blood pressure monitoring in elderly hypertensive patients, we have found that systolic blood pressure is consistenly higher than in younger hypertensive patients, and that diastolic blood pressures on average are lower [13]. Importantly, it has also been noted that the variability of systolic blood pressure is greater than that for diastolic blood pressure within older patients, and is significantly greater than the variability of systolic blood pressure in younger hypertensive patients. Unfortunately, similar data within a normotensive group of subjects are not available. It is likely that variability of systolic blood pressure in all older people is higher than in younger individuals, but this has not yet been established. Moreover, there is as yet no agreement as to the level of systolic blood pressure that separates normal subjects from those with hypertension, making it difficult to characterize normalcy of the whole-day blood pressure in older individuals.

The studies of the neuroendocrine profile of elderly individuals has shown that there is very little difference between normal subjects and hypertensives [14]. Although both groups of individuals had similar circadian patterns of blood pressure, the normotensive participants actually had higher levels of plasma norepinephrine concentrations throughout the day. Of interest, the usual nighttime decrease in plasma norepinephrine concentration which has been thought to explain the nocturnal decrease in blood pressure did not occur in either of the elderly groups, suggesting that factors other than the sympathetic nervous system may be important in determining the circadian patterns of blood pressure in elderly individuals. Similarly, the circadian patterns of plasma renin activity in elderly normotensive and hypertensive individuals were blunted.

Some studies in hypertensive elderly individuals have suggested further approaches that might be required in studying normal volunteers. For example, it has been noted that whereas approximately two-thirds of elderly hypertensive patients exhibit the usual nocturnal decreases in blood pressure, others maintain their high levels of blood pressure consistently throughout the 24-h period [15]. This may have cardiovascular prognostic significance, for it was found that the incidence of complications was significantly higher in those patients who fail to exhibit the nocturnal fall in blood pressure. Whether this differential pattern is a result of ongoing hypertension and its cardiovascular sequelae, or whether such differences in the blood pressure pattern may be of predictive value in normal subjects or those with minimally increased blood pressures, remains to be determined.

A collaborative study has attempted to characterize patterns of blood pressure in almost 200 normal volunteers subdivided into differing age groups [16]. Unfortunately, this study used the same entry criteria (systolic blood pressure less than 140 mmHg) for elderly participants as for the young, thereby making it difficult to evaluate potentially unique properties of the systolic blood pressure in the elderly. Nevertheless, it was noted that the increase in diastolic blood pressure during the hours of work was significantly greater in older than in younger individuals, even though both groups had similar resting blood pressures. There was also a tendency in the study for the variability of blood pressure throughout the day to be somewhat greater in older individuals.

Family history

Although hypertension, based on conventional blood pressure measurements, tends to aggregate in families, its mode of inheritance is poorly defined. The technique of ambulatory blood pressure monitoring may be of value in better defining familial characteristics of blood pressure. In studies of normotensive twins, using both multiple conventional measurements over periods of 3—4 weeks, as well as whole-day blood pressure monitoring, it has been found that both the absolute levels of blood pressure and indices of lability tend to be similar among co-twins [17]. These data thus support the likelihood that blood pressure characteristics are determined, at least in part, by genetic factors. Interestingly, the same study indicated that a family history of hypertension may also be suggested by the blood pressure monitoring technique, for it was noted that individuals with such a family history tended to have an increased lability of blood pressure (as indicated by whole-day blood pressure monitoring) even though their overall blood pressure averages were within the normal range. Similar findings were obtained in our own evaluation of 33 normal subjects [18]. Although the conventionally-measured blood pressures in 14 individuals with a family history of hypertension were similar to those in the 19 participants without a family history, systolic blood pressure values during ambulatory blood pressure monitoring were significantly higher both during daytime and nighttime in the individuals with a positive family history of hypertension.

Conclusion

There have been comparatively few studies of normotensive subjects using automated non-invasive portable equipment for the whole-day monitoring of blood pressure. It has not yet been possible to establish firm criteria for differentiating normal from hypertensive values, especially as the association between whole-day blood pressure values and evidence for cardiovascular complications is still awaiting definition. Preliminary studies have shown that the circadian patterns of blood pressure in normal subjects and hypertensive patients are parallel to each other, suggesting that in general the blood pressure difference between normals and hypertensives is quantitative rather than qualitative. It has also been demonstrated that the circadian patterns of blood pressure in normotensive subjects are reproducible. Blood pressure monitoring for 24 h appears to be of value in evaluating whether patients with conventionally-diagnosed hypertension truly have this condition; but it is also of interest to note that some individuals whose office blood pressure measurements appear normal may be found to be hypertensive when studied for the day as a whole. Monitoring in older hypertensive patients has shown variable patterns of blood pressure, especially at night, and has also revealed an increased lability of systolic blood pressure values. Further studies to better differentiate normal from hypertensive whole-day blood pressure patterns, especially in the elderly, might be of considerable practical value in identifying those patients who might best benefit from treatment.

References

1. The 1984 Report of the Joint National Committee on Detection, Evaluation and Treatment of High Blood Pressure: Arch Intern Med 144: 1045—1057
2. Devereux RB, Pickering TG, Harshfield GA, Kleinert HD, Denby L, Clark L, Pregibon D, Jason M, Kleiner B, Borer JS, Laragh JH (1983) Left ventricular hypertrophy in patients with hypertension: importance of blood pressure response to regularly recurring stress. Circulation 68: 470—476
3. Drayer JIM, Weber MA, De Young JL, Wyle FA (1982) Circadian blood pressure patterns in ambulatory hypertensive patients: Effects of age. Am J Med 73: 493—499
4. Drayer JIM, Weber MA, De Young JL (1983) Blood pressure as a determinant of cardiac left ventricular muscle mass. Arch Intern Med 143: 90—92
5. Drayer JIM, Weber MA, Hoeger WJ (1985) Whole-day blood pressure monitoring in ambulatory normotensive men. Arch Intern Med 145: 271—274
6. Drayer JIM, Weber MA, Nakamura DK (1985) Automated ambulatory blood pressure monitoring: A study in age-matched normotensive and hypertensive men. Am Heart J 109: 1334
7. Drayer JIM, Gardin JM, Brewer DD, Weber MA (1987) Disparate relationships between blood pressure and LV mass in patients with and without LVH. Hypertension 9 (Suppl 2) 61—64
8. Kobrin I, Dunn FG, Oigman W, Kumar A, Ventura HO, Messerli FH, Frohlich ED (1984) Essential hypertension in the elderly: circadian variation of arterial pressure. In: Weber MA, Drayer JIM (eds) Ambulatory Blood Pressure Monitoring. Steinkopff, Darmstadt, pp 181—185
9. Mancia G, Bertinieri G, Grassi G (1983) Effects of blood pressure measurement by the doctor on patient's blood pressure and heart rate. Lancet 2: 295—697
10. Perloff D, Sokolow M, Cowan R (1983) The prognostic value of ambulatory blood pressure. J Am Med Ass 249: 2793—2798
11. Rose RJ (1984) Familial influences on ambulatory blood pressure: studies of normotensive twins. In: Weber MA, Drayer JIM (eds) Ambulatory Blood Pressure Monitoring. Steinkopff, Darmstadt, pp 167—172
12. Stern N, Beahm E, Sowers J, McGinty D, Eggena P, Littner M, Nyby M, Catania R (1984) The effect of age on circadian rhythm of blood pressure, catecholamines, plasma renin activity, prolactin and corticosteroids in essential hypertension. In: Weber MA, Drayer JIM (eds) Ambulatory Blood Pressure Monitoring. pp 157—162
13. Waeber B, Jacot des Combes B, Porchet M, Brunner AR (1984) Accuracy, reproducibility and usefulness of ambulatory blood pressure recording obtained with the Remler system. In: Weber MA, Drayer JIM (eds) Ambulatory Blood Pressure Monitoring. pp 65—69
14. Wallace JM, Thornton WE, Kennedy HL, Pickering TG, Harshfield GA, Frohlich ED, Messerli FH, Gifford RW, Bolen K (1984) Ambulatory blood pressure in 199 normal subjects, a collaborative study. In: Weber MA, Drayer JIM (eds) Abmulatory Blood Pressure Monitoring. Steinkopff, Darmstadt, pp 117—127
15. Weber MA, Drayer JIM, Nakamura DK, Wyle FA (1984) The circadian blood pressure pattern in ambulatory normal subjects. Am J Cardiol 54: 115—119
16. Weber MA, Drayer JIM, Chard ER (1984) Blood pressure fluctuation and amplitude in normal human subjects. In: Weber MA, Drayer JIM (eds) Ambulatory Blood Pressure Monitoring. Steinkopff, Darmstadt, pp 43—50
17 Weber MA, Drayer JIM (1986) Role of blood pressure monitoring in the diagnosis of hypertension. J Hypertension 4 (Suppl 5) S 325—S 327
18. Weber MA, Drayer JIM, Brewer DD. Repetitive blood pressure measurements: clinical issues, techniques, and data analysis. In: Scheving LE, Halberg F, Ehret CF (eds) Chronobiotechnology and Chronobiological Engineering. Martinus Nijhoff, Netherlands (in press)

Casual readings, self-measurements, and indirect 24-hour profile of blood pressure in the assessment of an antihypertensive combination therapy. Results of a multicenter trial.

W. Meyer-Sabellek[1], R. Gotzen[1], K.-L. Schulte[1], B. Streitberg2

[1] Medizinische Klinik und Poliklinik, Klinikum Steglitz, Freie Universität Berlin, Berlin, FRG

[2] Institut für Statistik, Universität Hamburg, Hamburg, FRG

Introduction

Since the classic study of Ayman and Goldshine [2], it has been recognized that the casual measurement represents a single measurement of blood pressure that reflects this constantly changing parameter to only a limited degree. Frequently altering conditions, especially the presence of a physician or nurse [9], lead to only limited reproducibility [1] of the casual blood pressure measurement, which nevertheless routinely enters into the establishment of the diagnosis and the decision for therapy and has been accepted and recommended by the World Health Organization (WHO) [21]. Apart from repeated measurements, home blood pressure measurement by the patients is particularly considered [8, 13] in order to obtain everyday representative blood pressure values. Continuous invasive intraarterial [10, 12] long-term techniques for blood pressure measurement, particularly the discontinuously measuring noninvasive procedures recently developed, now make it possible for us to analyze the blood pressure variability and the intraindividual circadian blood pressure technique in hypertensive ambulant patients under placebo [7], as well as under conventional [5] and new [15] antihypertensive therapy.

Saluretics form the basis of practically any combination therapy and rank first in the graded therapy regimen of the German League for the Control of High Blood Pressure. The fixed combination of various antihypertensively active substances are discussed controversially. Thus, by exerting an additive antihypertensive influence, a common two-drug combination [saluretic and β-blocker] leads to a reduction of tablets and of possible subjective or metabolic side effects. While the effect of β-receptor-blockers and diuretics on resting blood pressure is equally strong on adequate dosage [4], the blood pressure in a lying or sitting position is reduced on the average by about 20 to 30 mmHg systolically, and about 10 to 15 mmHg diastolically, but the exclusive application of diuretics, in contrast to β-receptor-blockers, does not appear to clearly influence the stress-induced increase of blood pressure [3].

The aim of this outpatient study is to determine whether the effect of drug therapy with a fixed compound preparation can be enhanced by concomitant measures such as repeated supervision of home blood pressure measurement with intensive instruction and dietetic guidance. A comparative examination was done of the patient's home blood pressure measurement, a standardized casual blood pressure measurement by the attending physician and the 24-h blood pressure profile recorded on an outpatient basis.

Patients and methods

A multicenter test series is presently being performed in cooperation with 20 offices of internists and general practitioners in Berlin to examine the antihypertensive effect of a fixed combination therapy with the approved compound preparation Pertenso (one tablet contains 10 mg of bemetizide, 20 mg of triamterene, 20 mg of bupranolol and 20 mg of dihydralazine: Melusin Schwarz, Monheim, FRG.) in 120 patients. We present here the results of a preliminary evaluation. The study design is shown in Fig. 1. The results obtained in 69 hypertensive patients (diastolic value ≧ 95 and ≦ 120 mmHg corresponding to WHO I—II, mean value of three measurements at two different times), 39 women and 30 men (mean age 52.5 ± 12.1 [SD] years), were evaluated after inclusion in the study.

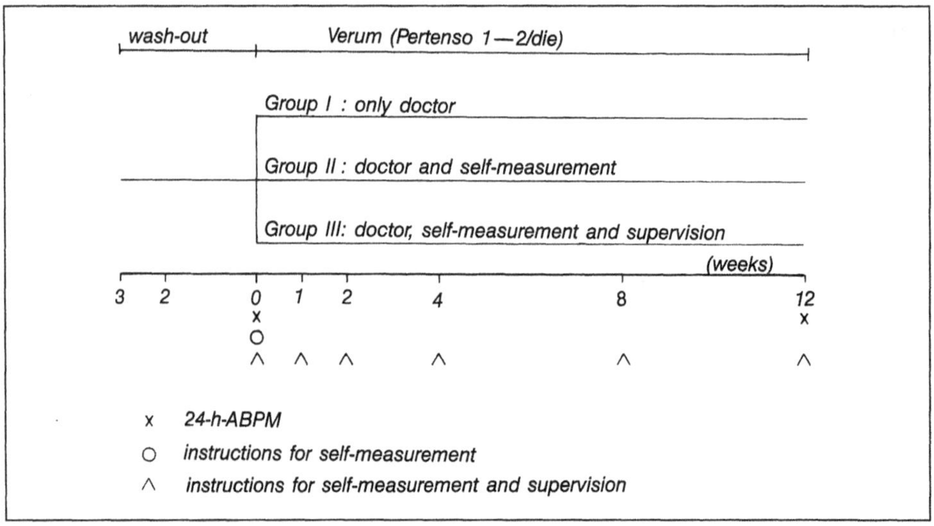

Fig. 1

Exclusion criteria:

— patient < 18 years of age
— patients with home blood pressure measurement
— hypochondria or neurosis
— impaired hearing
— cerebral sclerosis
— time after myocardial infarction ≦ 6 months
— circumference of upper arm > 40 cm

Further exclusion criteria based on the components of the preparation:
— secondary hypertension
— decompensated cardiac insufficiency

— AV-block II—III
— bradycardia 55 min$^{(-1)}$
— renal insufficiency (serum creatinine ≧ 1.8 mg%)
— chronic liver diseases
— alcohol or drug abuse
— obstructive lung disease
— pregnancy and nursing period

The target blood pressure was set at a diastolic value of ≧ 90 mmHg in a sitting position or a reduction of the diastolic value by at least 10 mmHg.
A one-week recruiting phase (see Fig. 1) was followed by a 2-week washout phase, if necessary, and then a 12-week treatment phase with the fixed compound preparation. For the treatment phase patients were assigned to three groups in a randomized manner:
Group I — conventional blood pressure measurement in the physician's practice;
Group II — as in Group I with home blood pressure measurement (after brief instruction);
Group III — as in Group I with regular home blood pressure measurement after intensive instruction and supervision, as well as dietetic guidance.
The therapeutic decision to change the dosis (doubling) was made after blood pressure measurement by the physician. The results of clinic, home and indirect 24-h long-term blood pressure measurements were assessed in a comparative analysis. It was planned to perform long-term blood pressure recordings with automated, programmable, portable monitors (SpaceLabs 5200 1.2 kg) in all groups before and at the end of the treatment phase. blood pressure was recorded at 15-min intervals during the day (0600—1200 hours), with the measurement being preceded by a signal, and a 30-min intervals at night (2400—0600 hours, without a signal). As a rule, long-term measurement was preceded by a 30-min control phase with measurements at five-min intervals in order to check the position of the cuff and the microphone (point of maximum impulse with Doppler stethoscope). The devices were calibrated via one side of an angle; deviations of ≦ 5 mmHg from a mercury manometer were accepted. A 24-h blood pressure profile was included in the assessment, if systolic and diastolic blood pressures were recorded at > 60% of the predetermined points of measurement. The SpaceLabs 5200 (formerly Squibb Pressuremaster) determines blood pressure by the conventional measuring procedure, i.e., auscultatory registration of Korotkoff's sounds, and additionally by oscillometric registration. This combination ensures a high assessment rate (approx. 91%). This system does not have ECG gating; heart rate is determined by auscultation. There were no significant differences between the randomly formed subgroups with regard to the most important anamnestic and diagnostic parameters. Initial diastolic blood pressure levels were likewise comparable between the groups, so that randomization can be regarded as successful.
The preliminary evaluation of our study allows only descriptive statistics. Differences in blood pressure changes between the individual groups were compared using the Mann-Wihtney test. The results obtained are preliminary ones intended to show tendencies only. Changes compared to the initial values within the groups were assessed by means of the Wilcoxon sign rank test. The asymptomatic Wilcoxon test was used for the statistical analysis of circadian blood pressure and heart rate profiles [19].

Results

A significant blood pressure decrease occurred in all patients under Pertenso therapy after single morning application of the drug. Statistic analysis showed no differences in the degree of blood pressure decrease within the randomized groups.
Figure 2 shows that the diastolic and systolic blood pressure at rest measured by the physician after 10 min in a sitting position did not differ within the subgroups.
In the first patient group, in which blood pressure was measured by the physician only, diastolic blood pressure returned to normal levels in 11 of the 15 monitored patients (from a mean of 167/105 to 142/90 mmHg, $p < 0.001$).
In the second patient group, in which the patients measured their own blood pressure without prior intensive instruction, normalization of blood pressure was achieved in 12 of the 18 monitored patients (from a mean of 171/105 to 140/89 mmHg, $p < 0.001$).
In the third patient group, in which the patients measured their own blood pressure after intensive instruction and guidance, blood pressure was normalized in 11 of the 12 continually monitored patients (from a mean of 170/106 to 139/88 mmHg, $p < 0.01$). Comparison of the repetitive blood pressure readings in group III patients shows no significant differences between the values measured by the patient and those measured by the physician. However, comparable measurements were available for only nine of the patients.
Figure 3 shows that mean blood pressure levels determined by the patients of group III (with intensive instruction for home blood pressure measurement) were lower (n. s.) compared to those measured by the physician. While the systolic levels were slightly higher during the inital phase of therapy, diastolic blood pressure determined by the physician was higher.
A statistical difference between the 24-h blood pressure profiles in the group of patients in whom such profiles were obtained could not be calculated because of the low number of cases. This remains to be reassessed after conclusion of the study. A 24-h profile could be evaluatated in a total of 69 patients in whom more than 60% of the predetermined measurement points, i.e., > 70 measurements per 24 h, were registered. A second measurement could not be performed in nine patients.
The antihypertensive effect on the systolic and diastolic 24-h profile led to a significant reduction of the waking and sleeping profiles. The mean blood pressure decrease observed in the entire study population was 13.9/8.3 mmHg (from 130.9/85.5) (SD to 117.0/77.4) during the wake-up phase at 0600 hours and 16.7/9.5 mmHg (from 152.2/99.3 to 135.5/89.8) at 1800 hours. The decrease was significant ($p < 0.001$).
The mean blood pressure value (especially the diastolic value in the evening) of an age-matched normotensive control group was not completely reached (Fig. 4). The blood pressure variation, as measured by standard deviation, remained unchanged under therapy as compared to the treatment-free period.
The heart rate showed a comparable profile and a biphasic course before and during therapy (Fig. 4).

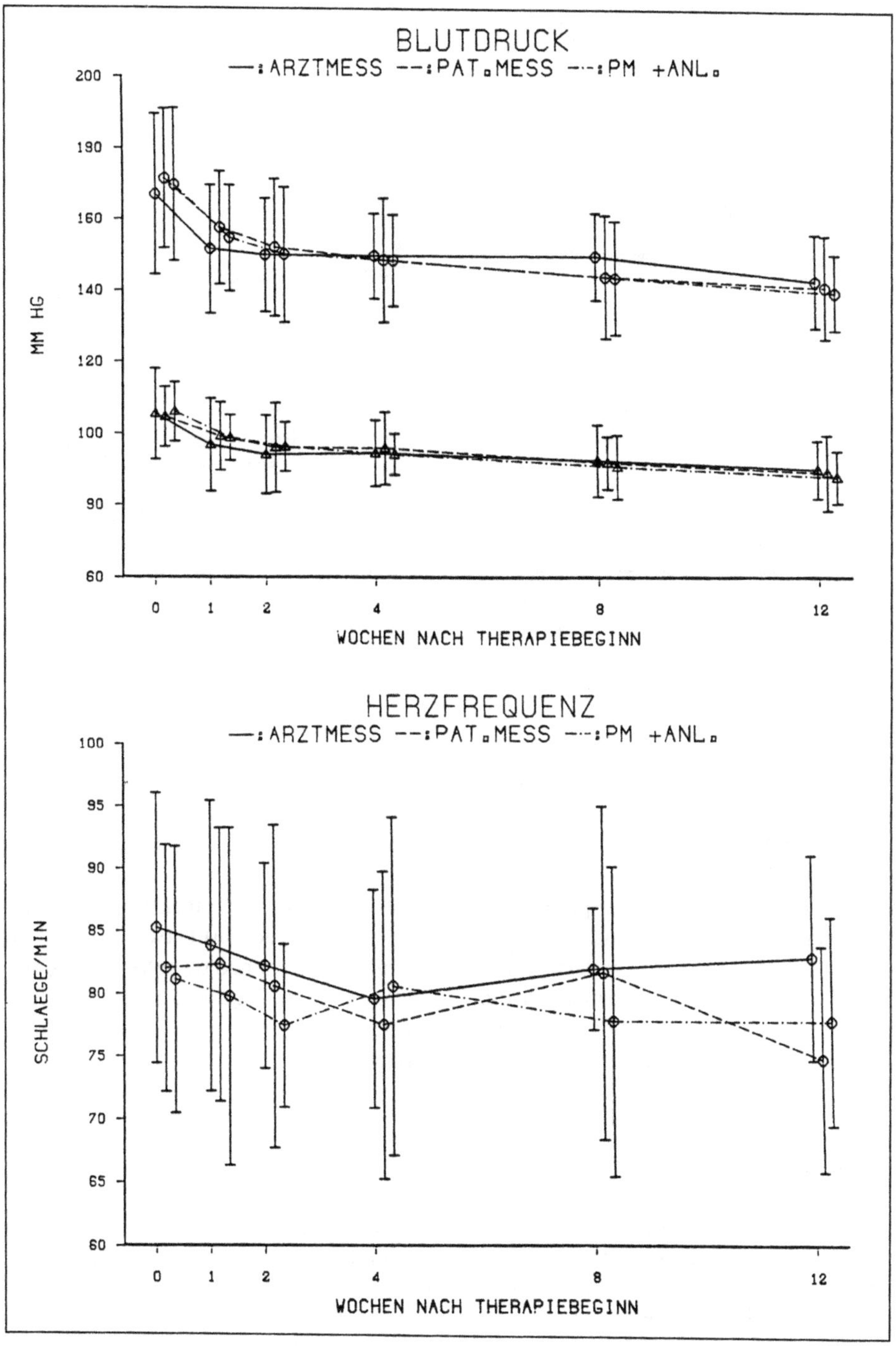
BLUTDRUCK
—: ARZTMESS --: PAT. MESS -·-: PM +ANL.
MM HG
WOCHEN NACH THERAPIEBEGINN
HERZFREQUENZ
—: ARZTMESS --: PAT. MESS -·-: PM +ANL.
SCHLAEGE/MIN
WOCHEN NACH THERAPIEBEGINN

Fig. 2

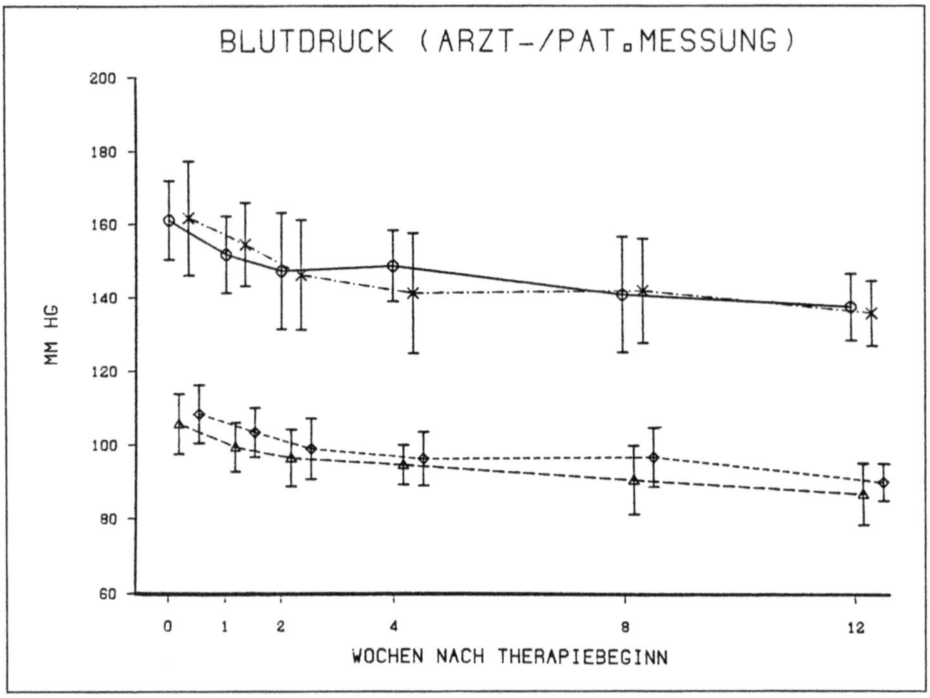

Fig. 3

The mean daily dose did not differ between the three groups:
Group I: 1.2 tablet/day
Group II: 1.2 tablet/day
Group III: 1.3 tablet/day.
At the end of the observation period, the values obtained by home measurement, i.e., the values measured by 23 patients (group III, intensive instruction) between 0700 and 0800 hours, were correlated with the mean hourly values determined by automated long-term blood pressure measurement on the day of registration. Figures 5a and 5b show that there is a marked significance during the morning and evening hours, whereas this does not hold true for noon and night blood pressure.

Conclusion

The preliminary results of our ongoing study reveal a significant decrease in systolic and diastolic blood pressure determined by clinic and home measurements after single application of the fixed compound preparation Pertenso in 69 hypertensives treated on an outpatient basis. The mean pressure determined by the physician, especially the systolic pressure measured by sphygmomanometer, is higher than that measured by the patient, a problem that has been described in the literature [8, 13]. While the value of home blood pressure measurement has been demonstrated in previous studies [11, 14],

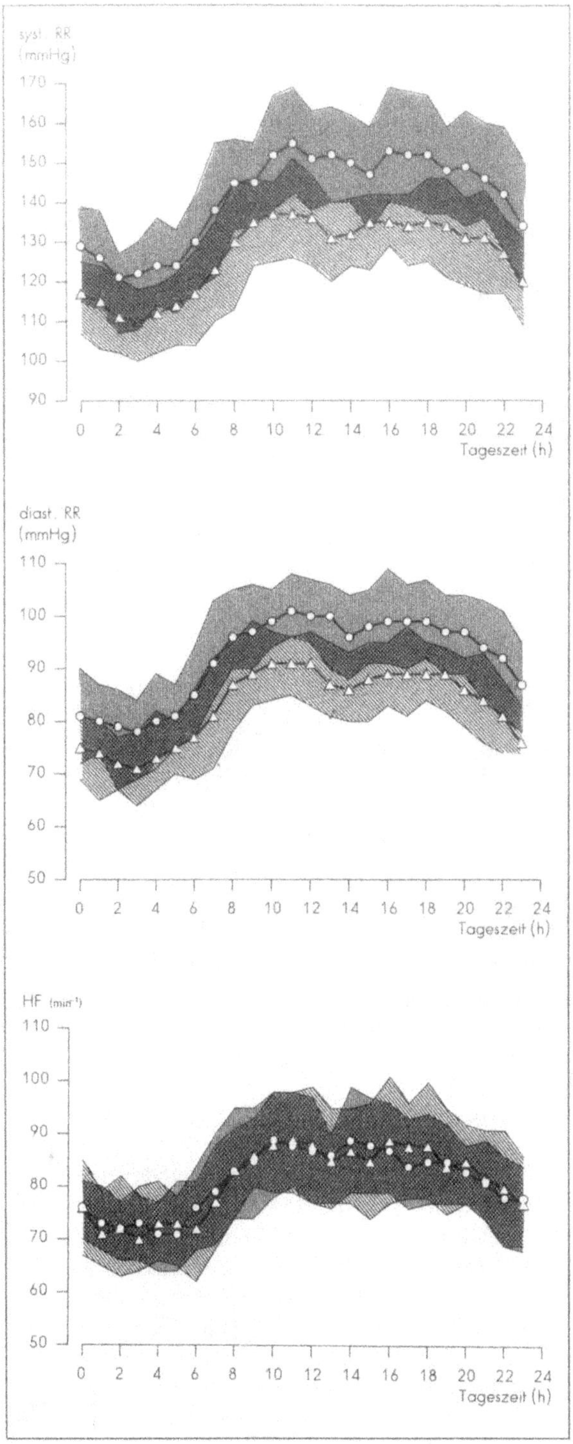

Fig. 4. 24-h systolic, diastolic blood pressure (RR) and heart rate (HF), before (O——O) and after treatment (Δ——Δ) of a combination therapy (Pertenso; hourly median and 25th and 27th percentiles are given) in patients (n = 69) with primary hypertension.

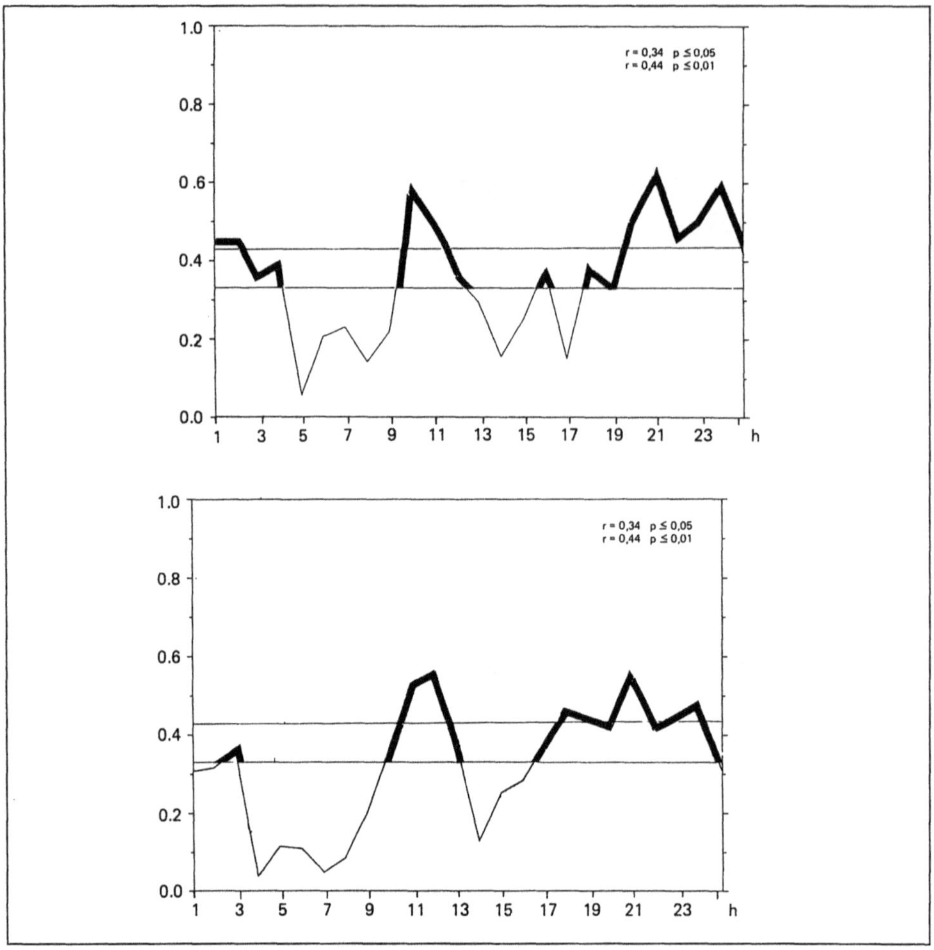

Fig. 5. Correlation of systolic (a) and diastolic (b) blood pressure by selfmeasurement (in the morning) to hourly mean during a 24-h blood pressure monitoring in ambulatory patients with primary hypertension (n = 29). Only blood pressure Values in the morning and in the evening are represented with statistically signification ($p < 0.01$).

the value of clinic blood pressure in the assessment of antihypertensive therapy has been questioned. The prognostic value of ambulatory blood pressure measurements has already been described in detail by Perloff et al. [15]. Home blood pressure measurements are recommended for the diagnostic and therapeutic monitoring of hypertensives [20]. Concomitant measures such as intensive instruction and repeated supervision of the measuring technique appear to have a positive influence on the therapeutic success. The rate of blood pressure normalization was markedly higher in the group of patients who received intensive instruction than in other groups. However, the differences were not significant. This finding should be verified in larger groups of patients.
The question as to whether standardized home blood pressure measurements reflect the

circadian, biphasic 24-h blood pressure profile, is discussed controversially. The present data show that the correlation was goode for the morning hours, relatively good for the early evening hours and that there was no correlation for afternoon and night blood pressure values (Fig. 5).
The assessment of blood pressure variability before and during therapy is improved by the use of indirect portable blood pressure recorders. The blood pressure variability (expressed as the degree of standard deviation) in all patients does not change under antihypertensive treatment with single application of the fixed compound preparation Pertenso. It remains to be elucidated whether there is a significant correlation between the lacking decrease in blood pressure variability and the prognosis of cardiovascular diseases. It was demonstrated, however, that left ventricular hypertrophy correlated with total daily blood pressure determined by indirect 24-h recording [6, 17, 18].

Acknowledgment

The study was supported by Melusin-Schwarz Corp., Monheim, FRG. We thank Mrs. Roswitha Günther for skilled technical assistance.

References

1. Armitage P. Fox W, Rose GA, Tinker CM (1966) The variability of measurements of casual blood pressure II. Survey experience. Clin Sci 30: 337—344
2. Ayman D, Goldshine AD (1940) blood pressure determinations by patients with essential hypertension: I. The difference between clinic and home readings before treatment. Am J Med Sci 200: 465—474
3. Distler A (1980) Beta-Rezeptorenblocker in der Hypertoniebehandlung. Nieren- und Hochdruck 9: 167—175
4. Weber MA, Drayer JIM (1989)
5. Drayer JIM, Weber MA, De Young JL, Brewer DD (1983) Long-term BP monitoring in the evaluation of antiypertensive therapy Arch Int Med 143: 898—901
6. Drayer JIM, Weber MA, De Young JL (1983) BP as a determinant of cardiac left ventricular muscle mass. Arch Inter Med 143: 90—92
7. Gould BA, Mann S, Davies AB, Altmann DG, Raftery EB (1981) Does placebo lower blood pressure Lancet II: 1377—81
8. Julius S, Mc Gin NF, Harburg E, Hoble SW (1964) Comparison of various clinical measurements of blood pressure with the self-determination technique in normotensive college males. J chron Dis 17: 391—396
9. Kleinert Hd, Harshfield GA, Pickering TG, Devereux RB, Sullivan PM, Marion RM, Marion RM, Mallory WK, Laragh JH (1984) What is the value of home blood pressure messurement in patients with mild hypertension? Hypertension 6: 547—578
10. Krönig B, Dufey K, Moergel K, Michaelis J, Jahnecke J (1974) Telemetrische Untersuchungen zur Wertigkeit eines Basalblutdruckes bei Hochdruckkranken Klin Wschr 52: 3054—61
11. Laughlin KD, Sherrard DJ, Fisher L (1980) Comparoson of clinic and home blood pressure levels in essential hypertension and variables associated with clinic-home differences. J Chronic Dis 33: 197—206
12. Littler WA, Honour AJ, Pugsley DJ, Sleight P (1975) Continous recording of direct arterial pressure in unrestricted patients. Its role in the diagnosis and management of high blood pressure. Circulation 51: 1101—1106

13. Mancia G, Bertinieri G, Grassi G, Parati G, Pomidossi G, Ferrari A, Gregorini L, Zanchetti A (1983) Efffects of blood pressure measurement by the doctor on patient's blood pressure and heart rate. Lancet II: 695—698
14. Marolf AP, Hany S, Bättig B, Vetter W (1987) Vergleich von Sprechstunden-, Langzeit-, und Selbstblutdruckmessung. Schweiz Rundschau Med (Praxis) 76,17: 459—461
15. Meyer-Sabellek W, Schulte K-L, Distler A, Gotzen R (1987) Circadian antihypertensive profile of carvedilol. J. Cardiovasc Pharm 10 (suppl 11): 119—123
16. Perloff D, Sokolow M, Cowan R (1983) The prognostic value of ambulatory blood pressures JAMA 249: 2792—98
17. Pessina AC, Palatini P, Sperti G, Cordone L, Libardoni M, Mos L, Mormimo P, Di Marco A, Dal Palu C (1985) Evaluation of hypertension and related target organ demage by average day-time blood pressure. Clin Exp Hypertension A7: 267—278
18. Sokolow M, Werdegar D, Kaim HK, Hinman AT (1966) Relationship between level of blood pressure measured casually and by portable recorders and severity of complications in essential hypertension. Circulation 34: 279—298
19. Streitberg B, Röhmel J (1987) Exakte Verteilung für Rang- und Randomisierungstests im allgemeinen C-Stichprobenproblem. In: Hrsg EDV in Medizin und Biologie, Val 18. Gustav Fischer, Stuttgart, S 12—19
20. Wilkinson PR, Raftery EB (1978) Patients attitudes to measuring their own blood pressure. Br Med J 1: 824—825
21. World Health Organization/International Society of Hypertension (1983) Guidelines for the treatment of Mild Hypertension. Hypertension 5: 394—397

Casual, ergometric and 24-h blood pressure in hypertensives after physical training

I.-W. Franz[1], R. Ketelhut[2], W. Meyer-Sabellek[3] and R. Gotzen[3]

[1] Klinik Wehrawald, Todtmoos, FRG
[2] Department of Internal Medicine, Section on Hypertensive Diseases, Ochsner Clinic and Alton Ochsner Medical Foundation, New Orleans, Louisiana, USA
[3] Medizinische Klinik und Poliklinik, Klinikum Steglitz, Freie Universität Berlin, Berlin, FRG

Introduction

The effective control of high blood pressure is essential in preventive medicine and public health. It must be asked, however, whether drug therapy for hypertension will continue to play the dominant role in hypertension management, given the large financial burden that is imposed by the use of antihypertensive drugs on a broad scale.

It has been stated previously that the reduction of blood pressure by endurance training depends on the group that is selected for study [1, 4, 5—8]. In most studies there are no data on the quality and quantity of training and the effect on body weight. However, this information is a prerequisite for the assessment if exercise can lower high blood pressure. Hypertensive patients have lower cardiac outputs and stroke volumes, higher heart rates and a markedly elevated peripheral resistance than normotensives at the same level of exercise [10, 11]. The question of whether endurance training has a positive effect on the high peripheral vascular resistance in hypertensive patients is unknown.

However, previously [9] we were able to show that the increased peripheral resistance could be reduced acutely during aerobic exercise under steady-state conditions, inducing a reduction in blood pressure up to 1 h after exercise. We will now try to answer four further questions:

1. Is the resting blood pressure of hypertensive patients positively influenced in the long run by regular aerobic exercise?
2. Is the blood pressure response of hypertensive patients to a standardized ergometry test (50—100 watts) reduced after aerobic training?
3. Is the drop in blood pressure during aerobic exercise also relevant during the recovery period after exercise?
4. Is the 24-h ambulatory blood pressure profile reduced after aerobic training?

Method

Ten male hypertensive patients (WHO I) aged 43.3 ± 3.1 years participated in the study. They had all mild hypertension at rest and during and after standardized ergometry [3].

The patients were examined on a work-free Saturday. In phase 1, the resting blood pressure was measured every 10 min for 1 h in a supine position. Then the patients were subjected to a standardized ergometric test (50—100 watts; 10 watt increments/min, 50 revolutions/min, half-sitting position) and 5 min after the ergometric work (phase 2). After that, phase 3 was conducted, which consisted of a 60-min steady-state endurance test on a bicycle ergometer in a sitting position. The workloads were adjusted in such a way that constant heart rates of 130—140 beats/min were achieved during the whole test. Finally in phase 4, following the endurance test, the blood pressure was measured every 10 min in a supine position for 2 h. All these tests were then repeated under identical conditions after 6 and 18 months of regular aerobic training twice a week.

Blood pressure was measured according to the Riva-Rocci-Korotkoff cuff method, using Korotkoff phase IV for diastolic blood pressure. Additionally, in five patients we investigated the 24-h ambulatory BP profiles before and after training, using a portable Pressurometer III (Delmar Avionics, USA).

Results

As previously reported [9], there was a significant and continuous reduction in systolic and diastolic blood pressure during the first 60 min of steady-state exercise before starting training (Fig. 1). Even 60 min after this exercise, the resting blood pressure was significantly ($p<0.01$) lower compared with preexercise values, which could not be shown 120 min after exercise (Fig. 1).

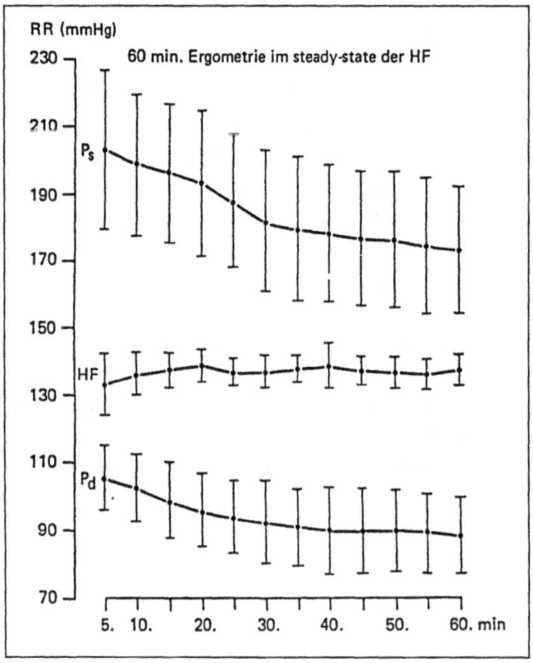

Fig. 1. Systolic (P_s), diastolic (P_d) blood pressure and heart rate (HF) during aerobic exercise of 60 min duration under steady-state conditions of heart rate.

After 6 months of training, the resting blood pressures (phase 1) of 125 ± 7/91 ± 7 mmHg were not significantly different from those before training (126 ± 6/92 ± 7 mm Hg). However, blood pressures 60 min (phase 4, 113 ± 7/82 ± 9 mmHg) as well as 120 min after exercise (118 ± 9/85 ± 9 mmHg) were significantly ($p<0.01$) lower (Table 1, Fig. 2).

Table 1. Means ± SD of blood pressure in hypertensive patients measured over a period of 60 min before and 120 min after a 60-min endurance exercise, before and after starting an aerobic training program (x p 0.05; xx p 0.01; xxx p 0.001)

Blood pressure (supine)

	Before exercise (min)			After endurance exercise (min)				
(mmHg) x ± SD	10	30	60	10	30	60	90	120
Before training	132 ± 8 92 ± 7	128 ± 7 91 ± 6	126 ± 6 92 ± 7	120 ± 10 87 ± 7	122 ± 7 88 ± 7	122 ± 7 87 ± 8	122 ± 7 88 ± 8	125 ± 9 90 ± 8
6 months training	128 ± 7 91 ± 8	125 ± 7 91 ± 7	125 ± 7 91 ± 7	116 ± 12 83 ± 9	113 ± 8 82 ± 8	113 ± 7 82 ± 9 xx	116 ± 10 84 ± 9	118 ± 9 85 ± 9 xx
18 months training	120 ± 11 86 ± 7	121 ± 9 88 ± 7	121 ± 8 86 ± 7 x	118 ± 7 80 ± 7	113 ± 8 79 ± 5	114 ± 8 79 ± 7 xx	118 ± 9 82 ± 7	121 ± 10 83 ± 7 xx

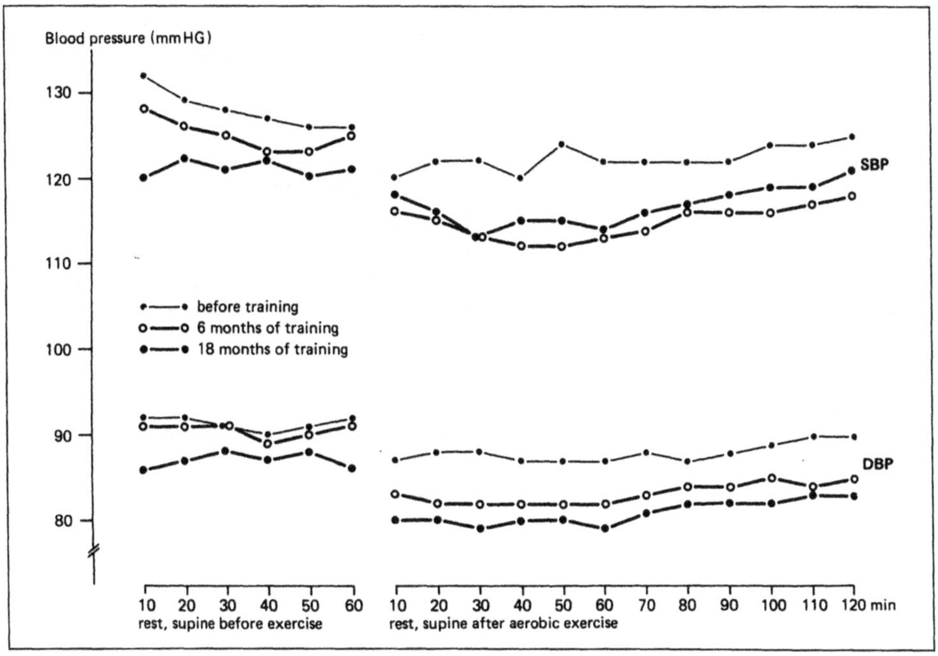

Fig. 2. Systolic (SBP) and diastolic (DBP) blood pressure before and up to 120 min after the aerobic exercise test of 60 min duration before and after long-term training.

During the standardized ergometry at 100 watts there was a significant ($p < 0.01$) decline in systolic and diastolic blood pressure from 184 ± 10/107 ± 6 mmHg to 170 ± 10/100 ± 7 mmHg even after 6 months of training (Table 2, Fig. 3). Simultaneously, heart rate dropped significantly ($p < 0.01$) from 116 ± 11/min to 106 ± 9/min and rate pressure product, as a measure of myocardial O_2 consumption, was significantly ($p < 0.01$) reduced (Fig. 4). After 18 months of training, the resting blood pressure (phase 1) was now significantly ($p < 0.05$) reduced to 121 ± 8/86 ±7 mmHg. Also resting blood pressures 1 h (124 ± 8/79 ± 9 mmHg) and 2 h (121 ± 10/83 ± 7 mmHg) after the endurance test were significantly ($p < 0.05$) decreased, even in comparison with the preexercise values (Table 1, Fig. 2).

Table 2. Means ± SD of blood pressure in hypertensive patients before, during and 5 min after a standardized ergometric test, before and after starting an aerobic training program (x $p<0.05$; xx $p<0.01$; xxx $p<0.001$)

Blood pressure						
(mmHg)	At rest		100 watts		5 min after work	
x ± SD	SBP	DBP	SBP	DBP	SBP	DBP
Before training	126 ± 7	92 ± 7	184 ± 10	107 ± 6	140 ± 7	96 ± 5
6 months training	125 ± 7	91 ± 7	170 ± 10 x	100 ± 7 xx	134 ± 10	92 ± 8 x
18 months training	121 ± 8 x	86 ± 8 x	172 ± 8 x	96 ± 7 xx	135 ± 10	88 ± 7 xx

Also, at the workload of 100 watts (phase 2) a further significant ($p < 0.05$) reduction in diastolic blood pressure (172 ± 8/96 ± 7 mmHg) was found (Table 2, Fig. 3).

The fall in blood pressure measured during the initial 60 min of steady-state exercise was not significantly changed after 6 and 18 months.

In all five patients with 24-h ambulatory BP profile available before and after long-term training, a reduction in systolic and diastolic blood pressure could be shown (Table 3). Although, the number of investigated patients was small, there was a significant ($p < 0.05$) reduction in diastolic blood pressure.

The mean body weight of 82.4 ± 10 kg prior to starting the training program was reduced to 80.9 ± 9.8 kg after 6 months, with no further change in the following 12 months (80.7 ± 8.8 kg).

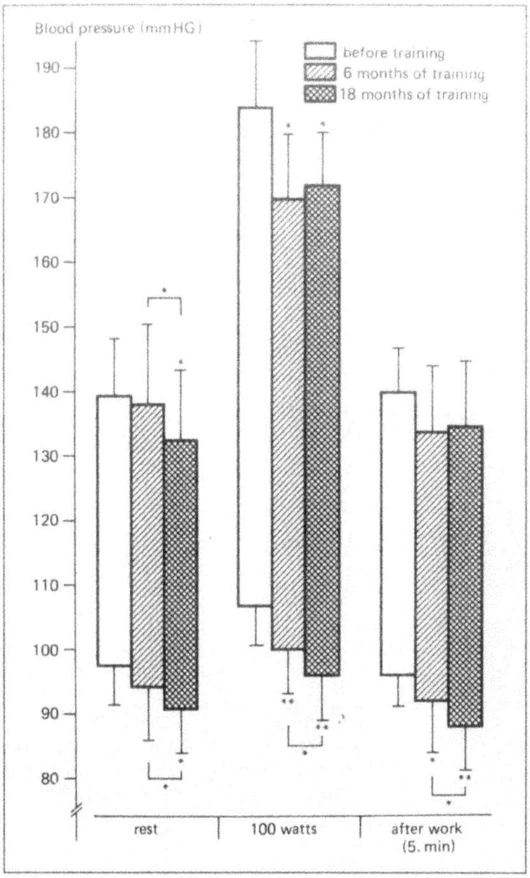

Fig. 3. Blood pressure at rest, during 100 watts and in the 5th minute of the recovery phase before and after long term training.

Table 3. 24-h ambulatory blood pressure monitoring before and after long term aerobic training in five hypertensive patients

		24-h Ambulatory blood pressure monitoring			
		total 24-h-SBP		total 24-h-DBP	
Patients	Age (years)	Before training	After training	Before training	After training
B.K.	42	131	136	91	81
H.K.	44	122	109	100	75
J.M.	44	135	143	89	82
A.M.	48	141	128	106	91
A.M.	47	126	140	87	83
$\bar{x} \pm s$	45 ± 4.1	131 ± 7.5	129.2 ± 12.7	94.6 ± 8.1	83.4 + 7.7 x

x = $p > 0.05$

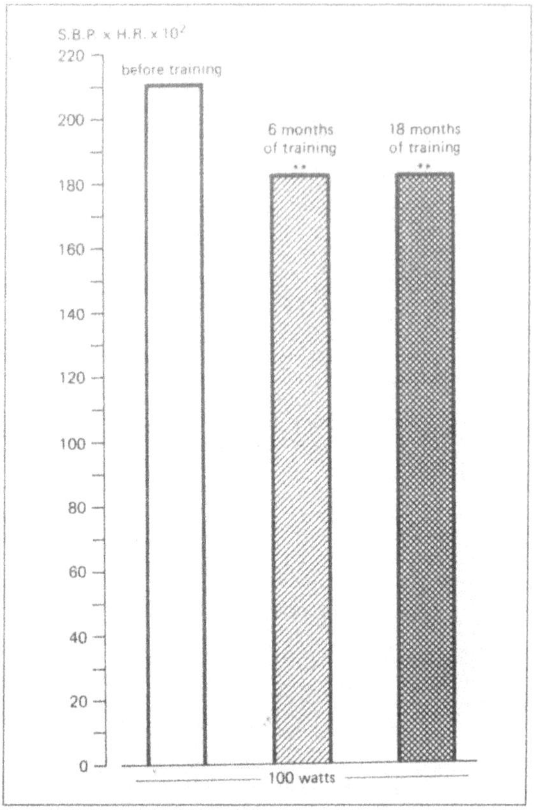

Fig. 4. Rate-pressure product (SBP x HR x 10^2) blood pressure at rest, during 100 watts and in the 5th minute of the recovery phase before and after long term training.

Discussion

The results show that in hypertensive patients, regular aerobic training can result in a significant reduction of blood pressure at rest and during and after exercise.

Physical aerobic training probably achieves this goal by effecting a redistribution of systemic blood flow and by increasing metabolic vasodilatation (which significantly lowers the total peripheral resistance). Furthermore an increase in the capillary bed in the skeletal muscle and functional changes in the arterioles are also under discussion [2], which would restitute the capacity for vasodilation, probably by changing the sensitivity and/or number of α-receptors of the vascular bed.

Bradycardia as a result of training points to the assumption that other factors, e.g., altering central circulatory regulation, may also play an essential role in the down-regulation of blood pressure.

It is unlikely that the blood pressure reduction in this study was attributable to weight reduction, because there was no significant change in weight during the last 12 months, but a significant reduction in blood pressure.

Conclusion

In hypertensive patients, long-term aerobic training leads to a reduction of blood pressure at rest and during exercise and prolongs the drop in blood pressure after exercise, implying a beneficial effect in the management of mild hypertension.

References

1. Blair SN, Goodyear NN, Gibbons LW, Cooper KH (1974) Physical fitness and incidence of hypertension in health normotensive men and women. J Am Med Ass 211: 1668
2. Blomquist CG, Saltin B (1986) Cardiovascular adaptations of physical training. Ann Rev Physiol 45: 169
3. Franz I-W (1986) Ergometry in Hypertensive Patients – Implications for Diagnosis and Treatment. Springer, Berlin Heidelberg New York Tokio
4. Franz I-W (1978) Therapie der hypertonen Kreislaufregulationsstörungen bzw. Hypertonie durch dosiertes Training. Schweiz Z Sportmed 3: 117
5. Franz I-W, Eismann D, Mellerowicz H (1983) Einfluß von Training und Gewichtsabnahme auf koronare Risikofaktoren. In: Heck H, Hollmann W, Liesen H, Rost R (Hrsg) Sport: Leistung und Gesundheit. Deutscher Ärzteverlag, Köln, S 373
6. Hanson JS, Nedde WH (1970) Preleminary observations on physical training for hypertensive males. Circ Res 26: 49
7. Johnson W, Grover J (1967) Hemodynamic and metabolic effects of physical training in four patients with essential hypertension. Canad Med Ass J 96: 842
8. Jokl E, Ball M, Frankel L (1967) Ergometry, Exercise and hypertension. In: Mellerowicz H, Hansen G (Hrsg) 2. Int Seminar für Ergometrie (Ergon)
9. Ketelhut R, Franz I-W (1985) Zur Wirkung einer akuten und chronischen Ausdauerleistung auf das Blutdruckverhalten bei Hochdruckkranken. In: Franz I-W, Mellerowicz H, Noack W (Hrsg) Training und Sport zur Prävention und Rehabilitation in der technisierten Umwelt. Springer, Berlin Heidelberg New York Tokio, S 704
10. Lund-Johansen P (1981) Hämodynamik bei der essentiellen Hypertonie in Ruhe und während Ergometrie und deren Beeinflussung durch Diuretika, β-Rezeptorenblocker und Vasodilatatoren. In: Franz I-W (Hrsg) Belastungsblutdruck bei Hochdruckkranken. Springer, Berlin Heidelberg New York, S 107
11. Sannerstedt R (1966) Hemodynamic response to exercise in patients with arterial hypertension. Acta Med Scand (Suppl) 180: 458

Antihypertensive effect of the new agent carvedilol: evaluation by 24-hour indirect blood pressure monitoring

K.-L. Schulte, W. Meyer-Sabellek, A. Distler, R. Gotzen

Medizinische Klinik und Poliklinik, Klinikum Steglitz, Freie Universität Berlin, Berlin, FRG

Introduction

Therapeutic intervention in hypertension is usually based on casual blood pressure (BP) readings and is predicted on the assumption that BP measured under standardized conditions represents the mean pressure over each 24-h period. Noninvasive ambulatory BP monitoring was recently introduced as a technique to define and quantify BP variability [1—3] and to assess the effects of antihypertensive therapy [4, 5] on the circadian pattern of BP.

The effect on BP of β-adrenergic blocking drugs is not well correlated with plasma levels of the agent. Automated indirect ambulatory devices may provide up to 200 BP and heart rate (HR) readings over 24 h and therefore may help to evaluate the dosage and the long-lasting antihypertensive effect of a new agent, and to compare the efficacy with commonly used β-blockers. Carvedilol (C) is a new vasodilating noncardioselective β-blocking agent [6] which exerts its relevant properties of direct precapillary vasodilating activity and β-blockade in the same dose range. The antihypertensive effect in essential hypertensive patients has been described previously [7—9] and compared in clinical trials with labetalol [10] and propranolol [11].

In the present study we evaluated the antihypertensive effect of C on casual and exercise-induced BP and HR and compared the effectiveness of a once and twice daily regimen to metoprolol (M). The antihypertensive effect of long-term treatment and single oral daily administration on the circadian BP and HR pattern was studied.

Patients and Methods

In a placebo-controlled double-blind randomized trial, 18 ambulatory patients, 10 males and eight females (the latter either postmenopausal or of child-bearing age who were not pregnant or not actively seeking pregnancy, but not on oral contraceptives), aged 25—57 years, with mild to moderate essential hypertension (WHO I-II) were included after informed consent was obtained.

After a 2-week washout and a 2-week placebo run-in period, chronic treatment with either C (25 mg/capsule) or M (100 mg/capsule) was randomly administered to the patients for 2 weeks in a single morning dose, for 3 weeks in twice daily regimen, and for 3 weeks in a single morning double dose.
Patients were considered for the active treatment period if three BP readings after 5

min at rest in the sitting position showed a Vth phase diastolic pressure of 95—110 mmHg. Other criteria for exclusion included ischemic heart disease, chronic obstructive pulmonary disease, diabetes mellitus, severe hepatic, renal or hematological diseases, cardiac failure and A-V block of more than the first degree. Casual systolic BP, diastolic BP (Korotkoff phase V) and HR were assessed using a regularly calibrated standard sphygmomanometer after each period in the morning (0700—0900 hours) before and 2 h after oral administration. In addition, hemodynamic variables were determined in standing and supine position at rest and during graded cycle ergometry (6 min, up to 100 W), followed by a recovery period. The antihypertensive effect of the two different antihypertensive agents was investigated not only casually and during ergometric work load, but also during daily activities and sleep, using a Pressurometer III (Del Mar Avionics, Calif., USA), an ambulatory noninvasive portable, automated monitor on two occasions: at the end of the placebo period and at the end of the treatment period. Systolic (sBP) and diastolic (dBP) pressure are monitored as well as HR at preset intervals (15 min). Data are stored by the 1.8 kg monitor including a solid memory and is evaluated via an interface to a programmed computer (Euromac II, FRG). One hundred measurements per 24 h were planned for computation.

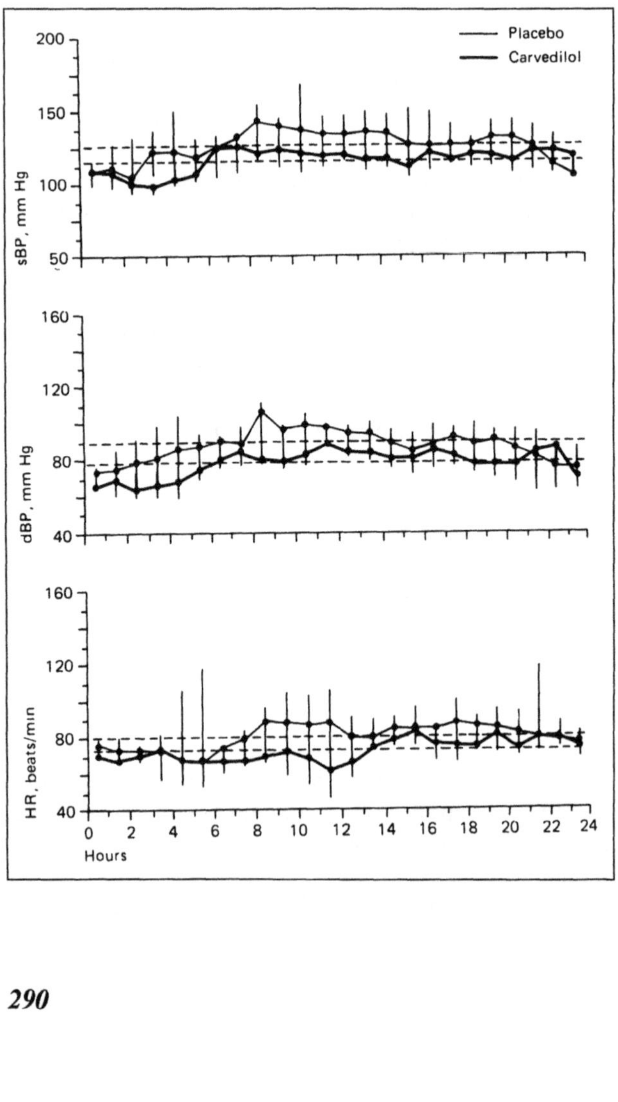

Fig. 1. 24-h noninvasive sBP, dBP, and HR before and after long-term application of C (hourly median and 25th and 75th percentiles). Time of day is shown on the abscissa. Dashed line represents overall median.

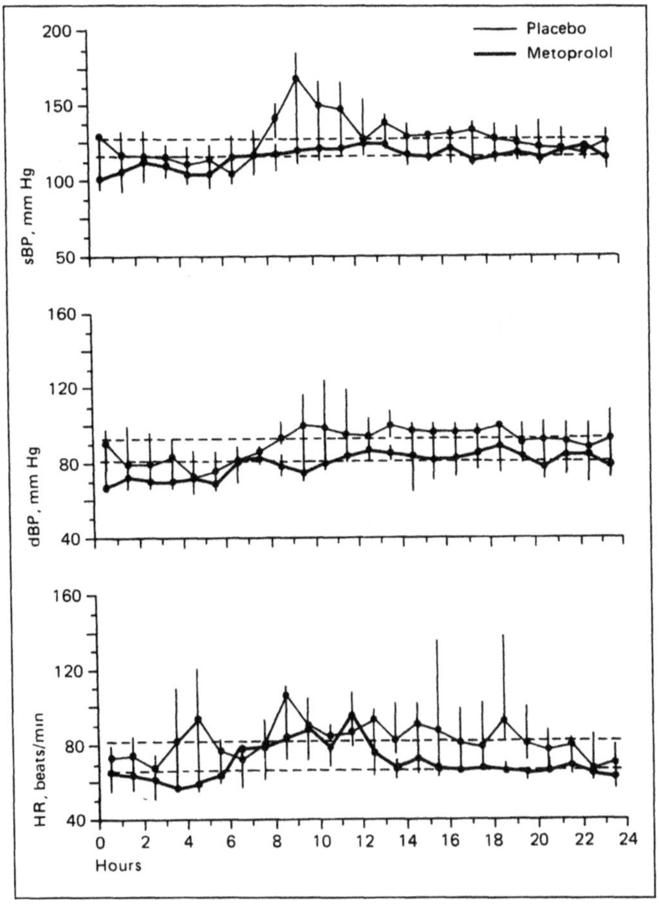

Fig. 2. 24-h noninvasive sBP, dBP, and HR before and after long-term application of M (hourly median and 25th and 75th percentiles). Time of day is shown on the abscissa. Dashed line represents overall median.

Compliance was measured by counting the tablets the patients returned at the end of each period as well as by measurement of plasma drug levels. Compliance during the study was good, although one patient had to be rejected because plasma levels of C were not detectable on two occasions.

Data analysis was performed using Wilcoxon's nonparametric rank sum and signed rank test at $p < 0.05$ as a level of significance. Means and standard deviation (SD) are given in the text. For intraindividual differences and drug comparison in the figures, the medians and the 25th and 75th percentiles are plotted.

Results

Automatically recorded BP and HR results under baseline (placebo) conditions and after three weeks of 50 mg C once daily are given in Fig. 1. The hourly averages of ambulatory BPs followed the usual pattern of being lower during sleep [5[and were similar in both groups when averaged for awake and asleep states for the entire 24 h. At the end of the

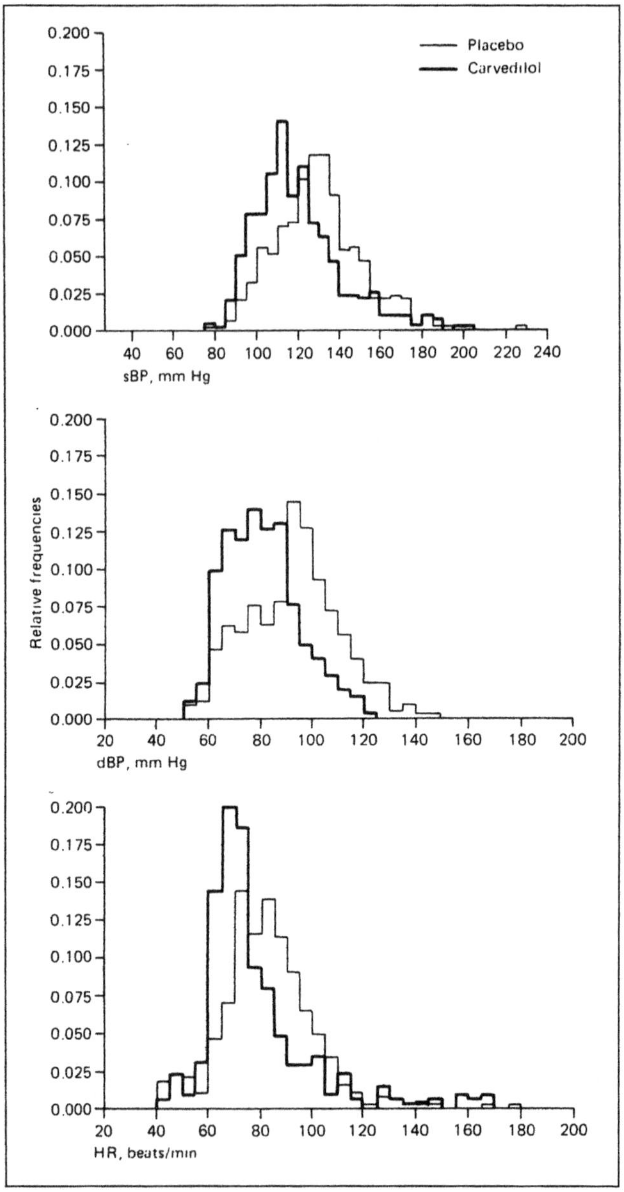

Fig. 3. Histograms of relative frequencies of sBP, dBP, and HR calculated from noninvasive 24-h monitoring (Pressurometer III) before and after long-term treatment of C.

study after 3 weeks of 50 mg C daily, the 24-h recording showed a significant fall for overall median of sBP (C: —10 mmHg). This was comparable to M (—11 mmHg; see Fig. 2).

As observed with intraarterial devices [12] there was an early morning increase in BP which was reduced more with M (—17 mmHg, before wakening) than with C (—7 mmHg). The median BP 2 h before, overall (C: —10; M: —8 mmHg) and 2 h after wakening was comparably reduced. There was an overlap in the late evening BP for both

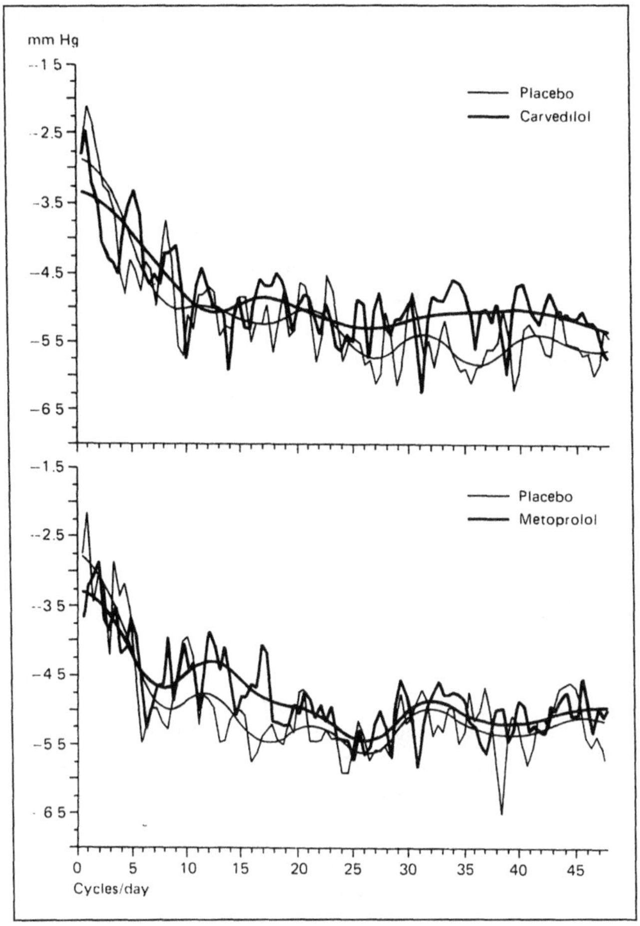

Fig. 4. Log-relative spectral power analysis vs cycles per day of sBP before (placebo) and after long-term antihypertensive treatment with C and M.

agents, whereas the BP during sleep, which was lowered during the placebo phase, was not affected. The overall median of HR was decreased by both M and C. M significantly ($p < 0.05$) decreased overall HR more (—17 beats/min) than did C (—5 beats/min). This effect was pronounced 2 h before wakening.

The histogram on relative frequencies of sBP, dBP and HR is given in Fig. 3, demonstrating a normal distribution before and after treatment, with less variability for the new drug C. Spectral analyses have been provided in a search for ultradian BP rhythms and for deterioration of circadian rhythm. In these patients, demonstrated in Fig. 4 for sBP, no patterns other than the previously described day and night patterns could be documented either before or after treatment for either antihypertensive agent.

A significant antihypertensive effect could be documented using standardized casual readings for the new antihypertensive agent on sBP, dBP standing 24 h after a once-daily administration, from a mean of 150/110 (SD $\pm 20/\pm 13$) mmHg to 125/95 (SD $\pm 20/\pm 14$). sBP and dBP were also significantly reduced at rest and at peak exercise levels of 100 W, whereas no significant alteration of HR at rest, standing, or supine could be observed. Body weight was comparable at the beginning for both groups and was constant throughout the study.

Discussion

Standardized casual BP measurements still represent a somewhat artificial condition. BT and HR under ergometric workload are influenced by inter- and intraindividual training conditions. The recent introduction of fully automated noninvasive ambulatory BP recorders has made it possible to evaluate BP under a variety of circumstances at the clinic and during normal daily activities including work and sleep.

The noninvasive devices used for ambulatory 24-h BP and HR monitoring have revealed that BP values form a characteristic circadian pattern in ambulatory normal [13] and hypertensive subjects [14, 15] and the reproducibility of circadian pattern in essential hypertension [16] has been evaluated. The availability of reliable equipment and the good validity of measurements have been used in drug trials comparing antihypertensive treatment [17, 18]. BP values recorded intermittently by a noninvasive device have been shown to reflect those determined continuously by monitoring from an intraarterial device [19]. Ambulatorily recorded BP was lower than casual BP measured in the clinic at the end of both the placebo and the treatment period. This has been reported using direct intraarterial [12] or different noninvasive methods [20, 21]. Intraarterial devices which record about 120000 measurements/24 h allow beat-to-beat analysis, whereas the Pressurometer III used in the present study does not allow sampling more often than every 7.5 min, providing less than 200 BP values/day. Di Rienzo et al. [19] confirmed the applicability of indirect techniques also at 10- and 15-min intervals. Computing at 15-min intervals in this study, 29 out of 36 profiles were available. Loss of data was due to technical problems (e. g., storing) and noncompliance (lack of sleep).

Casual reading using standardized methods at rest as well as during ergometric workload did show a good antihypertensive effect of both drugs in this trial. Despite this, there was no evidence of a significant effect on morning wakening BP. The overlap of BP recordings in the late evening raised the question as to whether a twice daily regimen might more adequately lower BP throughout the day. Additional BP lowering in the sleeping period could be ruled out.

In contrast to intraarterial devices, the present automatic method may be applied several times in a patient and thus be useful for evaluating both new antihypertensive regimens and commonly used antihypertensive agents.

Conclusion

Indirect automatic 24-h blood pressure monitoring has been found to be reliable and valid, and thus has been introduced for the evaluation of dosage and efficacy of antihypertensive drugs. The present double-blind placebo-controlled randomized long-term study reports the therapeutic results of the oral administration of a new β-adrenergic blocking agent, carvedilol, with direct vasodilator activity in patients with primary hypertension. The antihypertensive effect was acute at onset and comparable in the supine and standing position judged by casual blood pressure readings. Indirect automatic blood pressure monitoring demonstrated a good antihypertensive effect throughout daily activities after single oral dosage. Despite some technical problem with the apparatus (Pressurometer III, Del Mar Avionics), a circadian pattern could be documented in both untreated and treated patients. Blood pressure and heart rate were normally distributed but less variable during treatment. The long-lasting antihypertensive effect was comparable to the commonly used β-blocker metoprolol. A significantly reduced awakening blood pressure in the morning may indicate a beneficial effect on a possible prognostic factor in arterial hypertension.

Acknowlegdgements:

We thank Boehringer Mannheim for constant support to elaborate the method of 24-h blood pressure monitoring on the highest available standard, enabling us to maitain up-to-date data and statistics on drug monitoring.
We acknowledge with admiration and appreciation the technical assistance of Mrs. R. Günther.

References

1. Perloff D, Sokolow M, Cowan R (1983) The prognostic value of ambulatory blood pressure. J Am med Ass 249: 2792—2798
2. Sheps SG, Elveback LR, Close EL (1981) Evaluation of the Del Mar Avionics blood pressure recording device. Mayo Clin Proc 56: 740—743
3. Pickering TG, Harshfield GA, Kleinert HD (1982) Blood pressure during normal daily activities, sleep and exercise: comparison of values in normal and hypertensive subjects. J Am med Ass 247: 992—996
4. Messerli FH, Glade LB, Ventura HO (1983) Diurnal variations of cardiac rhythm, arterial pressure, and urinary catecholamines in borderline and established essential hypertension. Am Heart J 104: 109—114
5. Drayer JIM, Weber MA, De Young JL, Brewer DD (1983) Long-term blood pressure monitoring in the evaluations of antihypertensive therapy. Archs intern Med 143: 898—901
6. Möllendorff E, Abshagen U, Akpan W, Neugebauer G, Schröter E (1986) Clinical pharmacologic investigations with carvedilol, a new beta-blocker with direct vasodilator activity. Clin Pharmacol Ther 39: 677—682
7. Meyer-Sabellek W, Schulte K-L, Thiede HM, Gotzen R (1983) Acute hypotensive responsive to the new antihypertensive agent BM 14190 in essential hypertensive patients. J Hypertens I (suppl 2): 351—352
8. Eggertsen R, Sivertsson R, Denhart A, Hansson L (1984) Hemodynamic effects of carvedilol, a new beta-adrenoceptor blocker and precapillary vasodilator in essential hypertension. J Hypertens 2: 529—534
9. Kaski JC, Rodriguez-Plaza L, Brown J, Masers A (1985) Efficacy of carvedilol (BM 14190), a new beta-blocking drug with vasodilating properties in exercise-induced ischemia. Am J Cardiol 56: 35—40
10. Cubedan LX, Fuenmayor N, Varin F, Viuagra V, Colindres R, Powell JR. Mechanism of carvedilol in normal volunteers: a comparison with labetalol (pers. commun.).
11. Eggertsen R, Andrew L, Sivertsson R, Hansson L (1984) Acute hemodynamic effects of carvedilol (BM 14190), a new combined beta-andrenoceptor blocker and precapillary vasodilating agent in hypertensive patients. Eur J clin Pharmacol 27: 19—23
12. Raftery EB, Mann S, Bala Subramanian V (1982) Once-daily pindolol in hypertension: an ambulatory assessment. Am Heart J 104: 109—114

13. Weber MA, Drayer JIM, Nakamura DK, Wyle FA (1984) The circadian blood pressure pattern in ambulatory normal subjects. Am J Cardiol 54: 115—119
14. Messerli FH, Glade LB, Ventura HO et al. (1982) Diurnal variations of cardiac rhythm, arterial pressure, and urinary catecholamines in borderline and established essential hypertension. Am Heart J 104: 109—114
15. Pickering TG, Harshfield GA, Kleinert HD (1982) Blood pressure during normal daily activities, sleep and exercise: comparison of values in normal and hypertension subjects. J Am med Ass 247: 992—996
16. Weber MA, Drayer JIM, Wyle FA, De Young IL (1982) Reproducibility of the whole-day blood pressure pattern in essential hypertension. Clin exp Hypertens A4: 1377—1390
17. Berglund S, DeFaire U, Castenfors J, Andersson G, Hartford M, Liedholm H, Ljungman S, Thulin T, Wikstrand J (1985) Monitoring 24-hour blood pressure in a drug trial. Evaluation of a noninvasive device. Hypertension 7: 688—694
18. Rion I, Waeber B, Graf HJ, Jaussi A, Porchet M, Brunner HR (1985) Blood pressure response to antihypertensive therapy ambulatory versus office blood pressure readings. J Hypertens 3: 139—143
19. Di Rienzo M, Grassi G, Pedotti A, Mancia J (1983) Continuous versus intermittent blood pressure measurements in estimating 24-hour average blood pressure. Hypertension 5: 264—269
20. Jacot des Combes B, Porchet M., Waeber B, Brunner HR (1984) Ambulatory blood pressure recordings: reproducibility and unpredictability. Hypertension 6: 110—114
21. Drayer JIM, Weber MA, De Young JL, Brewer DD (1983) Long-term BP monitoring in the evaluation of antihypertensive therapy. Archs intern Med 143: 898—901
22. Meyer-Sabellek W, Schulte K-L, Streitberg B, Gotzen R (1989) Two years: follow-up of 24 hour indirect blood pressure monitoring: evaluation of once and twice daily regimen of carvedilol. Drugs.
23. Meyer-Sabellek W, Schulte K-L, Streitberg B, Gotzen R, Distler A (1988) 24-hour noninvasive oscillometric blood pressure monitoring: evaluation of the antihyertensive circadian profile of nitrendipine. J Cardiovasc Pharm 12 (Suppl. 4)

Chronobiologic blood pressure assessment with a cardiovascular summary, the sphygmochron

F. Halberg[1], E. Bakken[2], G. Cornélissen[1], J. Halberg[3], E. Halberg[1], W. Jinyi[1, 4], S. Sánchez de la Peña[1], P. Delmore[2] and B. Tarquini[5]

[1] Chronobiology Laboratories, University of Minnesota, Minneapolis, Minnesota, USA
[2] Medtronic Inc., Minneapolis, Minnesota, USA
[3] Department of Occupational Health, St. Paul-Ramsey Medical Center, St. Paul, Minnesota, USA
[4] Department of Physiology, Chengdu College of Traditional Chinese Medicine, Chengdu, Sichuan, People's Republic of China
[5] Istituto di Clinica Medica Generale e Terapia Medica II, Florence, Italy

Chronobiology and medicine

Chronobiology deals with rhythmic patterns that occur in all forms of life [1—5, 7—33, 35—38, 40—44, 47]. Virtually all organisms exhibit approximately daily (circadian) cycles. In human beings, prominent rhythms are found in blood pressure, circulatory pulse, body core and surface temperature and in chemical variables of blood, urine, and tissues. (Fig. 1). The medical section of this new science explores the relationships of rhythms to prediction, prevention, diagnosis, and treatment of diseases. Several decades of research worldwide have established that medical diagnoses can be subject to a much higher proportion of false positives (e.g., "office hypertension") and false negatives (e.g., "odd-hour" hypertension) when only single samples are taken at arbitrary times of the day instead of taking rhythms into account. Radiation, chemotherapy, and other treatments have been shown to have markedly different efficacy and safety depending upon the pattern of administration within the day. Without modern engineering tools, chronobiology had to rely on manual measurement series that were cumbersome to collect and required methods of analysis that were not generally available. Modern bioengineering with microcomputers can bring the findings of chronobiology on circadian and other rhythms into the mainstream of medicine. Chronobiology can thus provide new dimensions to an individualized, positive assessment of health complementing the current negative approach relying solely on the absence of unusual values or overt disease.

Medicine and health care more generally stand on the threshold of a new era in prevention as well as diagnosis and treatment, based on the combination of several emerging engineering technologies with an understanding and application of the health effect of life's rhythms. Through chronobiologic programs, modern engineering technologies can lead to:

— the large-scale use of portable, personal long-term ambulatory monitors of biologic variables such as blood pressure, pulse, ECG, EEG, respiration, body temperature, motor activity, gastric acidity and other variables that undergo large, spontaneously and reactively recurrent changes; — the availability of data base systems to acquire and analyze the considerable volumes of data obtained from personal monitors;

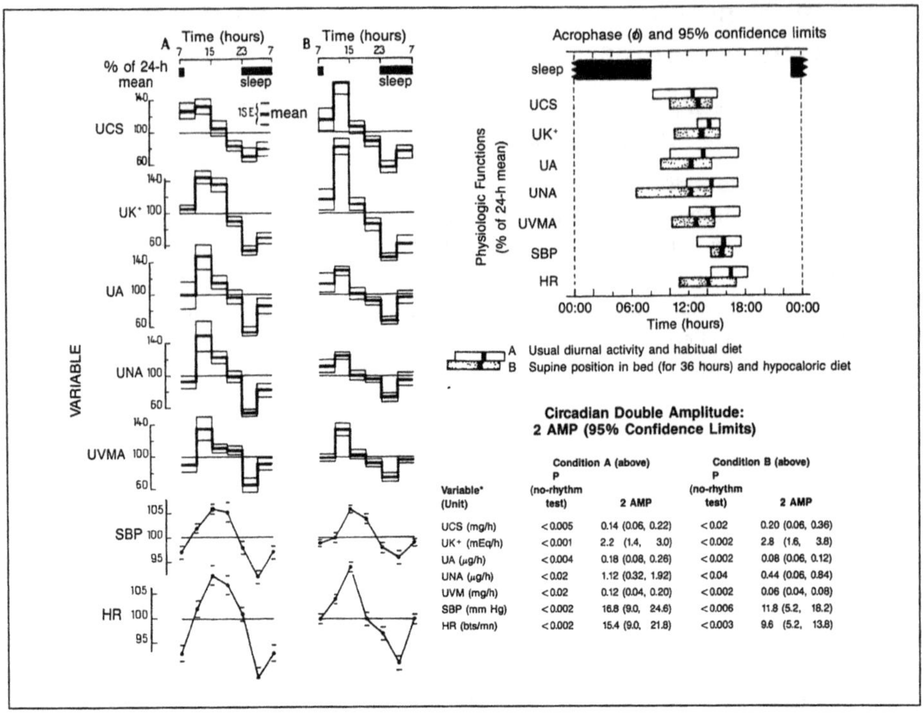

Circadian Double Amplitude: 2 AMP (95% Confidence Limits)

Variable* (Unit)	Condition A (above) P (no-rhythm test)	Condition A (above) 2 AMP	Condition B (above) P (no-rhythm test)	Condition B (above) 2 AMP
UCS (mg/h)	<0.005	0.14 (0.06, 0.22)	<0.02	0.20 (0.06, 0.36)
UK⁺ (mEq/h)	<0.001	2.2 (1.4, 3.0)	<0.002	2.8 (1.6, 3.8)
UA (μg/h)	<0.004	0.18 (0.08, 0.26)	<0.002	0.08 (0.06, 0.12)
UNA (μg/h)	<0.02	1.12 (0.32, 1.92)	<0.04	0.44 (0.06, 0.84)
UVM (mg/h)	<0.02	0.12 (0.04, 0.20)	<0.002	0.06 (0.04, 0.08)
SBP (mm Hg)	<0.002	16.8 (9.0, 24.6)	<0.006	11.8 (5.2, 18.2)
HR (bts/mn)	<0.002	15.4 (9.0, 21.8)	<0.003	9.6 (5.2, 13.8)

Fig. 1 Original data (left) and cosinor analyses (right) show that complete bedrest for 36-h and a 4-hourly hypocaloric diet do not abolish the circadian rhythmicity of physiologic functions such as systolic blood pressure (SBP), heart rate (HR), or the urinary excretion (U) of 17-hydroxycorticosteroid (CS), potassium (K^+), adrenaline (A), noradrenaline (NA) and vanilylmandelic acid (VMA), indicating that those variables are not directly dependent upon rest/activity cycles. Data and analyses from seven healthy adults from [36]).

— the availability of statistical procedures to analyze and model the biologic rhythms, and from them, to devise optimal dosage time patterns for specific individuals; and
— the availability of portable, programmable devices to administer therapy, e.g., by physiologic rate-adjusted cardiac pacemakers or drug pumps.

Such advances can be integrated as needed for the routine employment of chronobiologic methods in medical screening, diagnosis, prognosis, treatment and, most important, disease prevention. This challenge remains to be met, yet the importance of chronobiology in medicine, in light of the first three points listed above, can and will be illustrated here in the context of blood pressure assessment. The scope of chronobiology, however, is much broader. Thus, recent debates revolving around measuring cholesterol [39] may also benefit from a chronobiologic approach [28, 29, 43]. More than half of serious diseases and deaths occurring in middle-aged people could be prevented by changes in behavior. Three very important examples are smoking, a diet high in saturated fat, and our topic herein, deviant blood pressure.

Blood pressure measurements that miss the chronobiologic point

As an example of an application of chronobiology, health assessment of an individual should not rest only on a visit to the clinic. Visits are currently scheduled at a time convenient to both patient and physician, without taking into account the great variations that occur in all of our physiologic variables over a 24-h period, over a weekly period, and even over monthly and yearly periods. Since quite large variations take place in human blood pressure over 24-h periods, chronobiology is particularly pertinent to our way of handling blood pressure [3, 13, 15—18, 20, 24]. At present, (non-chronobiologic) blood pressure screening is usually based on casual measurements and the use of 24-h ambulatory cardiovascular monitoring is mostly restricted to cases posing diagnostic problems or to research.

Most health professionals and most of the general public ask only: What is your blood pressure? Official convention focuses upon "the" blood pressure, relying on casual measurements. Such measurements are recommended, among others, in the World Health Organization (WHO) Guidelines [6, 45, 49]. For a test of a mild blood pressure elevation (90—104 mmHg diastolic), without organ damage and "to provide a safe classification of patients", the International Society of Hypertension joins WHO in recommending the criterion of the average of two (casual) diastolic measurements. If the average of these is 90 mmHg or above, further measurement pairs on at least two more days over four weeks are recommended. If the average values of these are above 100 mmHg, drug treatment is to start (with a delay of treatment of one month). If in turn the means of two measurements on two occasions during the first 4 weeks are below 100 mmHg, further measurements over 3 months and behavioral intervention, but not drug treatment, are recommended. If the overall average is now above 95 mmHg, drug treatment is recommended (with a delay of four months after the first visit). If the average is below 95 mmHg, behavioral intervention is prescribed with further observations over 3 months (and, if indicated, drug treatment is instituted with a delay of 7 months). During all of this span, it is left to the individual's and/or the physician's convenience or experience to pick the intervals between visits and thus the times of day and of the week for the office visita.

Implicit in the convention of the WHO guidelines are the assumptions that **a)** variations in blood pressure and heart rate are the effect of changes in posture, responses to meals, exercise or other stimuli, emotional or physical, and that b) a short span of sitting or lying down of, say, 5 min or so, in the setting of a medical office, is a better standardization than no standardization whatsoever, in order to somehow "control" the stimuli of daily life and thus to approximate the (true) blood pressure.

The recommendation of only 24-h ambulatory blood pressure and heart rate monitoring does not take full advantage of the data in light of chronobiologic facts. Assumption a) above is the excuse for refraining from a consideration of the dynamics of blood pressure. These continue to be regarded as trivial effects of changes in posture, notably exercise and other stimuli. With most ambulatory monitoring instruments, it remains necessary to stop what one does physically during the actual measurement, but with this qualification, assumption b) is changed into endeavor c) namely into the aim of obtaining a reflection of average pressure in "real life" by a 24-h, and perhaps also by a daytime and nighttime average pressure. Since all variations are treated as responses to external stimuli, one does not do much if anything about them, except perhaps for asking that changes in posture, meals, etc., be recorded. In debates about nonchronobiologic ambulatory 24-h records vs casual measurements, it should be realized that both approaches present serious shortcomings. Built-in rhythms and their characteristics such as a measure of the extent of regular 24-h change (circadian amplitude) and of the timing of high values (acrophase) are ignored. Definitions of some rhythm characteristics are provided in Fig. 2. That three of these characteristics of heart rate are partly inherited is

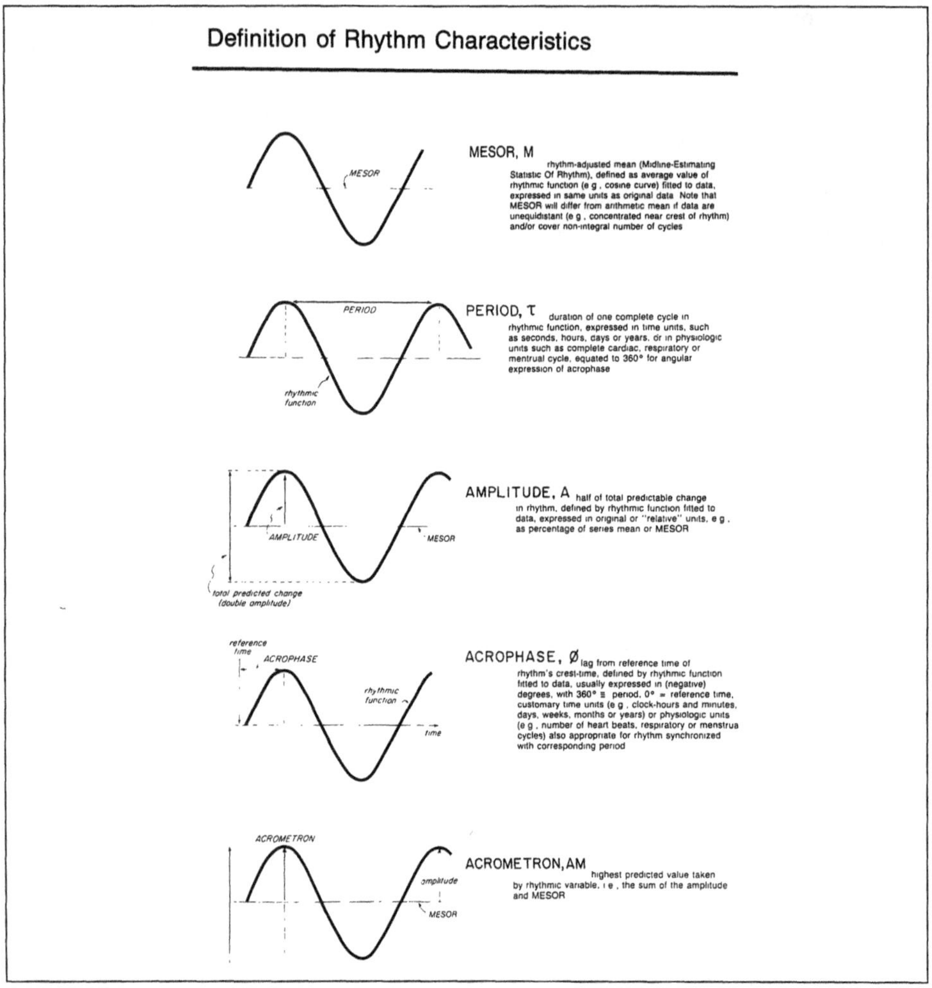

Fig. 2 Definition of rhythm characteristics. (© Halberg, 1981.)

shown by studies on twins reared apart [26]). Indirect evidence for the endogenicity of the human heart rate and blood pressure rhythms is available from their free-running with natural periods differing from environmental ones in social isolation [2] and under certain other conditions [21]. The fact is also demonstrated that responses to external stimuli depend upon the circadian rhythm stage of partly endogenous circadian rhythms. Cases in point are the blood pressure change in response to the immersion of the hand in ice water [22] or simply reading aloud (unpublished data).

Table 1. Chronobiologic approaches include descriptive statistics and inferential opportunities

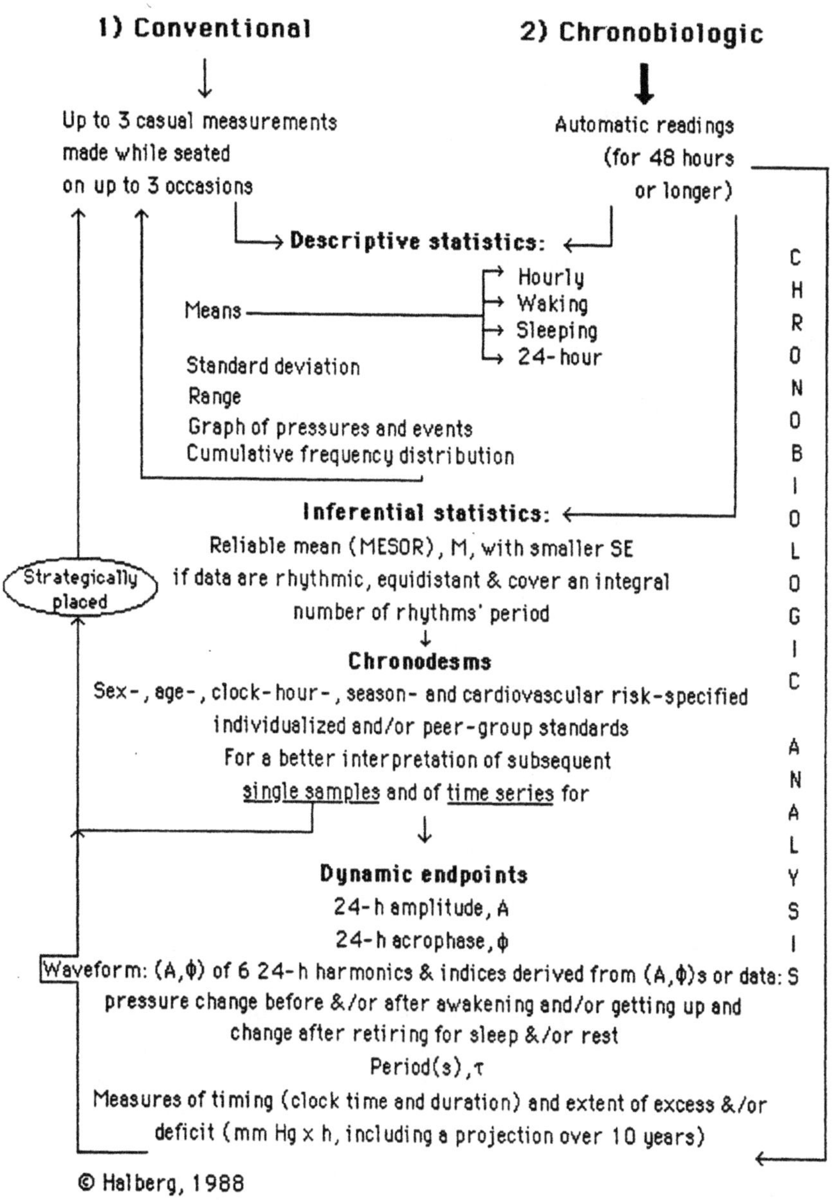

Table 2. Chronobiologists compute novel dynamic characteristics that may work (in providing information of medical interst) when the conventional mean and dispersion indices fail, as for instance in cardiovascular disease risk detection on groups of newborns monitored during the first two days of life. The MESOR, computed by curve-fitting to systematically obtained data, also is usually more reliable than the mean of casual measurements.

Chronobiologic endpoints, e.g., of human blood pressure (© Halberg, 1981)

1. MESOR, M: Midline-Estimating Statistic **O**f Rhythm, based on systematic sampling, taking dynamics into account; replaces mean of casual measurements at arbitrary times.

2. Range, R:	total partial, e.g., 90%, 50% circadian range (e.g., of hourly mean values)
3. Standard deviation, SD	
4. Trends:	Intercept and slope of linear trend; coefficients of higher-order (e.g., quadratic of cubic) polynomials
5. Periodicities:	Rhythm characteristics, e.g. circadian amplitude, A circadian acrophase, ∅ circadian waveform, (A,∅) of harmonics
6. Non-periodic, non-tred components	Parameters describing shape of spectrum, eg., high frequency dominant over low frequency or vice versa

All of the above endpoints may or may not be deviant. Other endpoints, related to cumulative deviation, are:

7. Excess:	short-term: extent: hyperbaric index duration and timing of elvation long-term projection; e.g., 10-year excess
8. Deficit:	short-term: extent: hypobaric index duration and timing of deficit long-term projection; e.g., 10-year deficit

The cost-effectiveness of non-chronobiologic 24-h ambulatory monitoring has been scrutinized thus far without considering what can be learned from the spontaneous and reactive blood pressure and heart rate dynamics. The investment in new machines has not been accepted as justified on the basis of an improved 24-h average or of averages for fractions of the day, such as the waking, sleeping, or other spans. Thus far, the health profession's response has been guarded. Whatever their data source, whether they rely upon conventional manual or ambulatory automatic measurements, most health care personnel continue to act according to what "the", or "the average" blood pressure of a given person is. This inquiry only into "the", or "the average" blood pressure is insufficient when a more reliably defined mean and added dynamic information can be extracted from the same data. There *is* indeed another alternative to the guidelines of WHO [6, 45, 49], one that adds a new dimension to blood pressure assessment: the *chronobiologic* approach, as summarized in Tables 1 and 2. The message of this note is that there is a need for chronobiologic monitoring in order to improve the sensitivity of screening, the reliability of diagnosis, the accuracy of prognosis and the timing and efficacy of treatment. But first and foremost, there is a need to emphasize approaches for the prevention of high blood pressure.

Chronobiology of blood pressure

Blood pressure chronobiology focuses upon both the predictable and the global dynamics of *the variation in* this variable and detects blood pressure deviations that are likely to be missed if one measures at only one or another convenient time of day. As in the case of the 24-h profile, some treated or untreated cases of high blood pressure show elevations at times when casual measurements are not taken as a rule, as for instance in the evening or during sleep (Fig. 3), [18]. To detect such cases, systematic manual or preferably automatic around-the-clock measurement is required. Chronobiologic evaluation also reveals that a 24-h profile does not suffice for a first screen. Thus, in a majority of cases, statistically significant differences are found in the 24-h average of two 24-h profiles repeated within a few weeks, even when each profile is based on relatively dense (7.5-min.) measurements. A 48-h average, more reliable than the 24-h average, is not necessarily the sole and major merit of the chronobiologic approach. An important point in the chronobiologic approach is the need to start any screening with around-the-clock measurements rather than carrying out such a monitoring profile only in the case of suspicion of deviant blood pressure. The contribution by chronobiology is, further, the ability, by the methods of this new science, to account for a usually large circadian variation, encountered over 24-h under ambulatory conditions, by resolving part of the overall variation as predictably rhythmic, and by assessing any changes in rhythm characteristics while also assessing any cumulative excess or deficit. By the fit of cosine functions with periods of 24 h and submultiples thereof, computer software resolves the characteristics of variation, as shown in Fig. 2. Chronobiologic methods can be applied to measurements taken manually, with a sampling schedule shown to be useful for a given purpose and adopted with a discipline that has to be taught in the context of early formal as well as adult education. The use of presently available modern automatic, fully ambulatory recording systems, (Fig. 4) however, greatly facilitates data collection and, in combinaton with proper software, renders the chronobiologic approach to blood pressure variation much more practical than reliance only upon a few casual measurements.

Methods

If one measures any of the body's physical variables continuously or at frequent intervals around-the-clock (preferably for at least 2 days), the plotted data invariably show rises and falls that have an obvious 24-h periodicity, as shown on the left of Fig. 1. By submitting these data to mathematical analysis, one can pull out the fundamental frequency and plot it as a sinusoidal function. The cosine curve can be used for convenience. From this plotted cosine, one can see the amplitude of the fundamental variability and the timing

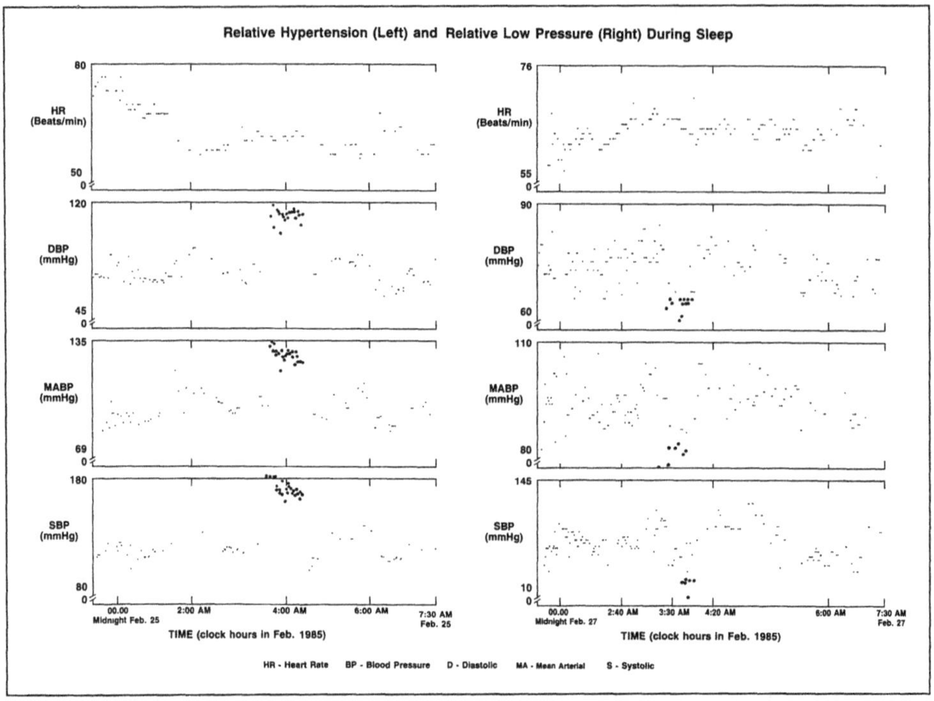

Fig. 3. Unsolved problem: A rise in systolic mean arterial and diastolic blood pressure (BP) at night, for about 50 min, is seen on the left, in rows 2—4, in the absence of corresponding changes in heart rate (top row). This fact suggests that the changes in blood pressure are not due to changes in movement. In the absence of a concomitant electroencephalographic tracing, one can only speculate as to whether the subject had a panic episode in a dream. If indeed he dreamt, one would also have to account for the mechanisms that under certain conditions, in a dream, bring about an increase in BP (left) and under others a decrease in BP (right), as observed during another sleep episode [18] on the same subject. Whether the changes noted, (the hypertensive episode in particular), are related to the medication (Nardil [Rx]) which the subject took, must be explored. The changes in BP may reflect states-of-mind of interest to those concerned about brain-heart interactions. The 2.325 values/variable monitored on this man (not all shown) allow the isolation in his BP spectrum of 1.6- and 1.8-h components. Certainly, the data during the 50-min episode exceed the range of change usually encountered for BP ultradians. The 50-min duration of the episode is in keeping with the possibility that it is an exacerbation lasting for half the duration of an underlying ultradian (~ 1.7-h) rhythmicity. Such episodes would not be detected by sole reliance upon daytime measurements. The episode may pose a threat if it is maintained for longer than half of an ultradian cycle (about 50 min), a period actually isolated for this particular subject and/or if it represents more than an isolated episode in the particular BP series examined. (From Wendt H., et al. (1986). Circadian and ultradian blood pressure rhythmometry also reveals nocturnal episodic elevation of BP but not of heart rate J. Minn, Acad, Sci, 51: 14; © Halberg, 1981.)

of the peak(s) and valley(s) and can also plot the midline for the variability. These mathematically calculated features, Fig. 2, some shown on the right of Fig. 1, are often sensitive indicators of present or potential disease that cannot be found in a few casual measurements, e.g., of blood pressure and heart rate, taken at an arbitrary time in a physician's office. In many cases, this chronobiologic approach yields meaningful information when casual readings do not.

Hardware: Until recently, the taking of blood pressure readings every 10 min or so around-the-clock on a large scale for screening has not been clinically practical. Now, automatic blood pressure recording equipment has become available. The stationary equipment is good. Increasingly smaller, wearable equipment for fully ambulatory recording is being developed [18]. Today, extensively used instruments include, in addition to the nearly noiseless and hence less sleep-disturbing miniaturized ambulatory monitor (Fig. 4), manufactured by Colin Medical Instruments (Komaki, Japan); the pioneer

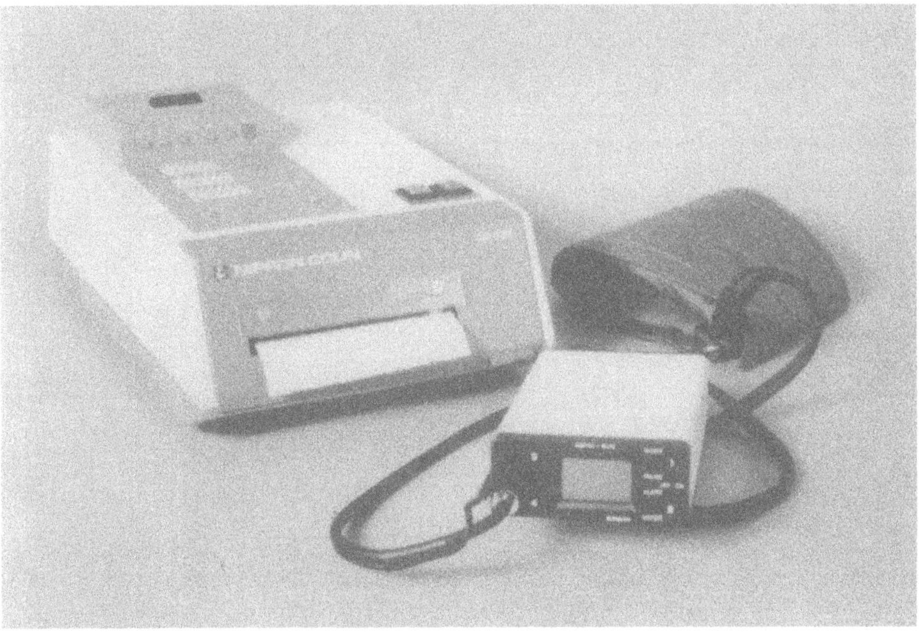

Fig. 4 Illustrative ambulatory monitor manufactured by Colin Medical Instruments (South Plainfield, New Jersey, USA) in front. Larger data analyzer providing printout and amenable to connection with a personal computer shown in back. For details, see text.

Pressurometer III (Del Mar Avionics, Irvine, California, USA); the Ambulatory Blood Pressure Monitor (Instruments for Cardiac Research, Liverpool, New York, USA, a subsidiary of Squibb); and the Acutracker Model 103C, (Oxford Medilog, Clearwater, Florida, USA). In their present form, the large-scale, long-term use of these monitors is difficult and costly. The Pressurometer demands the placement of electrodes that are a nuisance for the patient and, after long-term use, may cause skin rashes; the Squibb requires battery changes; and the Colin requires CO_2 cartridges. There are also limitations to data storage in solid-state memory, although the Colin holds over 600 measurements that can easily accomodate more than one week of data with a sampling interval of 20 min. The Colin instrument has the added merit of providing both auscultatory (a) and oscillometric (o) measurements, first and foremost as backup, when one or the other method fails, e.g., in the case of movement or acoustical noise. Moreover, the a-o difference is in itself, under certain conditions, a rhythmic phenomenon and may provide complementary information. With the qualification that it is subject to movement artifact, the Colin-type of equipment begins to give us data that represent real life and take into account what happens to the blood pressure during most of the range of life experiences from different stages of sleep to various kinds of experience in wakefulness on weekends as well as weekdays.

Recordings over at least 48 h (Tables 3 and 4), and preferably over a week's time show the effects of emotional, physical and *time* impactors that cannot be assessed in single

Table 3. Percentage of statistically significant differences in circadian rhythm characteristics between two consecutive 24-h cardiovascular* profiles

site	N	MESOR			Amplitude			Acrophase		
		%**		P+	%		P	%		P
SBP										
MStP	36	25.0	(8.3)	>0.5	19.4	(11.1)	≦0.05	27.8	(5.5)	≦0.01
K	170	17.7	(9.4)		7.1	(7.1)		7.1	(4.1)	
MAP										
MStP	36	27.8	(13.9)	>0.1	16.7	(13.9)	>0.1	22.2	(11.1)	≦0.001
K	170	20.6	(5.9)		10.0	(6.5)		4.7	(6.5)	
DBP										
MStP	36	33.3	(2.8)	≦0.05	16.7	(8.3)	>0.2	19.4	(16.7)	≦0.001
K	170	15.3	(7.6)		8.2	(5.9)		4.1	(4.7)	
HR										
MStP	36	27.8	(5.6)	>0.1	16.7	(2.8)	>0.1	11.1	(11.1)	>0.1
K	170	15.9	(2.4)		7.1	(7.1)		6.5	(4.7)	

* Of systolic (S), mean arterial (MA) and diastolic (D) blood pressure (BP) in Minneapolis-St. Paul, Minnesota (MStP, urban USA, and Komaki (K), suburban Japan.

** Number in ( ) is percentage of differences between series of borderline statistical significance (0.10 > P > 0.05).

\+ Inter-site comparison.

Table 4. Comparison of circadian characteristics in 2 consecutive 24-h cardiovascular profiles of Japanese adults of both genders

Variable	P from parameter test	Total	MESOR Increase	Decrease	Same
	≦ 0.05	30	10	20	
SBP	> 0.05 ≦ 0.10	16	7	9	
	> 0.10	124	64	60	
	≦ 0.05	35	10	25	
MAP	> 0.05 ≦ 0.10	10	4	6	
	> 0.10	125	54	70	1
	≦ 0.05	26	8	19	
DBP	> 0.05; ≦ 0.10	13	3	10	
	> 0.10	131	59	72	
	≦ 0.05	27	15	12	
HR	> 0.05; ≦ 0.10	4	3	1	
	> 0.10	139	56	83	

Variable	P from parameter test*	Amplitude			Acrophase			
		Total	Increase	Decrease	Total	Advance	Delay	Same
SBP	≦ 0.05	12	7	5	12	3	9	
	> 0.05; ≦ 0.10	12	6	6	7	3	4	
	> 0.10	146	70	76	151	78	70	3
MAP	≦ 0.05	17	9	8	8	4	4	
	> 0.05; ≦ 0.10	11	6	5	11	5	6	
	> 0.10	142	63	79	151	66	84	
DBP	≦ 0.05	14	8	6	7	4	3	
	> 0.05; ≦ 0.10	10	7	3	8	2	6	
	> 0.10	146	72	74	155	82	69	4
HR	≦ 0.05	12	7	5	11	4	7	
	> 0.05; ≦ 0.10	12	8	4	8	5	3	
	> 0.10	146	72	74	151	70	76	5

* Of the equality of the MESOR, amplitude or acrophase of systolic (S), mean arterial (MA) and diastolic (D) blood pressure (BP) in the two 24-h recordings. Second 24-h recording started immediately after first. Table shows that numerically, MESOR decreases appear to be more frequent than increases. χ^2 tests did not reveal differences in incidence of MESOR increase vs decrease, considering the three categories of statistical significance in comparing the two profiles. Similarly, no difference in increase vs decrease was found for the circadian amplitude and no difference in delay vs. advance was found for the circadian acrophase.

readings as, for instance, the episodes of relatively high or low pressure occurring during sleep (Fig. 3), [18]. During one night, the blood pressure rose for ~ 50 min, without a concomitant change in heart rate. In another night, in the same subject [18], an episode of a relatively low blood pressure occurred, as can be seen on the right of Fig. 3 [18]. It is important to know the duration of episodes of such hyper- or hypotension and what their extent might be, whenever they occur. A chronobiologic approach is particularly rewarding when it uncovers events that are not seen in casual measurements.

Analyses: chronobiologic blood pressure assessment relies on both parametric and non-parametric approaches. For either approach, the reference standard is best derived from data of living age- and sex-matched peers, as a superior standard, as compared to the insurance statistics relating blood pressure to mortality of a previous generation (Fig. 5). The fit of a cosine curve, e.g., with a period of 24 h, serves for a "zero amplitude" or "no rhythm" test (Fig. 6). When time-varying reference limits are unavailable, the excess can be referred to the sum of the circadian amplitude and the rhythm-adjusted mean or MESOR. This sum, the acrometron, (Fig. 2) based upon around-the-clock sampling on healthy peers, is preferred to an arbitrary limit such as 140 and 90 mmHg for systolic and diastolic blood pressure, respectively. The reference limits used here solely for illustrative purposes are derived from only 39 clinically healthy ambulatory North American men, each monitored at 7.5-min-intervals around-the-clock. This sample size

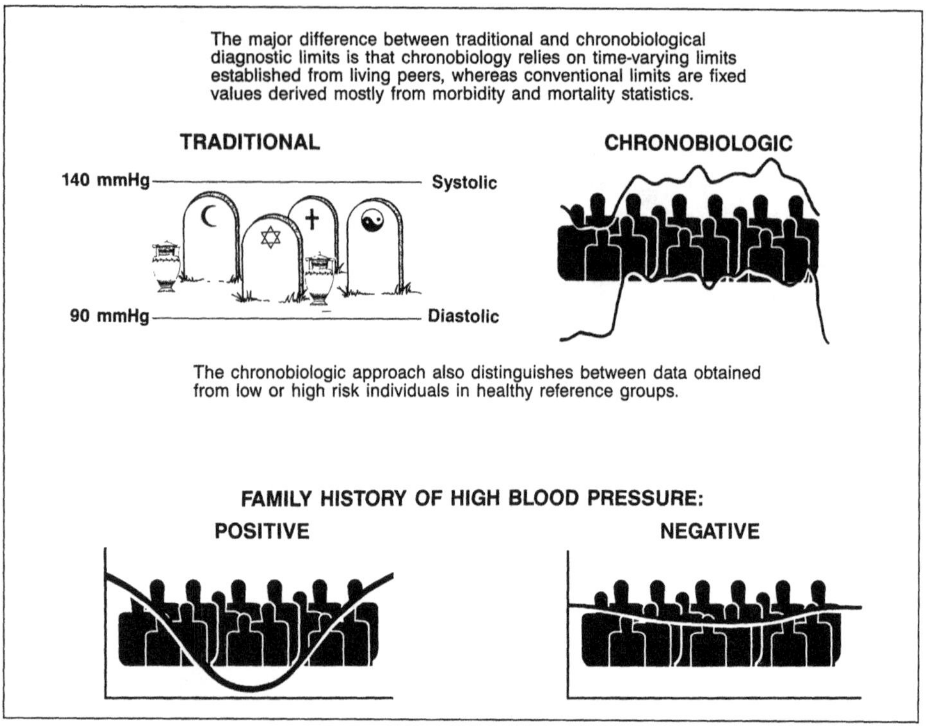

Fig. 5. A 24-h profile interpreted conventionally must not be confused with the chronobiologic approach. The automatic monitoring is usually *added* in the case of suspicion of high blood pressure by some internists. In a chronobiologic procedure, automatic blood pressure monitoring is the *initial* approach to diagnosis. The chronobiologic procedure starts with *48-h* rather than *24-h* monitoring and continues monitoring, as need be, rather than monitoring for an arbitrarily fixed span. But the principal difference between the conventional 24-h profile and a chronobiologic approach lies in the concepts and methods of parametric and nonparametric analyses. (© Halberg, 1988.)

of a reference standard is to be replaced by one based on several thousand series to be obtained by non-invasive 48-h monitoring at 15-min to 1-h intervals on both genders from now-planned international studies. The recommended monitoring span has been extended to a minimum of 48-h, to be continued for a week if need be, so that a decision about the institution of non-drug or drug therapy is not delayed for months, as in the case of the recommendations by WHO, among others.

Sphygmochrons: monitoring profiles over time for comparison with peers Special forms have been designed to report the blood pressure status of patients chronobiologically (Figs. 7, 8). These forms focus on circadian features of blood pressure variability, such as the MESOR, amplitude, and acrophase (Fig. 2), and also take into consideration the waveform of the blood pressure rhythm by assessing the 24-h and other ultradian components of variability. Results from the fit of harmonics are given on the back of the sphygmochrons, except that those from the fit of a 12-h cosine curve are also shown on the face of the long form, as seen in Fig. 8. Indices of blood pressure change before and/or just after awakening and/or getting up and after retiring for sleep and/or rest can also be derived from the data or from the computed waveform approximated by harmonics.

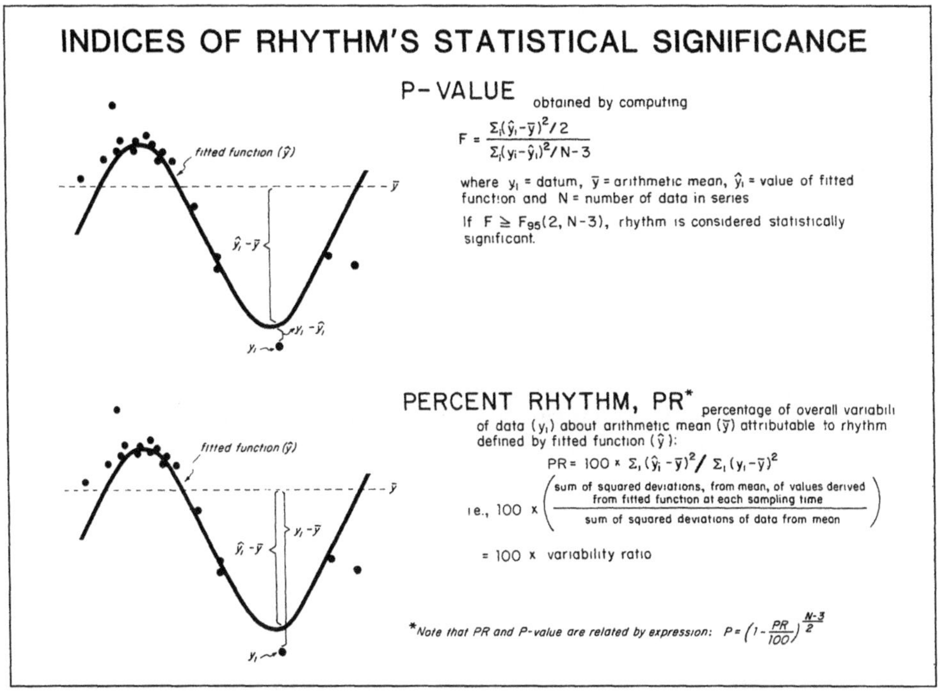

Fig. 6 Parametric blood pressure assessment involves the fit of a mathematical model consisting of a set of cosine curves (only one shown on graph) for both the detection of a rhythm and the description of the parameters in Fig. 2. (© Halberg, 1973.)

In addition, indices of blood pressure excess (or deficit) are evaluated by comparing the patient's own record with the characteristics of healthy peers. These forms assist in the proper detection and treatment of patients and can be used as a convenient tool in clinical practice. This data summary chart, developed by us, has been dubbed a *sphygmochron,* a blood pressure and heart rate monitoring profile over time (18). It represents a computer comparison of a person's data with clinically healthy peer group limits. These sphygmochrons describe a number of chronobiologic characteristics that result from an approach summarized in Table 2.

Results

When one records blood pressure around-the-clock, one can observe even larger changes than those that occur from moment to moment, both in systolic and diastolic readings. Figure 9 shows the distribution of blood pressures of a clinically healthy woman, ranging systolically from 73 to 153 mmHg and diastolically from 51 to 91 mmHg. The overlap between the two distributions is shown as black dots. It may be foolhardy to disregard circadian changes which are as large as the difference between the systolic and diastolic pressure or even larger, as Fig. 9 documents. Healthy individuals can have an average dispersion of 60 mmHg in systolic and 50 mmHg in diastolic pressure. By submitting

MONITORING PROFILE OVER TIME; COMPUTER COMPARISON WITH PEER GROUP LIMITS

SPHYGMOCHRON™-S (short form)

BLOOD PRESSURE (BP) AND RELATED CARDIOVASCULAR SUMMARY.

(Circadian Sphygmochron, from *sphygmo-*, of or relating to the circulation, notably blood pressure, as well as pulse and *chronos*, time)

Name ______ Patient # ESCH 8610 No of Profiles 1

Age 63 Sex (M) F Monitoring From October 8 To October 24, 19 86

TIME OF AWAKENING (A) 06^{30} (~ 06^{30}) **FALLING ASLEEP (S)** 23^{00} (~ 23^{00})
Day of Profile (Habitually) Day of Profile (Habitually)

Rx: Dyazide 1 p.o., qA & q 15:30; Hydralazine 75 mg pp. qA & q 15:30;
Aldomet 260 mg p.o., q 15:30; Proventil 2 mg pp., qA, q 15:30 & qS;
Theo-Dur 300 mg p.o., qA, q 15:30 & qS.

COMMENTS[1,2] ______

CHRONOBIOLOGIC CHARACTERISTICS

	SYSTOLIC BP (mmHg)		DIASTOLIC BP (mmHg)		HEART RATE (bpm)	
	PATIENT VALUE	NUMBER OF SD* FROM PEER GROUP MEAN	PATIENT VALUE	NUMBER OF SD* FROM PEER GROUP MEAN	PATIENT VALUE	NUMBER OF SD* FROM PEER GROUP MEAN
ADJUSTED 24-h MEAN (MESOR)	145.0	+ 2.60	88.3	+ 1.85	83.7	+ 0.96
PREDICTABLE CHANGE (DOUBLE AMPLITUDE)	19.5	− 0.46	19.8	+ 0.11	6.3	− 1.53
TIMING OF OVERALL HIGH VALUES (ACROPHASE) (hr:min)**	17:00	1.43 L	16:32	1.52 L	16:56	1.76 L

*SD = STANDARD DEVIATION; ** L MEANS LATER; E EARLIER

	SYSTOLIC BP	DIASTOLIC BP	HEART RATE
PERCENT TIME OF ELEVATION	64.5%	23.5%	4.3%
TIMING OF EXCESS	22:43 (hr:min)	17:04 (hr:min)	02:15 (hr:min)
EXTENT OF EXCESS DURING 24 HOURS	132 (mmHg x hour)	32 (mmHg x hour)	< 1 (bpm x hour)
10-YEAR CUMULATIVE EXCESS	483 (mmHg x hour) (in 1,000's units)	118 (mmHg x hour) (in 1,000's units)	< 1 (bpm x hour) (in 1,000's units)

INTERVENTION NEEDED

- [ ] No
- [x] Yes [ ] Drug [x] Non-Drug

MORE MONITORING NEEDED

- [ ] Annually
- [x] As soon as possible
- [ ] Other specify ______

PREPARED BY [signature] DATE 86 / 10 / 25

1) Unusually long standing or lying-down during waking unusual activity, such as exercise, emotional loads, or schedule changes, e.g., shiftwork, etc., 2) Salt, calories, kind and amount, other, etc

Chronobiology Laboratories, University of Minnesota, 5-187 Lyon Labs., 420 Washington Ave S.E., Minneapolis, MN 55455. For questions, call F Halberg or G Cornelissen at 612-624-6976

Fig. 7. The short form of the sphygmochron-S, a monitoring profile over time for a computer comparison of a person's data with peer group reference standards (and also with any available prior personalized reference standard). (© Halberg, 1981.)

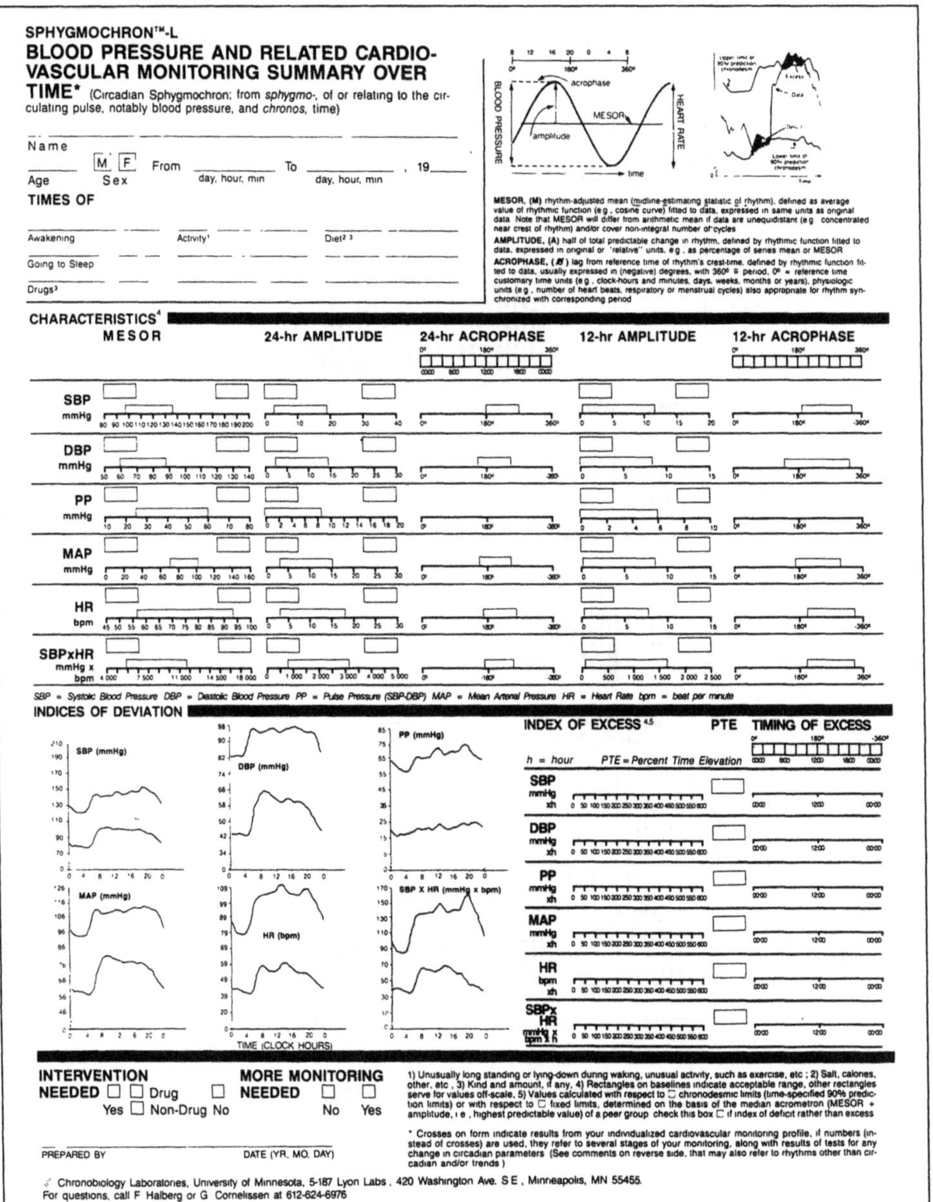

SPHYGMOCHRON™-L

BLOOD PRESSURE AND RELATED CARDIO-VASCULAR MONITORING SUMMARY OVER TIME* (Circadian Sphygmochron; from *sphygmo-*, of or relating to the circulating pulse, notably blood pressure, and *chronos*, time)

Name

Age Sex M F From (day, hour, min) To (day, hour, min) , 19

TIMES OF

Awakening Activity[1] Diet[2,3]

Going to Sleep

Drugs[3]

MESOR, (M) rhythm-adjusted mean (midline-estimating statistic of rhythm), defined as average value of rhythmic function (e g , cosine curve) fitted to data, expressed in same units as original data Note that MESOR will differ from arithmetic mean if data are unequidistant (e g concentrated near crest of rhythm) and/or cover non-integral number of cycles

AMPLITUDE, (A) half of total predictable change in rhythm, defined by rhythmic function fitted to data, expressed in original or "relative" units, e g , as percentage of series mean or MESOR

ACROPHASE, (Ø) lag from reference time of rhythm's crest-time, defined by rhythmic function fitted to data, usually expressed in (negative) degrees, with 360° ≡ period, 0° = reference time customary time units (e g , clock-hours and minutes, days, weeks, months or years), physiologic units (e g , number of heart beats, respiratory or menstrual cycles) also appropriate for rhythm synchronized with corresponding period

CHARACTERISTICS[4]

	MESOR	24-hr AMPLITUDE	24-hr ACROPHASE	12-hr AMPLITUDE	12-hr ACROPHASE
SBP mmHg					
DBP mmHg					
PP mmHg					
MAP mmHg					
HR bpm					
SBPxHR mmHg x bpm					

SBP = Systolic Blood Pressure DBP = Diastolic Blood Pressure PP = Pulse Pressure (SBP-DBP) MAP = Mean Arterial Pressure HR = Heart Rate bpm = beat per minute

INDICES OF DEVIATION

INDEX OF EXCESS[4,5] **PTE** **TIMING OF EXCESS**

h = hour PTE = Percent Time Elevation

	INDEX OF EXCESS	PTE	TIMING OF EXCESS
SBP mmHg xh			
DBP mmHg xh			
PP mmHg xh			
MAP mmHg xh			
HR bpm xh			
SBPx HR mmHg x bpm x h			

INTERVENTION NEEDED ☐ Yes ☐ Drug ☐ Non-Drug ☐ No

MORE MONITORING NEEDED ☐ No ☐ Yes

1) Unusually long standing or lying-down during waking, unusual activity, such as exercise, etc ; 2) Salt, calories, other, etc , 3) Kind and amount, if any, 4) Rectangles on baselines indicate acceptable range, other rectangles serve for values off-scale, 5) Values calculated with respect to ☐ chronodesmic limits (time-specified 90% prediction limits) or with respect to ☐ fixed limits, determined on the basis of the median acrometron (MESOR + amplitude, i e , highest predictable value) of a peer group check this box ☐ if index of deficit rather than excess

* Crosses on form indicate results from your individualized cardiovascular monitoring profile, if numbers (instead of crosses) are used, they refer to several stages of your monitoring, along with results of tests for any change in circadian parameters (See comments on reverse side, that may also refer to rhythms other than circadian and/or trends)

PREPARED BY DATE (YR, MO, DAY)

© Chronobiology Laboratories, University of Minnesota, 5-187 Lyon Labs , 420 Washington Ave. S E , Minneapolis, MN 55455. For questions, call F Halberg or G Cornelissen at 612-624-6976

Fig. 8. The long form of the sphygmochron-L, including results of both a 24-h and 12-h cosine curve fit and time-specified peer-group reference limits. (© Halberg, 1981.)

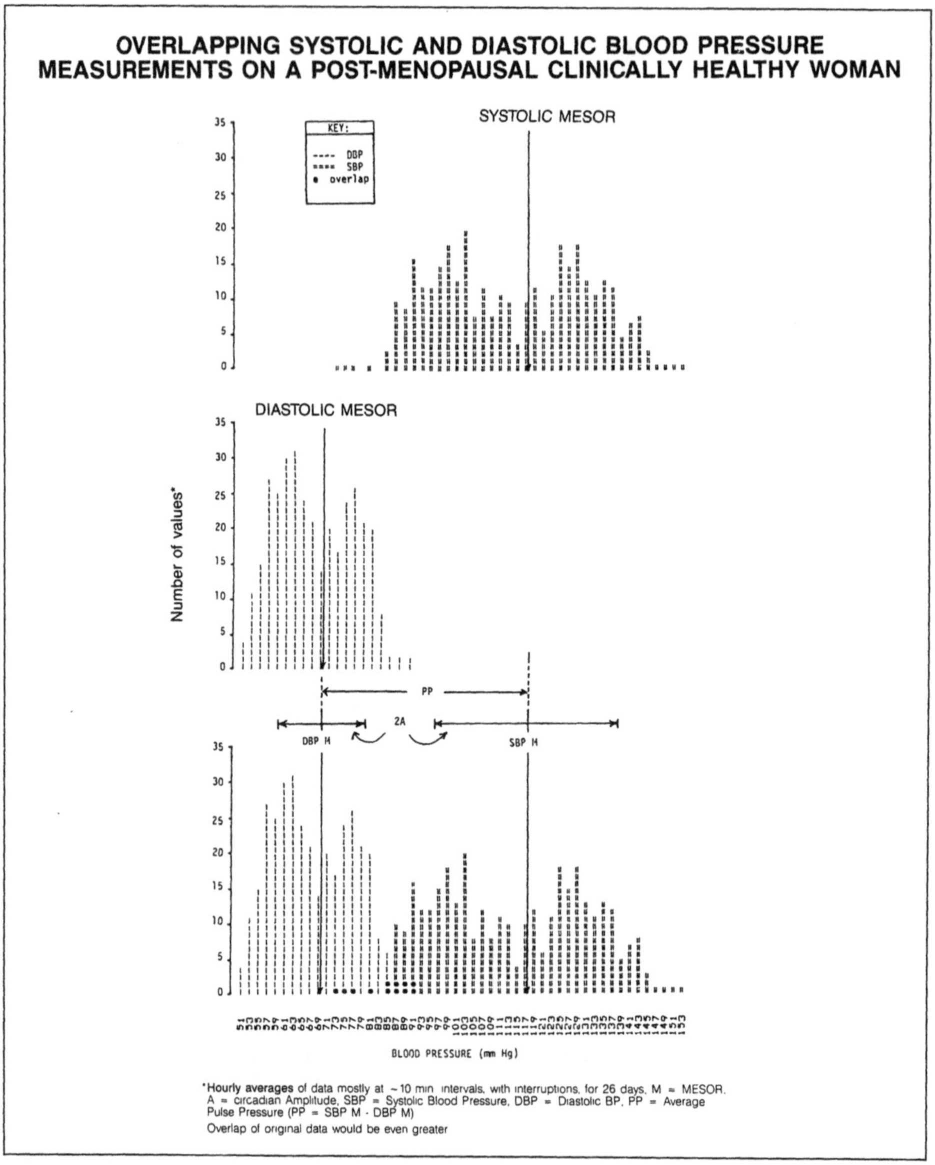

Fig. 9. Fully ambulatory automatic monitoring of a clinically apparently healthy woman (EH, age 64 years) reveals a wide range of cardiovascular variability. Questions about *the blood pressure* (BP) of a patient are rhetorical. The cost-effective recording and interpretation of variation are mandatory. Note bimodal rather than bell-shaped distribution of systolic and diastolic BP of the subject and the large overlap between the two distributions. (© Halberg, 1981.)

these data to a computer program, one can plot not only the time-course of the blood pressure, but one can also derive characteristics of an approximating curve (consisting of a fundamental such as a 24-h cosine plus, e.g., five harmonics) [20]. This curve for the individual can then be compared with upper and lower limits of a standard profile for a large peer group [20]. If the individual plot strays outside of the limits of the peer group at a given point in the 24 h, this may be termed an excess as defined for that person with respect to the peer group. If, for example, the patient's plot is above the upper limit of the peer group for, say 2 h by 10 mmHg, then the area between the curve and the limit represents the pressure x time excess. To get the area accurately, it can be integrated by computer. Therefore, even if the person is normotensive for 22 h of the day, there will be a 2-h x 10 mmHg excess day after day. Over time, this excess could explain possible increases in morbidity and mortality. Replotting this curve after taking corrective action (drugs, sodium restriction or addition where indicated, etc.) will adequately show the results of the therapy, as compared to sole reliance upon measurements at office visits. Based on the studies done using the chronobiologic approach to blood pressure recording and analysis, it has become clear that many people are being treated for high blood pressure who need not be [18] and that there are probably many others who should receive treatment but whose blood pressure elevation has not been detected by present methods.

False positive diagnoses: That the traditional approach is unsatisfactory can be suggested on the basis of a scholarly analysis of data published by Wilcox et al. [48[. These authors raise the question whether clinical practice should be based on the results of clinical trials and provide an answer in the negative. On the basis of the same results from these same clinical trials, the authors of another paper instead advocate the use of a "smorgasbord" of drugs [34]. Moreover, whereas Wilcox et al. [48] emphasize the discrepancies in the

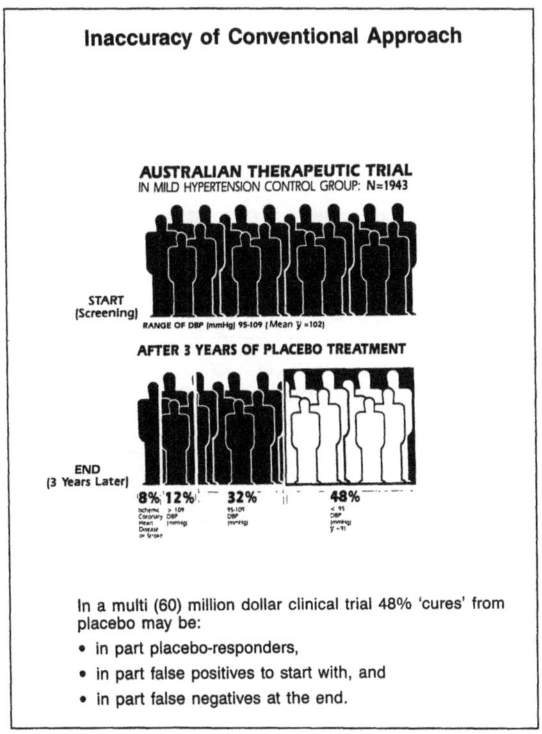

Fig. 10. The large proportion in clinical trials of "placebo responders" may be explained in part by entering individuals with "office" or "white coat" hypertension, i. e., by false-positive diagnoses, relying on one or a few casual BP measurements. (© Halberg, 1987.)

results from different large-scale clinical trials, the title of the paper by Pötschke-Langer and Apfelbach [34] reads "Mild hypertension — toward an international-national consensus". The chronobiologically unacceptable design of the reviewed studies may be considered.

More specifically, the outcome of large-scale clinical trials such as the Australian Therapeutic Trial in Mild Hypertension reflects the situation best. As shown in Fig. 10, out of nearly 2000 individuals in this study who received a placebo, almost half responded to this "treatment", most of them within less than a year [18]. The high percentage of responders to placebo (or responders to medical attention in other studies) renders it likely that "office-hypertension", associated with the excitement of one or a few visits to a physician's office leads to the entry into large-scale studies of many false-positive cases. This point is also apparent from Fig. 11.

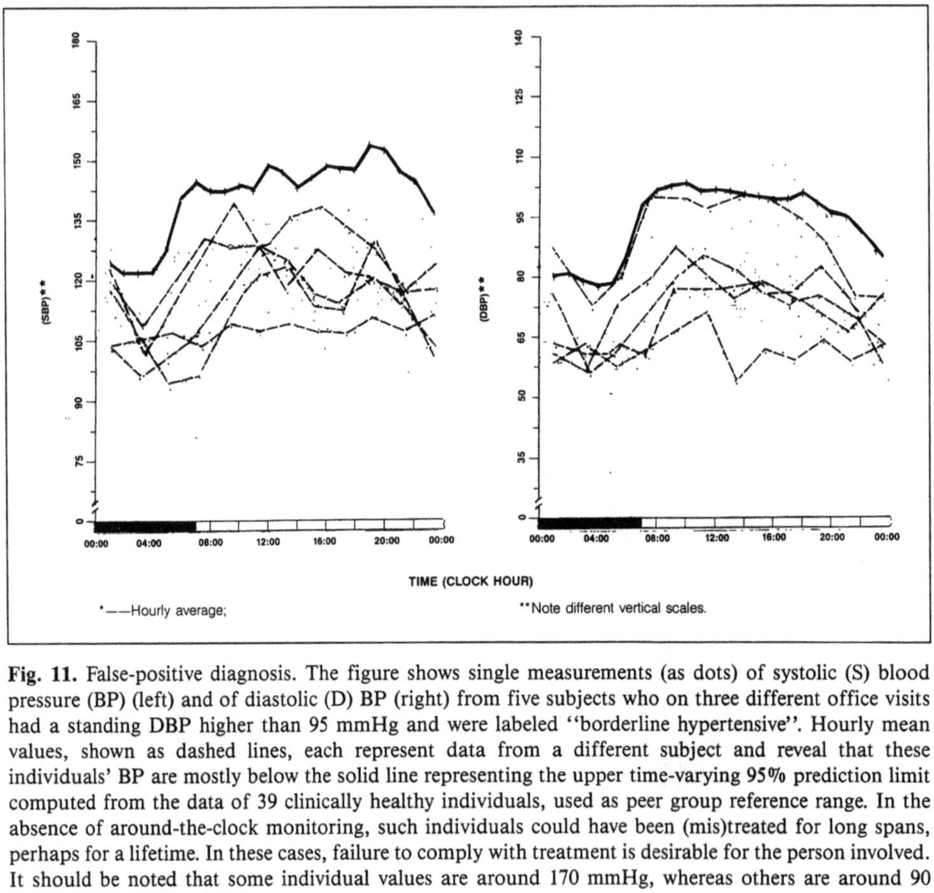

Fig. 11. False-positive diagnosis. The figure shows single measurements (as dots) of systolic (S) blood pressure (BP) (left) and of diastolic (D) BP (right) from five subjects who on three different office visits had a standing DBP higher than 95 mmHg and were labeled "borderline hypertensive". Hourly mean values, shown as dashed lines, each represent data from a different subject and reveal that these individuals' BP are mostly below the solid line representing the upper time-varying 95% prediction limit computed from the data of 39 clinically healthy individuals, used as peer group reference range. In the absence of around-the-clock monitoring, such individuals could have been (mis)treated for long spans, perhaps for a lifetime. In these cases, failure to comply with treatment is desirable for the person involved. It should be noted that some individual values are around 170 mmHg, whereas others are around 90 mmHg. (© Halberg, 1987.)

The numbers of "patients" treated with placebo and "converted" from "hypertension" to "normotension" deserve comment. In addition to the very real placebo and, in other studies, "bedside-manner" effects, occurring even in the absence of a placebo, as emphasized at the bottom of Fig. 10, it is certain that a considerable number of false-positives were accepted into a study they never should have entered. An unknown number of false-negatives at the final evaluation further biases the result. Substantial errors in diagnosis may well be made in clinical trials and otherwise, not only at the outset of a study in terms of many false-positives entering the study, but also at the final evaluation in which the ratio of "cured normotensives" is likely to be complicated by a substantial number of false-negative diagnoses. The outcome is somewhat less ambiguous in those studies that rely on endpoints such as mortality and incidence of heart attack, stroke, etc., that are directly related to actual cardiovascular disease, irrespective of any blood pressure measurement; but in these cases as well, the uncertainty associated with the diagnosis at the entry into the study may greatly complicate or even invalidate the outcome.

False negative diagnoses: In Fig. 12 (left), a patient's systolic blood pressures (SBPs), shown as dots, are mostly within the reference interval of peers during midday (when the patient is usually examined by his physician). At other times, however, notably at night, many of his SBPs are above the upper chronobiologic reference limit. The treatment of this patient was assumed to be satisfactory on a casual midday measurement basis. It is not, however, adequate in a chronobiologic perspective. The right side of Fig. 12 also shows why the same misdiagnosis applies to the same patient's diastolic blood pressures.

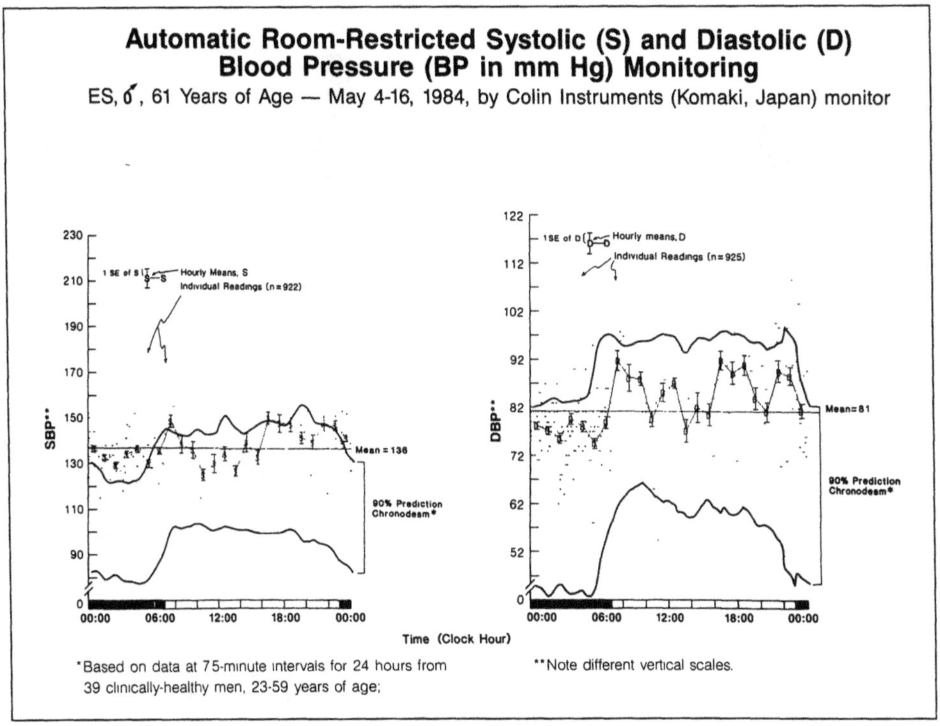

Fig. 12. High blood pressures (BPs) at odd times contrast with mostly acceptable BPs around noon in a patient believed to be well-treated on the basis of a casual examination at midday. Systolic BPs shown on the left; diastolic BPs on the right. (© Halberg, 1987.)

Therapy

Both the timing of treatment and the assessment of treatment effects are a chronobiologic matter. Fig. 13 exemplifies a successful treatment insofar as it is judged by the reduction to zero of both the circadian percent time elevation of blood pressure and the circadian hyperbaric index, a measure of BP excess.

The patient is a clinically healthy-appearing man who had no symptoms when he got a sphygmomanometer as a gift in February, 1981. On self-measurement, his pressures were elevated above conventional standards. After confirmation of a conventional measurement, his physician initiated treatment with 25 mg hydrochlorothiazide each morning. In late December, 1981, and early January, 1982, when the patient was monitored with an automatic instrument off treatment for eight days and back on treatment for six days, the rhythm-adjusted blood pressure mean off treatment was 128 mmHg systolic and 82 mmHg diastolic. Back on treatment, his blood pressure MESOR was lower: 122/79. Checkups in the ensuing four years demonstrate his MESORs to be even lower.

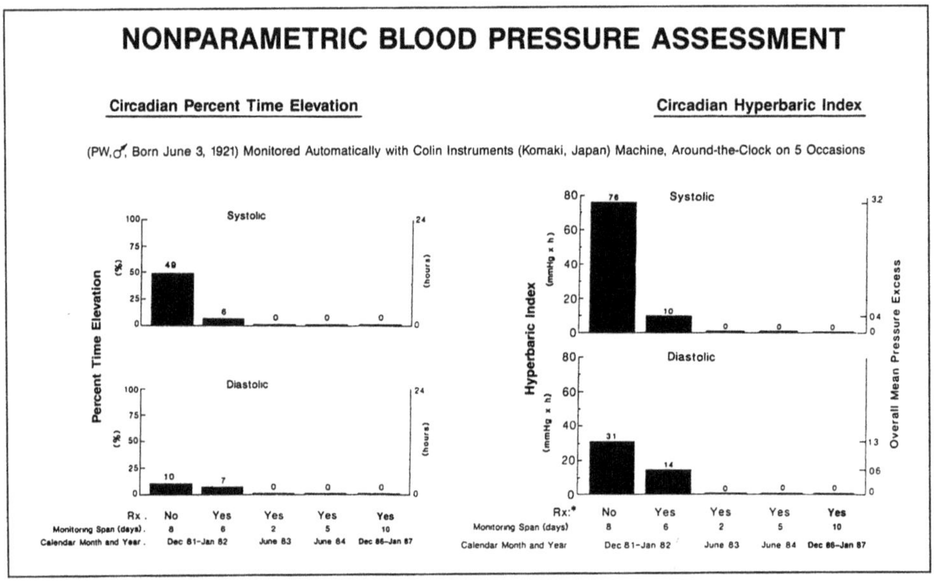

Fig. 13. The question may be debated as to whether one should treat, by drugs, a systolic and a diastolic blood pressure (BP) of 128 and 82 mmHg, respectively. In the case summarized by the figure, treatment was instituted with 25 mg of hydrochlorothiazide by mouth during the morning. The BPs were reduced by treatment at an apparently appropriate time. Off treatment, the BPs were above peer-group limits 49% (SBP) or 10% (DBP) of the time; after treatment, excess was eventually eliminated (left). The corresponding reduction and eventual disappearance of blood pressure excess, measured in mmHg x h, denoted as "hyperbaric index", is also shown (right). (© Halberg, 1987.)

The first column in the left-hand section of Fig. 13 shows that when the patient was off treatment, even though his means were below conventional limits, he was actually above a chronobiologic limit 49% of the time for systolic and 10% for diastolic BP. This percentage time was reduced thereafter to small, negligible values and to zero by treatment with hydrochlorothiazide, 25 mg orally in the morning.

Once there is excess, it is also important to know when it occurs so that treatment can be given at the proper circadian stage. Indeed, the excess occurred during the daytime, and therefore treatment at breakfast was properly timed.

The right side of Fig. 13 shows the BP excess and is presented as a change in concept from mmHg to mmHg x h. It can be seen that the patient's blood pressure excess became small if not negligible on treatment and disappeared on continued treatment.

In this case then, a snapshot in mmHg was replaced by the estimate of an index of excess expressed in mmHg x h. Future work will have to provide for respite and a nonlinear accumulation of harm without thresholds by postulating the existence of an increasing harm function of blood pressure. Such a harm function should estimate the pressure-related cardiovascular disease risk by a pressure-related health index (PRHI), time-qualified as discussed elsewhere [15, 18]. By using this PRHI, one might refer to a relatively low population percentile of the PRHI at which to intervene by non-drug treatment while also using a criterion of excess pressure if not in mmHg, then in some more appropriate unit that takes care of non-linearities in risk and provides some reasonable limit at which drug treatment is indicated. The need for such improvements notwithstanding, the step from mmHg to mmHg x h, from the use of a fixed to that of a variable threshold, and the use of parameter tests to assess the statistical significance of a change in the indices used herein ($P < 0.01$) may represent a step toward reducing harm associated with diseases related to a high blood pressure [12, 18]. Although many are content in demonstrating a lowering of blood pressure with antihypertensive medication, we have taken the data one step further to demonstrate a preventive approach to high blood pressure, which is the topic of another chapter in this book, by Cornélissen et al.

Discussion

The uncertainty of an elevated blood pressure is usually discussed on the assumption that blood pressure variability is mainly due to measurement error, to the patient's posture, and to responses to external stimuli. This view disregards the fact that part of the variation in blood pressure is spontaneous and accounted for by rhythms of several frequencies, among which the 24-h (or circadian) rhythms are most prominent. In order to assess the variation in blood pressure, repeated measurements should be taken, preferably at strategically selected times so as to quantify and exploit more reliable mean values and novel dynamic endpoints. Although presently available automatic recorders greatly facilitate data collection, the analytical methodology available as computer software for resolving the characteristics of rhythm can also be applied to measurements taken manually, once a proper sampling schedule is adopted. The methodology offered by chronobiology allows the assessment of the extent and timing of rhythmic change and the establishment of time-varying norms for healthy peer groups and/or individuals. By comparing these dynamic indices of blood pressure variation of a given individual with those of peers, one seeks to recognize the risk of deviant behavior (e.g., of blood pressure), both early and in a time-dependent fashion to prompt preventive action. When such methods are applied to MESOR- or amplitude-hypertensive patients, they serve to assess their response to treatment.

The sphygmochron, a blood pressure and related cardiovascular monitoring summary, presents, illustrates, and interprets the circadian rhythm characteristics of blood pressure and heart rate. When many measurements are taken around-the-clock, one likely finds values above or below reference limits, not only the fixed limits recommended by WHO, but also outside chronobiologic limits, the so-called chronodesms. In addition to providing an estimate of such deviant single values, the sphygmochron also addresses new and more pertinent questions such as "How long does blood pressure remain above a given time-varying threshold?"; "To what extent does the blood pressure exceed the threshold at a given time?"; "What is the total excess and its projection over a lifetime?", and "When does most of the excess occur?". On this rational basis, treatment (when needed) can be timed more appropriately and its effects can be objectively monitored and tested statistically, not only on a population basis, but also for the given individual. In summary, characteristics of rhythms and of blood pressure excess (or deficit) serve several purposes:

1) to initiate treatment if needed;
2) to time treatment when it is most effective and least harmful in terms of undesired effects;
3) to help in prognosis and diagnosis with a better assessment of health status;
4) to screen for early recognition of risk before disease sets in, so as to intervene by preventive measures such as exercise, diet, or other non-drug treatment.

We are at the threshold of a constructive evolution in medicine, in particular with respect to blood pressure and heart rate. We recognize variability, not as a foe to medical diagnosis and treatment, but as the source of information to be extracted by special hardware and software for use in a refined screening and prevention as well as diagnosis and cure. Automatic recorders are available at a cost that will decrease as their use increases. Algorithms analyze dense and long records for dynamic characteristics. Accumulating evidence from the use of modern hardware and software reveals the health effects of rhythmic changes and some of their mechanisms. Rhythm characteristics include a better mean, the MESOR, than that of one or a few casual measurements.

We believe that the chronobiologic method of blood pressure analysis will lead to more accurate and successful diagnosis and treatment. If large numbers of today's "false-positives" can be removed from therapy and if a substantial percentage of today's "false-negatives" can receive the appropriate treatment, the reduction in morbidity and mortality will be considerable. Getting people into the right treatment category will clearly cut health costs while improving health care for millions.

The chronobiologic components in blood pressure variation reflect but one end-result of the body's coordinating systems, involving almost certainly intermodulations among three or more physiologic entities, such as the brain — notably the hypothalamus and the pineal — and glands such as the pituitary and the adrenal — actors, and reactors, respectively — in a network characterized by "feedsideward" mechanisms [11] that link the body systems into one harmonious symphony.[b)]

Intermodulating rhythms occur at all levels from the single cell to the whole organism. The synchronization of these changes is done via the central and autonomous nervous system and is influenced by the social regimen. Our getting up and going to bed at the times set by society each day resets our free-running internal rhythm setters into step with worldtime. The brain, or rather the chronobiologically challenging entity, the mind, is therefore a vital link in the time region's coordination of the heart, the rest of the cardiovascular system and the whole person. Looking at all biophysical and psychological

variables from a chronobiologic viewpoint will greatly enhance diagnosis, therapy, and prevention in nearly all facets of medicine, but the application to blood pressure can be used already now with great service to the quality of life for many patients.
The chronobiologic views is that circadian and other rhythms, notably in blood pressure and heart rate, are endogenous components that are synchronized by physico-chemical as well as socio-ecologic factors. The existence of an underlying intrinsic rhythmic mechanism is supported by the observation, which is validated statistically, that blood pressure rises before awakening and cannot thus result only from a change in posture or activity [7, 18, 44]. It was also shown that the circadian amplitude in blood pressure may decrease, yet it is not obliterated under conditions of bedrest [18, 36]. Halberg in 1953 documented the phenomenon of an activation of both the adrenal cortex [8] and medulla, codetermining a rise in blood pressure prior to awakening, and postulated that the rise occurs perhaps in preparation for the start of each day's motor activities. [c)]
Chronobiologic blood pressure monitoring can be started by evaluating the mother during pregnancy [18] and is indicated as early in life as possible, certainly immediately after birth [17, 18], when it is easily implemented and can already serve as an index for cardiovascular risk assessment. During schooling, blood pressure self-monitoring and rhythm analysis can be part of instruction for acquiring both the competence and the discipline for medically-guided self-help in preventive health care [13].

Conclusions

The extreme variation of human blood pressure can be cost-effectively recorded by ambulatory monitoring devices under conditions of real life. The issue at hand in such records **for the individual** is to separate short-lived, presumably useful blood pressure increases in the course of physical or mental activity, that can be beneficial if not long maintained, from cumulative excess with an impact upon the vessel wall, that is reflected **for the group** in a correlation of increases in blood pressure and mortality, revealed by insurance statistics. For the individual, chronobiologic software extracts from records of variation more representative means with smaller standard deviations than those obtained from conventional measurements or even from ambulatory monitors that print out conventional summaries. Chronobiologic software yields, in addition, dynamic (e. g., circadian rhythm) characteristics for a comparison of the individual's profile over time and of its characteristics with those of a standard profile and the corresponding characteristics with peers. Chronobiologic endpoints may work for risk or excess assessment when the mean does not. Indices of a 10-year projection of excess are proposed, as are reference limits for rhythm characteristics and single values. One of the rhythm characteristics, the circadian amplitude (but not the mean) correlates in 14-year-olds with target organ involvement, as evaluated by the thickness of the interventricular cardiac septum. Accordingly, focus upon **the** casual or average blood pressure, the current endpoints from measurements or 24-h profiles in medical practice has to be complemented (and eventually replaced) by focus upon the more complete and more reliable chronobiologic, static (MESOR) and dynamic characteristics of blood pressure variation. In medical practice on adults, systematic chronobiologically designed self-measurement or automatic monitoring is warranted. Almost certainly, a number of false-positive and false-negative diagnoses of high blood pressure can be eliminated by a chronobiologic analysis of such data. More specifically, undue side effects from unwarranted medication and cost are prevented by the reduction of wrongly diagnosed "hypertension". Furthermore, by eliminating false-negative diagnoses, a root of devastating illnesses is removed, with the savings in suffering and in cost for care after heart attack or stroke. Prevention promises to render chronobiologic health care most cost-effective.

To be healthy, to be seriously handicapped, or to die in the prime of life: these are the outcomes that prompt a dynamic, that is chronobiologic, approach to blood pressure and heart rate measurement. With traditional sphygmomanometers, but preferably with automatic monitors, we can take advantage of modern computer technology and knowledge gained from chronobiologic studies with automatic instrumentation to prevent the diseases and deaths caused by a preventable problem: high blood pressure.

Summary

The diagnosis and treatment of deviant blood pressure can be undertaken with greater accuracy and higher success if one uses the "dynamic" characteristics of the pressure rather than just the present "static" viewpoint based primarily on an average pressure. In lieu of sole reliance upon repeated casual measurements, as recommended by the WHO, and also in lieu of inspecting only records from automatic 24-h monitoring, we advocate a third alternative, namely a chronobiologic exploitation of data collected systematically. These can be obtained by traditional sphygmomanometers or by means of automatic monitoring devices. Modern ambulatory monitors become cost-effective once the merit of chronobiologic endpoints, such as a measure of excess or deficit, each assessed in relation to time-varying limits derived from peer groups, are recognized. The information obtained by additional endpoints describing the extent and timing of change, all presented in a computer-prepared profile over time, the sphygmochron, is documented by illustrative examples and by reference to a more detailed presentation and bibliography. Indications for the use of the chronobiologic approach to blood pressure evaluation are also succinctly presented. By these examples from the field of blood pressure evaluation, we have tried to document the need for awareness of the broader scope of the science of physiologic variation in relation to time: chronobiology, for medical practitioners as well as researchers.

Acknowledgement

This paper is a slightly modified version of a manuscript in press in the proceedings of a meeting on "Heart & Brain/Brain & Heart" held at Tromsø, Norway, in June, 1987. The work summarized herein was supported by the U. S. National Institutes of Health, in particular GM-13981 and HL-40650; the Fontazione Hoechst, Milan, Italy; Medtronic Inc., Minneapolis, Minnesota, USA; Colin Medical Instruments, Komaki, Japan; the Minnesota Medical Foundation and the Dr. Betty Sullivan Fund. Dr. Donald W. Marquardt (Consultant Manager, Applied Statistics, E. I. DuPont de Nemours & Co. Engineering Department, Louviers Bldg., Wilmington, Delaware, USA) contributed to the formulation of the status of chronobiology and medicine as presented in the first several paragraphs of the body of this paper dealing with chronobiology and medicine. Michael Moore (Science Writer, University of Minnesota) kindly edited part of this manuscript.

Footnotes

a) By contrast, a rigorous assessment is obtained much sooner by a chronobiologically assessed 48-h profile, extended to a week of monitoring in case of doubt and, of course, to yet longer spans in case of a suspicion of certain secondary blood pressure deviations, such as the intermittent elevations associated with a pheochromocytoma.

b) Feedsideward mechanisms supersede simplistic feedbacks, feedforwards, feedups or feeddowns, as long as the latter, in practice, are documented only by the interaction of homeostatic entities. The feedsideward recognizes the *a priori* periodic nature of each of at least three intermodulating physiologic entities. For the sake of defining a testable situation, one refers to an actor and a reactor — such as adrenal, producing corticosteroid — and the pituitary, producing ACTH — both influenced by a modulator, such as pineal-producing melatonin, all contributing their products with rhythms of several frequencies [11]. In this respect, one can document the rhythmic effect of the pineal on corticosterone production by the adrenal and the equally rhythmic pineal effect upon ACTH production by the pituitary. These periodic intermodulations at several frequencies, notably with circadian and about-7-days (circaseptan) components, result in sequences of stimulation, no-effect, or inhibition by a third entity, such as the pineal, upon the interaction of the other two, such as the adrenal and pituitary.

c) The adrenal cortex is a critical node in the interdigitating networks coordinating metabolic and adjusting networks as well as complementary networks for growth, repair, and reproduction. The adrenal cortical cycle has been described as the pacemaker of circadian rhythms in circulating blood eosinophil cells and of acting at the cellular level upon rhythms in phospholipid labelling and mitosis [35]. The adrenal cycle was shown to persist in the histologically validated absence of the suprachiasmatic nuclei [41].
The persistence of adrenal cortical bioperiodicity in rodents was documented directly by corticosterone determinations after stepwise brain ablation [5] and in vitro [1]. Indirectly, on human beings, the persistence of circadian adrenal periodicity has also been documented by counts of circulating blood eosinophils after hemispherectomy [18], during regressive electroshock [8], and in coma [30].
Robel and Baulieu have shown that, apart from the long-known contribution of major steroidogenic glands, dehydroepiandrosterone and its sulfate (both abbreviated as D) are also made in the brain [37]. These authors also showed that D undergoes a circadian cycle in the brain, as do other steroids, and that following adrenalectomy and orchidectomy in rats, i.e., after removal of the steroidogenic endorine glands, D not only continues to be found in respectable amounts, but it continues to exhibit a circadian rhythm in the brain, whereas corticosterone nearly disappears and no circadian rhythm can be detected [38]. These results support the hypothesis about the existence of an autonomous cerebral

mechanism coordinating the production of Δ5-3β-hydroxysteroids. It is also pertinent to note that the acrophase of pregnenolone in brain precedes, with statistical significance, the acrophase of corticosterone in rats [46], as does the acrophase of D in plasma. Moreover, in the rat, the circadian rhythm of corticosterone, pregnenolone, and D are in phase between their variation in plasma and brain. This is not the case for the adrenal phase relations of cortisol and D-sulfate in humans, the rise of cortisol preceding that of D-S by about 6 h [19]. The differences in phase relations between the two kinds of steroids observed between the two species (rodents and humanbeings) describes internal phase relations and are therefore independent of the difference in rest/activity cycle between the two species. These differences may result in part from a modulatory effect exerted by the CNS. The pineal gland is a logical candidate to intervene in such a coordinating mechanism by means of its feedsideward action [35].

Methodologic appendix

To recognize the variability in blood pressure, largely as part of a broad rhythmic structure, is to admit that the question of whether "the" blood pressure is too high or too low should be replaced by some other, more pertinent questions such as how long are pressures elevated above a given threshold, what is the excess blood pressure, and when does most of the excess occur.* Several steps of sophistication can be considered to answer such questions. First, one could count how many measurements in an around-the-clock blood pressure profile are above a given limit. Taking chronobiologic considerations into account, one may prefer to replace the admittedly arbitrary limits now recommended by WHO (140/90), based on morbidity and mortality statistics from a previous generation, by a reference value reflecting data on age- and gender-matched healthy peers (Fig. 5). The median acrometron, the sum of the MESOR and circadian amplitude (Fig. 2) representing the highest predicted value for any individual profile, may represent such a chronobiologic threshold. In approximating an individual's blood pressure data with a 24-h cosine curve, fitted by least squares, answers to the above questions are easily obtained.

To evaluate the duration of elevation, one has to find the times, t_1 and t_2, when the fitted cosine curve, y(t), intersects the threshold, y_c. This amounts to solving the equation

$$y(t) = M + A\cos(\omega t + \Phi) = y_c, \text{ with } \omega = 2\pi/\tau; \tag{1}$$

solving for t yields

$$t = \frac{\tau}{2\pi}\left[\arccos\left(\frac{y_c - M}{A}\right) - \Phi\right]. \tag{2}$$

Provided $M - A < y_c < M + A$, there are two solutions to (2), one, t_1, corresponding to the upslope, and the other, t_2, corresponding to the downslope of y(t). The duration of the elevation (DE) and percent time elevation (PTE) are then given by:

$$DE = \begin{cases} 0 & \text{if } y_c > M + A \\ (t_2 - t_1) & \text{if } M - A < y_c < M + A \\ \tau & \text{if } y_c < M + A \end{cases} \tag{3}$$

$$PTE = \frac{DE}{\tau} \times 100 \qquad (4)$$

As a measure of the total load exerted upon the arterial walls, the hyperbaric index (HBI) is computed as the total area, within one cycle, of blood pressures above the threshold y_c

$$HBI = \begin{cases} 0 & y_c > M + A \\ \int_{t_1}^{t_2} [M + A\cos(\omega t + \Phi) - y_c]\, dt & M - A < y_c < M + A \\ \tau (M - y_c) & y_c < M + A \end{cases} \qquad (5)$$

* The considerations herein of an elevated blood pressure can easily be adapted for the case of a lowered blood pressure.

It may be argued that a 24-h cosine curve is only a rough approximation of the blood pressure waveform. Primarily when dense data are collected around the clock, to derive the percent time elevation and the hyperbaric index, it is preferable to use the raw data rather than any fitted models that unavoidably smooth the profile. This can easily be achieved by numerical integration. In the case of a fixed threshold, the problem amounts to a summation of trapezoidal areas delineated by the limit y_c and straight lines connecting successive data points. Since only the area of pressures above the critical limit is of interest, whenever consecutive data points lie on opposite sides of the threshold, the time when the blood pressure exceeds y_c needs to be computed. This can easily be done by linear interpolation. Results obtained on the basis of the original data or the fitted cosine curve are usually similar, although the latter tend to be slightly smaller than the former, in keeping with the smoothing effect of the fitted cosine model.

With the availability of instrumentation to collect data around the clock, one would also like to account for the prominent rhythmic structure in blood pressure (and many other physiologic variables) in defining reference limits. It is therefore proposed to replace the fixed threshold, y_c, by reference limits that vary as a function of rhythm stage. In order to determine such chronodesmic limits, large data bases from age- and gender-matched peers are needed. A critical threshold curve can then be defined, for instance, as the upper 95% prediction limit computed over short intervals (1 or 2 h) that are displaced in increments (15 or 30 min) along the 24-h scale. Such prediction limits account for both inter- and intra-individual variation and offer the advantage of considering both changes in mean and variance as a function of rhythm stage. Once such limits are defined, both the duration of excess and the hyperbaric index can be obtained by numerical integration. The procedure is similar to that explained above, except that successive segments are determined not only by the sampling times, but also by the discrete timepoints at which the chronodesmic limits have been defined.

Whenever a fixed threshold is considered, the time when, on the average, most excess occurs corresponds roughly to the circadian acrophase. This is no longer the case when chronodesmic limits are used. Depending on the relative values of the MESOR and circadian amplitude of the patient as compared to those of the reference population, excess can occur near the patient's acrophase or at any other circadian stage, even when the patient's acrophase is in keeping with that of the reference population. For instance, in cases of "borderline hypertension"; when the MESOR is only slightly elevated, one may frequently find excess by night since the blood pressure in these patients tends to drop less than expected by night. Whenever chronodesmic limits are used, the timing of excess can be computed as the "center of gravity" of the area of excess

$$tg = \arctan(s/c), \qquad \text{where } s = \Sigma_j hbi_j \sin\varphi_j / \Sigma_j hbi_j \quad (6)$$
$$\text{and } c = \Sigma_j hbi_j \cos\varphi_j / \Sigma_j hbi_j,$$
$$\text{with } \varphi_j = -\omega t_j,$$

where t_j represents the midpoint of the area of excess (between consecutive sampling times) and hbi_j is the corresponding area of excess; the summation over j corresponds to the need to cover an entire cycle.

Although, in most cases, this approach is validated by the observation that most of the excess occurs during a given portion of the day, there may be cases where this estimate of timing may be misleading, for instance when the excess is split more or less equally between two different portions of the day. This may be the case, for instance, when a patient is treated with short-acting anti-hypertensive drugs. In order to avoid any misinterpretation on this basis, for instance, when adjusting the timing of medication for a given patient, it is recommended to compute a fractionated hyperbaric index, say over consecutive 3-h intervals, to cover the 24-h cycle, to check on any occurrence of "split excess". Unless such split excess occurs, one often finds that a cosine curve fits the 3-h values for excess sufficiently well to reject a zero-24-h amplitude assumption. Thus, one can determine not only the amplitude and the acrophase of the blood pressure values themselves, but one can get parameters for the rhythm in excess as such.

References

1. Andrews RV (1968) Temporal secretory responses of cultured hamster adrenals. Comp Biochem Physiol 26: 179—193
2. Carandente F, Halberg F(eds) (1984) Chronobiology of blood pressure in 1985. Chronobiologia 11, *3, 152 pp.
3. Cornélissen G (1987) Instrumentation and data analysis methods needed for blood pressure monitoring in chronobiology. In: Scheving LE, Halberg F, Ehret CF (eds), Chronobiotechnology and Chronobiological Engineering, Martinus Nijhoff, The Netherlands, 1987, pp. 241—261
4. Croppi E, Livi R, Scarpelli L, de Leonardis V, de Scalzi M, Halberg F, Romano S, Cagnoni M, Scarpelli PT (1987) Chronobiologically assessed blood pressure and left ventricular wall thickness in children with and without a family history of a high blood pressure. In: Tarquini B, Vergassola R (eds), Social Diseases and Chronobiology: Proc. III Int Symp Social Diseases and Chronobiology, Florence, Nov. 29, 1986, Società Editrice Esculapio, Bologna, pp. 135—144
5. Galicich JH, Halberg F, French LA, Ungar F (1965) Effect of cerebral ablation on a circadian pituitary adrenocorticotropic rhythm in C mice. Endocrinology 76: 895—901
6. Gross F, Strasser T (eds) (1983) Mild Hypertension: Recent Advances. Raven Press, New York
7. Halberg E, Halberg F, Shankaraiah K (1981) Plexo-serial linear-nonlinear rhythmometry of blood pressure, pulse and motor activity by a couple in their sixties. Chronobiologia 8: 351—366
8. Halberg F (1960) Temporal coordination of physiologic function. Cold Spr Harb Symp quant Biol 25: 289—310
9. Halberg F (1969): Chronobiology. Ann Rev Physiol 31: 675—725

10. Halberg F (1981): Biologic rhythms, hormones and aging. In: Vernadakis A, Timiras PS (eds), Hormones in Development and Aging, Spectrum Publications, New York, pp. 451—476
11. Halberg F 1983): Quo vadis basic and clinical chronobiology: promise for health maintenance. Am J Anat 168: 543—594
12. Halberg F (1987) Perspectives of chronobiologic engineering. In: Scheving LE, Halberg F, Ehret CF (eds): Chronobiotechnology and Chronobiological Engineering. Dordrecht, The Netherlands, Martinus Nijhoff, pp 1—46
13. Halberg F, Ahlgren A, Haus E (1984) Circadian systolic and diastolic hyperbaric indices of high school and college students. Chronobiologia 11: 299—309
14. Halberg F, Barnum CP, Silber RH, Bittner JJ (1958) 24-hour rhythms at several levels of integration in mice on different lighting regimens. Proc Soc exp Biol (N.Y) 97: 897—900
15. Halberg F, Bingham C (1987) The scope and promise of chronobiology and biostatistics: interpenetrating, inseparable disciplines. Proc Biopharmaceutical Section, American Statistical Association, Chicago, Illinois, Aug 15—18, 1986, 11—32
16. Halberg F, Carandente F, Montalbetti N (1986) The sphygmochron, a cardiovascular summary, illustrates rhythmometry for advanced technology. Biochim Clin 10: 939—942.
17. Halberg F, Cornélissen G, Bingham C, Tarquini B, Mainardi G, Cagnoni M, Panero C, Scarpelli P Romano S, März W, Hellbrügge T, Shinoda M, Kawabata Y. 1986 Neonatal monitoring to assess risk for hypertension. Postgrad Med 79: 44—46
18. Halberg F, Cornélissen G, Halberg E, Halberg J, Delmore P, Bakken E (1987) Chronobiology of human blood pressure. Medtronic Continuing Medical Education Seminars, 208 pp
19. Halberg F, Cornélissen G, Sothern R.B, Wallach L.A, Halberg E, Ahlgren A, Kuzel M, Radke A, Barbosa J, Goetz F, Buckley J, Mandel J, Schuman L, Haus E, Lakatua D, Sackett L, Berg H, Wendt HW, Kawasaki T, Ueno M, Uezono K, Matsuoka M, Omae T, Tarquini B, Cagnoni M, Garcia Sainz M, Perez Vega E, Wilson D, Griffiths K, Donati L, Tatti P, Vasta M, Locatelli I, Camagna A, Lauro R, Tritsch G, Wetterberg L (1981) International geographic studies of oncological interest on chronobiological variables. In: Kaiser H (ed), Neoplasms-Comparative Pathology of Growth in Animals, Plants and Man, Williams and Wilkins, Baltimore, pp. 553—596
20. Halberg F, Drayer JIM, Cornélissen G, Weber MA (1984) Cardiovascular reference data base for recognizing circadian MESOR- and amplitude-hypertension in apparently healthy men. Chronobiologia 11: 275—298
21. Halberg F, Good RA, Levine H (1966) Some aspects of the cardiovascular and renal circadian system. Circulation 34: 715—717
22. Halberg F, Kausz E, Winter Y, Wu J, März W, Cornélissen G (1986) Circadian rhythmic response in cold pressor test. J Minn Acad Sci 51: 14
23. Halberg F, Montalbetti N (1983) Chronobiologic specification of reference values. Bull Molec Biol Med 8: 75—103
24. Halberg F, Reale L, Tarquini B (eds) (1986) Proc. 2nd Int. Conf. Medico-Social Aspects of Chronobiology, Florence, Oct. 2, 1984, Istituto Italiano di Medicina Sociale, Rome
25. Halberg F, Sánchez de la Peña S, Fernandes G (1983): Immunochronopharmacology. In: Hadden J, Chedid L, Dukor P, Spreafico F, Willoughby D (eds): Advances in Immunopharmacology. Pergamon Press, Oxford, pp. 463—478.
26. Hanson BR, Halberg F, Tuna N, Bouchard TJ Jr, Lykken DT, Cornélissen G, Heston LL (1984) Rhythmometry reveals heritability of circadian characteristics of heart rate of human twins reared apart. Cardiologia 29: 267—282
27. Hermida RC, Halberg F, Halberg E (1986) Closer to a psychoneuroendocrine hemopsy? Biochem Clin 10: 1053—1066
28. Kanabrocki EL, Scheving LE, Halberg F, Brewer RL, Bird TJ (1973) Circadian variations in presumably healthy men under conditions of peace-time army reserve unit training. Space Life Sci 4: 258—270
29. Kanabrocki EL, Scheving LE, Halberg F, Brewer RL, Bird TJ (1974) Circadian variation in presumably healthy young soldiers. Department of the Army, Document *PB228427, 56 pp.
30. Levine H, Ramshaw WA, Halberg F (1967) Least-squares spectral analyses on core temperature and blood pressure of a comatose girl (abstract). Physiologist 10: 230
31. Mainardi G, Maggioni C, Halberg F, Hurley P, Panero C, Tarquini B, Cariddi A, Sorice V, Cornélissen G, Bingham C, Scarpelli P, Scarpelli L, Livi R, Romano S, Cagnoni M (1986) Family history of high blood pressure (BP) and diabetes and newborn‘s circadian BP amplitude. In: Tarquini B,

Vergassola R (eds), III Int. Symposium, Social Diseases and Chronobiology, Florence, Nov. 29, 1986, pp. 64—65
32. Meyer-Sabellek W, Gotzen R (eds) (1988) Indirekte 24-Stunden-Blutdruckmessung: Methodik und klinische Bedeutung. Steinkopff Verlag, Darmstadt, 243 pp.
33. Panero C, Maggioni C, Halberg F, Hurley P, Mainardi G, Tarquini B, Cariddi A, Sorice V, Cornélissen G, Bingham C, Scarpelli P, Scarpelli L, Livi R, Romano S, Cagnoni M (1986) Beta-adrenergics in pregnancy and maternal high blood pressure (BP) increase newborn's circadian BP amplitude — In: Tarquini B, Vergassola R (eds), III Int. Symposium, Social Diseases and Chronobiology, Florence, Nov. 29, 1986, pp. 67—68
34. Potschke-Langer M., Apfelbach J (1986) Milde Hypertonie — auf dem Wege zu einem internationalen und nationalen Konsens. Fortschr. Med. 44: 852—856
35. Redfern PH, Campbell I, Xavier JA, Martin KF (eds) (1985) Circadian Rhythms in the Central Nervous System. Macmillan, 1985 (cf Halberg F, Sánchez de la Peña S, Cornélissen G: Circadian rhythms and the central nervous system, pp. 57—79)
36. Reinberg A, Ghata J, Halberg F, Gervais P, Abulker Ch, Dupont J, Gaudeau C (1970) Rythmes circadiens du pouls, de la pression artérielle, des excrétions urinaires en 17-hydroxycorticostéroïdes, catécholamines et potassium chez l'homme adulte sain, actif et au repos. Ann Endocrinol (Paris) 31: 277—287
37. Robel P, Bourreau E, Corpéchot C, Dang DC, Halberg F, Clarke C, Haug M, Schlegel ML, Synguelakis M, Vourch C, et al (1987) Neuro-steroids: 3β-hydroxy-Δ5-derivatives in rat and monkey brain. Proc 7th Int Cong Hormonal Steroids, Madrid, Sept 21—29, 1986. J Ster Biochem 27: 649—685
38. Robel P, Synguelakis M, Halberg F, Baulieu EE (1986) Neurophysiologie. — Persistance d'un rythme circadien de la déhydroépiandrostérone dans le cerveau, mais non dans le plasma, de rats castrés et surrénalectomisés. CR Acad Sci Paris 303, Série III, *6: 235—238
39. Roberts L (1987) Measuring cholesterol is as tricky as lowering it. Science 238: 482—483
40. Scheving LE, Halberg F (eds) (1980): Chronobiology: Principles and Applications to Shifts in Schedules. Sijthoff and Noordhoff, Alphen aan den Rijn, The Netherlands.
41. Scheving LE, Tsai TS, Powell EW, Pasley JN, Halberg F, Dunn J (1983) Bilateral lesions of suprachiasmatic nuclei affect circadian rhythms in ^{3}H thymidine incorporation into deoxyribonucleic acid in mouse intestinal tract, mitotic index of corneal epithelium, and serum corticosterone. Anat Rec 205: 239—249
42. Schweiger H-G, Berger S, Kretschmer H, Mörler H, Halberg E, Sothern RB, Halberg F (1986) Evidence for a circaseptan and a circasemiseptan growth response to light/dark cycle shifts in nucleated and enucleated *Acetabularia* cells, respectively. Proc Natl Acad Sci USA 83: 8619—8623
43. Smolensky M, Halberg F, Sargent F II 1972 Chronobiology of the life sequence. In: Itoh S, Ogata K, Yoshimura H (eds), Igaku Shoin Ltd., Tokyo, pp. 2281—2318
44. Stadick A, Bryans R, Halberg E, Halberg F (1987) Circadian cardiovascular rhythms during recumbency. In: Tarquini B, Vergassola R (eds), Social Diseases and Chronobiology: Proc. III Int. Symp. Social Diseases and Chronobiology, Florence, Nov. 29, 1986, Società Editrice Esculapio, Bologna, pp. 191—200
45. Strasser T, Ganten D (eds) (1987) Mild Hypertension: From Drug Trials to Practice. Raven Press, New York, 298 pp.
46. Synguelakis M, Halberg F, Baulieu EE, Robel P (1985) Evolution circadienne de $\Delta_5$3ß-hydroxystéroïdes et de glucocorticostéroides dans le plasma et le cerveau de Rat. CR Acad Sci Paris 301: 823—826
47. Tarquini B (ed) (1987) Social Diseases and Chronobiology: Proc. III Int. Symp. Social Diseases and Chronobiology, Florence, Nov. 29, 1986. Societá Editrice Esculapio, Bologna, 521 pp.
48. Wilcox R G, Mitchell J F A, Hampton J R (1986) Treatment of high blood pressure: should clinical practice be based on results of clinical trials? Brit. Med. J. 296: 433—437
49. 1986 Guidelines for the treatment of mild hypertension: Memorandum from a WHO/ISH meeting. J. Hypertension 4: 383—386

Prediction of cardiovascular morbidity from ambulatory blood pressure monitoring

T.G. Pickering and R.B. Devereux

Cardiovascular Center, The New York Hospital-Cornell University Medical Center New York, New York, USA

Introduction

The relationship between blood pressure and cardiovascular morbidity has been appreciated for many years and is based both on actuarial studies [26] and on population surveys [14]. This relationship is based on a relatively small number of blood pressure readings taken from each individual in an office or clinic setting. It is also well known that blood pressure varies considerably within individuals, both for measurements taken in similar circumstances on different occasions [2, 3], and when taken in different circumstances, e.g., at home rather than in the clinic [4]. It is generally assumed that the damage done by hypertension is related to the average level of pressure over time, although this assumption should not go unchallenged, because it is conceivable that the peaks of pressure and the shape of the arterial pressure waveform could also contribute [22]. Recent findings from the Framingham survey indicate that the average pressure over 30 years gives a closer correlation with left ventricular hypertrophy (LVH) measured by echocardiography [8], which is the most reliable measure of target organ damage available at the present time [7].

The need for improved prediction of individual risk

The Veterans Administration trial of the treatment of hypertension demonstrated that the treatment of patients with severe hypertension resulted in a significant reduction of cardiovascular morbidity [35]. Since that time, a number of other clinical trials have examined the benefits from treating patients with mild hypertension [5, 12, 19, 20]. Although the results have generally been positive, they have been disappointing in three respects. First, although myocardial infarction is the biggest risk for patients with mild hypertension, the reduction of morbidity as a result of treatment is relatively low as compared to the reduction in strokes (approximately 7% vs 40%). Second, when the results are viewed from the point of view of the individual patient rather than the population, the probability of benefit from treatment is very low. Third, there is as yet no evidence that treatment confers benefit in white women.

Given that an individual's level of blood pressure is not a fixed entity, a good case can be made for supposing that a more representative estimate of the "true" or average level of pressure than is possible by a small number of clinic measurements will improve the prediction of risk and hence the need for treatment. This can be done in two ways: either by measuring blood pressure in situations outside the clinic or by measuring target organ damage that is itself dependent on the overall level of blood pressure.

The relationship between blood pressure, target organ damage and morbidity

The relationships between blood pressure and other risk factors affecting cardiovascular morbidity are illustrated in Fig. 1, with target organ damage viewed as an intermediate risk factor resulting from the interactions of blood pressure and other primary risk factors, and which directly contributes to cardiovascular morbidity. At the present time, echocardiography gives the most sensitive measurement of target organ damage. The best established echocardiographic index is left ventricular hypertrophy (LVH), but diastolic dysfunction may be an even more sensitive marker of the effects of hypertension on the heart [32]. Although the major brunt of the effects of hypertension is borne by the arteries, there is unfortunately no good clinical method for the evaluation of the structural changes in the arteries. The relationships between blood pressure and morbidity can be examined in three ways (A, B and C in Fig. 1). Studies relating blood pressure and target organ damage have been mainly cross-sectional, while studies relating these variables to morbidity are of necessity longitudinal.

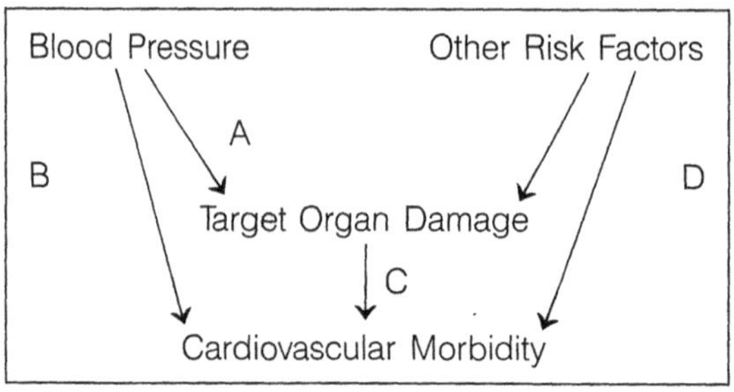

Fig. 1. Shows a conceptual relationship between primary risk factors (blood pressure and others), intermediate risk factors (target organ damage) and cardiovascular morbidity.

Studies relating blood pressure and target organ damage

Several studies have compared the correlation between different measures of blood pressure and target organ damage. The first was the classic paper by Sokolow et al. [33], in which three measures of target organ damage were used: LVH evaluated from the ECG, heart size from the chest X-ray, and fundal changes. This aggregate measure of target organ damage was more closely related to ambulatory daytime blood pressures ($r = 0.63$ for systolic and 0.65 for diastolic) than to casual pressures.

A similar composite index of target organ damage was used in a more recent study by Parati et al. [23], who also found a closer correlation between target organ damage with 24-h than with casual blood pressure.

Other studies have used echocardiography for evaluating LVH, which has the advantage of being both more sensitive and specific than the ECG. Thus, the prevalance of LVH by ECG criteria may be as low as 5% in patients with mild hypertension, while by echocardiographic criteria it may be between 20% and 50% [16].

The results of these studies are summarized in Table 1. In 50 patients studied in hospital using continuous intra-arterial blood pressure monitoring, Rowlands et al. [30] found higher correlations between LVH and ambulatory pressure than with casual pressure. In a smaller series of 12 patients, Drayer et al. [10] obtained similar results. In our own study of 100 patients [9], we, too, found higher correlations with ambulatory pressures.

We also found that this correlation was closer when blood pressure was measured on a working than on a nonworking day, which is analogy with the effects of physical conditioning on LVH, raises the possibility that intermittent elevations of pressure, such as occur during working hours, may be important in the development of LVH. Further evidence favoring this view is provided by studies which have related exercise blood pressure and LVH and shown a better correlation than with casual pressure (Table 1).

Table 1. Correlations between different measures of systolic blood pressure and LVH

Author	Ref	n	Casual SBP	Ambulatory SBP	Exercise SBP
Rowlands	30	50	0.51	0.59	—
Drayer	10	12	0.55	0.82	—
Devereux	9	100	0.24	0.50	—
Antivalle	1	84	0.26	0.45	—
Gosse	11	61	0.40	0.53	0.53
Ren	29	67	0.16	—	0.58
Nathwani	21	20	0.21	—	0.68

It has been known since the classic study of Ayman and Goldshine [4] that home blood pressures tend to be lower than clinic pressures. We subsequently demonstrated that home pressures taken by the patients show a closer agreement to the average 24-h pressure than do clinic readings taken by the physician [15]. Despite the growing and widespread use of home blood pressures, there is relatively little information about their predictive value. In one study it was reported that regression of LVH from the ECG correlated more closely with changes of home pressure than with clinic pressures [13]. Two studies have indicated that the correlation between echocardiographically determined LVH and blood pressure is better for home than for clinic readings [15, 36].

So far, all the published studies have shown that ambulatory pressures are superior to clinic pressures, and even that post-exercise and home pressures may be better in predicting target organ damage. There are several possible reasons for these findings. One is that ambulatory and home measurement give a bigger number of readings than clinic measurement, so that the averaged value is likely to be a closer approximation to the true level of pressure. Another may be that clinic pressures are less representative of the true level of blood pressure than the other measures. The reason why clinic pressures are generally higher than home pressures is presumed to be that the clinic situation itself provokes a pressor response which may initially be related to anxiety, but which may also be a conditioned response. Thus, the pressure is typically higher when taken by a physician than by a nurse or technician [27, 17]. This effect is variable from one patient to another, so that clinic pressures are a relatively poor predictor of pressures at other times. Another point worthy of consideration is whether measurement of pressure at one particular time of day will give a better prediction than another. It is theoretically possible, for example, that there might be a threshold effect of blood pressure on LVH and that pressures at the upper end of the range give a better prediction of LVH than pressures at the lower end. It is not possible to draw definitive conclusions on this point at the present time, but what evidence there is would be consistent with this view, as exemplified by our finding that work pressure gives the best correlation, and the fact that most studies have found that waking pressures are more closely related to LVH than sleeping pressures, which are, of course, lower. One proviso must be mentioned here, and is that the sleep pressure may not be reliably recorded by noninvasive recorders because of the effects of intermittent arousal occurring as a consequence of cuff inflation. The fact that clinic pressures tend to be higher than pressures at other times, and yet be relatively poor predictors of LVH does not necessarily invalidate this idea because they correlate relatively weakly with pressure at other times, e.g., while at work [28].

Studies relating target organ damage and morbidity

While clinical evidence of target organ damage is strongly associated with an increased risk of morbidity in hypertensive patients [27], this is of relatively little help in the evaluation of patients with mild hypertension, in most of whom elevation of blood pressure is the only abnormal finding. The same applies to abnormalities in the chest x-ray and ECG results. Devereux et al. [8] found that the sensitivity of echocardiography for detecting LVH (85%) is much higher than for the ECG (43% by the Cornell criteria) so that many cases which would be otherwise missed will be detected if an echocardiogram is included as part of the evaluation. This fact makes the echocardiogram a more cost-effective test than the ECG in hypertensive patients despite its higher cost [8].
So far, there is only one study has been published relating echocardiographically determined LVH to morbidity, which was conducted by our group, but others are likely to follow. In a prospective evaluation of 140 hypertensive men followed for 4.8 years, LVH was a predictor of cardiovascular morbidity, which was independent of other risk factors, such as clinic blood pressure, smoking and cholesterol level [6].
Preliminary data from the Framingham Study have been presented, which also indicate that LVH is a powerful risk factor independent of other major risk factors [31].

Studies relating blood pressure and morbidity

There have so far been two attempts to relate clinical outcome to ambulatory blood pressure. In the first, Perloff et al. [24] followed 1076 patients for an average duration of 5 years. Ambulatory and office pressures were significantly correlated with each other, although ambulatory pressures were on average 16/9 mmHg lower. Patients were classified according to whether their ambulatory pressures were high or low relative to their office pressures. Those with higher ambulatory pressures had a higher mortality and incidence of cardiovascular morbidity than those with lower ambulatory pressures. Ambulatory pressures had the greatest predictive value in patients who were less than 50 years old, whose diastolic pressure at the time of entry was less than 105 mmHg, and who had no prior cardiovascular event. They were not helpful in defining the prognosis of patients with more severe hypertension, however. These results are encouraging because it is the borderline patients in whom the decision to start treatment is most controversial.
The second study was performed by Mann et al. [18], who followed 137 patients for a mean of 2 years, during which time 14 subjects experienced cardiovascular events. Com-

bining the results of ambulatory monitoring with clinic pressures significantly improved the prediction of morbid events.

One important question that remains unanswered is whether the variability of blood pressure is also a determinant of target organ damage independently of the average level. The studies of Sokolow et al. [33] and Rowlands et al. [30] did not find any correlation between blood pressure variability and target organ damage, although Pessina's study did [25]. Parati et al. [23] reported that 24-h blood pressure variability was related to target organ damage. This finding must be interpreted with caution, however, because many of their patients had relatively advanced hypertension, and the increased blood pressure variability may have resulted from target organ damage, as a consequence of impaired baroreceptor reflexes. In the prognostic study of Mann et al. [18], blood pressure variability also did not appear to contribute to the prediction of morbid events. The currently available evidence would therefore suggest that the average level of pressure is more important than variability.

Do these findings apply to both men and women?

A number of findings suggest that different criteria should be adopted for men and women when defining the risks associated with hypertension. As shown by the MRC trial [19] and other studies [5], the risks associated with any given level of blood pressure are lower for women than for men. We have estimated the frequency of white coat hypertension, defined as elevated clinic pressure and normal ambulatory 24-h pressure, in our patients with mild hypertension, and found it to be about 20% [27]. This phenomenon seems to be more common in women than in men, and hence may contribute to the more benign course of hypertension in women.

The prevalence of LVH is also different in hypertensive men and women: when a single value of LV mass is used to define LVH for both sexes, LVH occurs more commonly in men, but if sex-specific criteria are used (men normally have bigger hearts), it is more common in women [7]. The meaning of these differences is unclear. Our finding relating echo LVH to morbidity applies only to men [6].

Most of the studies relating 24-h blood pressure to target organ damage have not discriminated between the sexes. Antivalle et al. [1] found that the relationship between ambulatory pressure and LVH was significant only in men, who had higher blood pressures, and more LVH. In the prospective study by Perloff et al. [24], ambulatory pressures predicted morbidity in both men and women.

Conclusions

In all of the studies so far reported, measurements of blood pressure made outside the clinic, whether by ambulatory or home monitoring, have proven superior in their ability to predict target organ damage or cardiovascular morbidity. This may in part be due to the fact that, for a function as variable as blood pressure, the bigger the number of measurements, the more reliable the characterization. It is not yet possible to reach any definite conclusion as to whether the average level of pressure is solely responsible for the changes, or whether the variability of blood pressure also contributes. These considerations are important because the physiological regulation of the two is not necessarily the same [34], and antihypertensive medications may affect the average level of pressure without affecting the variability [37]. The results reported here offer the possibility of improving the risk stratification in patients with mild hypertension beyond what can be achieved using clinic pressures. This is important because it means that it may be possible to reserve treatment for patients judged to be at highest risk. Both echocardiography and ambulatory monitoring offer promise in this regard. In theory, the best prediction might come from a combination of the two, although this is not yet proven, and the extra costs would have to be outweighed by the extra benefits. In addition, more data are needed concerning the prognostic value of home blood pressures, which might be able to substitute for ambulatory pressures in this respect, at a fraction of the cost.

References

1. Antivalle M, Lattuada S, Paraviani M, Rindi M, Libretti A (1986) Twenty-four hour noninvasive ambulatory blood pressure monitoring in the assessment of early hypertension. J Hypertension 4, (Suppl 5): 322—324
2. Armitage P, Rose GA (1966) The variability of measurements of casual blood pressure I. A laboratory study. Clin Sci 30: 325—335
3. Armitage P, Fox W, Rose GA, Tinker CM (1966) The variability of measurements of casual blood pressure II. Survey experience. Clin Sci 30: 337—344
4. Ayman D, Goldshine AD (1940) Blood pressure determinations by patients with essential hypertension I. The difference between home and clinic readings before treatment. Am J Med Sci 200: 465—474
5. Australian National Blood Pressure Study Management Comittee (1980) The Australian Therapeutic Trial in Mild Hypertension. Lancet 1: 1251—1267
6. Casale PN, Devereux RB, Milner M, Zullo G, Harshfield GA, Pickering TG, Laragh JH (1986) Value of echocardiographic measurement of left ventricular mass in predicting cardiovascular morbid events in hypertensive men. Ann Int Med 105: 173—178
7. Devereux RB, Pickering TG, Alferman MH, Chien S, Borer JS, Laragh JH (1987) Left ventricular hypertrophy in hypertension. Prevalence and relationship to pathophysiologic variables. Hypertension 9 (Suppl II): 53—60
8. Devereux RB, Casale PN, Wallerson DC, Kligfield P, Hammond IW, Liebson PR, Campo E, Alonso DR, Laragh JH (1987) Cost-effectiveness of echocardiography and electrocardiography for detection of left ventricular hypertrophy in patients with systemic hypertension. Hypertension 9 (Suppl II) II—69, II—76
9. Devereux RB, Pickering TG, Harshfield GA, Kleinert HD, Denby L, Clark L, Pregibon D, Jason MN, Kleiner B, Borer JS, Laragh JH (1983) Left ventricular hypertrophy in patients with hypertension: Importance of blood pressure response to regularly recurring stress. Circulation 68: 470—476
10. Drayer JIM, Weber MA, DeYoung JL (1983) BP as a determinant of cardiac left ventricular muscle mass. Arch Int Med 143: 90—92
11. Gosse P, Campello G, Aouizerate E, Roudaut R, Broustet JP, Dallochio M (1986) Left ventricular hypertrophy in hypertension: Correlation with rest, exercise and ambulatory systolic blood pressure. J Hypertension 4 (Suppl 5): S297—S299
12. Hypertension Detection and Follow-up Program Cooperative Group (1979) Five-year findings of the Hypertension Detection and Follow-up Program. J Am Med Ass 242: 2562—2571
13. Ibrahim MM, Tarazi RC, Dustan HP, Gifford RW (1977) Electro-cardiogram in evaluation of resistance to antihypertensive therapy. Arch Int Med 137: 1125—1129
14. Kannel WB (1974) Role of blood pressure in cardiovascular morbidity and mortality. Progr Cardiovasc Dis 17: 5—23

15. Kleinert HD, Harshfield GA, Pickering TG, Devereux RB, Sullivan PM, Marion RM, Mallory WK, Laragh JH (1984) What is the value of home blood pressure measurement in patients with mild hypertension? Hypertension 6: 547—578
16. Levy D, Anderson K, Savage DD, Kannel WB, Castelli WP (1987) Influence of 30 year mean blood pressure levels on left ventricular mass: The Framingham Heart study. J Am Coll Cardiol 9 (Suppl A): 115A—
17. Mancia G, Parati G, Pomidossi G, Grassi G, Casadei R, Zanchetti A. Altering reaction and rise in blood pressure during measurement by physician and nurse. Hypertension 1987 9, 209—215
18. Mann S, Millar-Craig MW, Raftery EB (1985) Superiority of 24-hour measurements of blood pressure over clinic values in determining prognosis in hypertension. Clin Exp Hyp 17 (2 & 3): 179-281
19. Medical Research Council Working Party (1985) MRC Trial of treatment of mild hypertension: Principal results. Brit Med J 291: 97—104
20. Multiple Risk Factor Intervention Trial Research Group (1982) Multiple Risk Factor Intervention Trial: Risk Factor changes and mortality results. J Am Med Ass 248: 1465—1476
21. Nathwani D, Reeves RA, Marquez-Julio A, Leener FHHH (1985) Left ventricular hypertrophy in mild hypertension: Correlation with exercise blood pressure. Am Heart J 104: 386—387
22. O'Rourke M (1985) Basic concepts for the understanding of large arteries in hypertension. J Cardiovasc Pharmacol 7: S14—S21
23. Parati G, Pomidossi G, Albini F, Malaspina D, Mancia G (1987) Relationship of 24-hour blood pressure mean and variability to severity of target-organ damage in hypertension. J Hypertension 5: 93—98
24. Perloff D, Sokolow M, Cowan R (1983) The prognostic value of ambulatory blood pressures. J Am Med Ass 249: 2792—2798
25. Pessinia AC, Palatini P, Sperti G, Cordone L, Libardoni M, Mos L, Mormino P, DiMarco A, Del Ralo C (1985) Evaluation of hypertension and related target organ damage by average day-time blood pressure. Clin Exp Hypertension A7 (2 & 3): 267—278
26. Pickering GW (1968) High Blood Pressure. Churchill, London
27. Pickering TG, Boddie C, James GD, Blank S, Harshfield GA, Laragh JH. How common is white coat hypertension? (in press)
28. Pickering TG, Harshfield GA, Kleinert HD, Blank S, Laragh JH (1982) Blood pressure during normal daily activities, sleep, and exercise. Comparison of values in normal and hypertensive subjects. J Am Med Ass 247: 992—996
29. Ren JF, Hakki AH, Kottler MN, Iskandriam AS (1985) Exercise systolic blood pressure: A powerful determinant of increased left ventricular mass in patients with hypertension. J Am Coll Cardiol 5: 1224—1231
30. Rowlands DB, Glover DR, Ireland MA, McLeay RAB, Stallard TJ, Watson RDS, Littler WA (1982) Assessment of left ventricular mass and its response to antihypertensive treatment. Lancet 1: 467—470
31. Savage DD, Garrison RJ, Castelli WP, Kannel WB, Anderson SJ, Feinlieb M (1985) Echocardiographic data from Framingham and newer studies of echocardiography. AHA Council on Cardiovascular Epidemic Newsletter, Abstract, p 33
32. Smith VE, White WB, Karimeddini MK (1987) Echocardiographic assessment of left ventricular diastolic performance in hypertensive subjects: Correlation with changes in left ventricular mass. Hypertension 9 (Suppl II) 81—84
33. Sokolow M, Werdegar D, Kaim HK, Hinman AT (1966) Relationship between level of blood pressure measured casually and by portable recorders and severity of complications in essential hypertension. Circulation 34: 279—298
34. Talman WT, Snyder D, Reis DJ (1980) Chronic lability of arterial pressure produced by destruction of A2 catecholamine neurons in rat brainstem. Circ Res 46: 842—853
35. Veterans Administration Cooperative Study Group on Antihypertensive Agents (1967) Effects of treatment on morbidity in hypertension: Results in patients with diastolic blood pressure averaging 115 through 129 mmHg. J Am Med Ass 212: 1028—1034
36. Verdecchia P, Bentivoglia M, Providenza M, Savino K, Corea L (1985) Reliability of home self-recorded arterial pressure in essential hypertension in relation to the stage of the disease. In: Germano G(ed) Blood Pressure Recording in the Clinical Management of Hypertension. Ediziono Pozzi, Rome, pp 40—42

37. Watson RDS, Stallard TJ, Littler WA (1979) Influence of once-daily administration of β-adrenoceptor antagonists on arterial pressure and its variability. Lancet 1: 1201 — 1213

Subject index

M

N

O

P

R

S

T

V

W

www.ingramcontent.com/pod-product-compliance
Lightning Source LLC
Chambersburg PA
CBHW061157240926
51846CB00006B/1042
* 9 7 8 3 6 4 2 7 2 4 2 5 1 *